BEHIND THE ONE-WAY MIRROR

BEHIND THE ONE-WAY MIRROR

Psychotherapy and Children

KATHARINE DAVIS FISHMAN

BANTAM BOOKS
NEW YORK • TORONTO • LONDON • SYDNEY • AUCKLAND

BEHIND THE ONE-WAY MIRROR
A Bantam Book / June 1995

Some portions of this book are drawn from an article by the author in the
June 1991 issue of *The Atlantic*, © 1991 by Katharine Davis Fishman.

Library of Congress Cataloging-in-Publication Data

Fishman, Katharine Davis.
    Behind the one-way mirror : psychotherapy and children / by
Katharine Davis Fishman.
        p.   cm.
    Includes bibliographical references and index.
    ISBN 0-553-07886-0
    1. Child psychotherapy.   2. Child psychiatry.   I. Title.
RJ504.F57   1995
618.92′8914—dc20   95-5446
                                                                    CIP

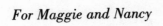

For Maggie and Nancy

Listen! you hear the grating roar
Of pebbles which the waves draw back, and fling,
At their return, up the high strand,
Begin, and cease, and then again begin,
With tremulous cadence slow, and bring
The eternal note of sadness in.

Sophocles long ago
Heard it on the Aegean, and it brought
Into his mind the turbid ebb and flow
Of human misery; we
Find also in the sound a thought,
Hearing it by this distant northern sea.

—Matthew Arnold,
"Dover Beach" (1867)

History suggests that the road to a firm research consensus is
extraordinarily arduous.

—Thomas S. Kuhn,
The Structure of Scientific
Revolutions (1962)

CONTENTS

PART V
THE RIGHT STUFF: BIOLOGICAL PSYCHIATRY

PART VI
PUTTING IT ALL TOGETHER

PREFACE

This book began as an article for *The Atlantic Monthly*. Its simple purpose was to find out what children experience in therapy. It started from the premise that clinicians approach the case at hand according to the particular theories in which they've been trained and the collegial communities (therapeutic tribes, as I came to regard them) in which they work. My goal then was not to explore theoretical or scholarly differences but merely to describe, briefly, how those differences determine clinical practice.

Two things happened in the course of writing the article. First, not surprisingly, I felt the need to learn more about the beliefs that shaped the clinicians' work, and I assumed that readers would feel that same need. Second, I wanted to convey the pace and feel of the therapy, in which a story unfolds bit by bit like a novel, and in the middle of it all, the clinician has to keep making small decisions on the basis of fragmentary information. Yes, the therapists are schooled and supervised for many years; their bookshelves overflow; and much of this information is now deep in their bones, as is the knowledge all professionals use to do their work. But they don't receive carefully sculpted, organized, digested case histories and then pull down the relevant volume: rather, they fly on very good instruments. We know this, but we often forget it. The upshot for me was to become ever more intrigued by the juncture of decades of theoretical history and the human tensions of the clinical moment. I was hooked.

I am not a therapist, nor (despite the light references to tribes) am I an anthropologist. My profession is journalism, and when thoughtfully pursued, it too draws on training, experience, and a set of received practices and tribal beliefs. The journalist hopes to be an intermediary between subject and reader: to sense what questions the reader wants to ask, to know who has the answers, to have the skill to draw the answers out, and to report those answers in clear and interesting language.

Probably the most useful quality I bring, as a reporter, to this study of therapists at work is that my tribe is wholly different from all of theirs. For an individual in any profession to claim absolute objectivity or neutrality is silly; nonetheless, while I often felt a common ground with the therapists—journalistic and therapeutic interviews, for example, have some similarities—I viewed them, ultimately, with the eye of a foreigner. My personal biases (many of them acquired during the course of this research) should become clear as the story unfolds. Readers who do not share them will either correct individually or vote with their feet.

For the past three years, in order to write this book, I have been observing and talking with psychotherapists, psychopharmacologists, their students, their patients (or clients, the term some clinicians prefer), and the patients' (or clients') families. I asked the therapists how they solved problems, and I watched and listened to children (in the flesh or on tape) in therapeutic sessions. Confidentiality was a concern. Accordingly, some of the children I observed were clinic patients with student therapists under supervision; this arrangement—in which the therapy was offered free or at a low rate—included the right to be observed by researchers. Some other families agreed, individually, to let me watch when the therapist offered them a free session. In all cases the names of patients and their family members have been changed and some identifying details altered to protect privacy, and with this understanding many compassionate parents and children were pleased to provide information that might help families with similar problems.

The clinicians I met came highly recommended: they represented the best the field has to offer, and their gifts were apparent to the observer. The creamy view I skimmed off these experiences was thinned by conversations with parents whose adventures with child therapy were rather more erratic and by my own efforts to elicit what the best therapists didn't know or felt unsure of. I also asked them to tell me about times when success had eluded them.

To learn what assumptions underlie the different types of treatment, I read volumes of theory and research findings that ranged from the classical and seminal to what I was told was the cutting edge. Because of the breadth of this report, it was necessary to choose some readings and leave out equally worthy others. I asked the therapists who lead each part of the book to supply reading lists. From those lists I began with the names I thought would be most familiar to readers outside the field and added others whose writings seemed—in my highly subjective judgment—to convey different information or to illuminate best where the field had been and where it was now going. Certainly some people might differ with my choices; I would defend them.

A book is first of all a literary entity: if it is exhaustive, it will exhaust the reader, and so the author must also make innumerable choices from the live material that's available. Mental health professionals reading this book ought not, therefore, to assume that because I have not reported every single step in the treatment of a case that the step was not taken. When the subject is diagnosis, for example, I have not covered the social work done on that particular case, because I am aiming to keep the reader's eye on the ball. Where the clinician appears not to have dotted every *i* and crossed every *t,* it may be my omission, not his or hers.

Finally the term *mental health professional* has such a bureaucratic flavor that I have avoided it whenever possible. Therefore the term *professional,* used hereafter, applies to professionals in the field of mental health. The term *nonprofessional* or *lay person* applies not only to parents and relatives but also to people in other fields, even if they're reading this book in the line of work. It applies, for example, to educators, pediatricians, policymakers, and indeed, journalists like me.

PART I

STATING THE PROBLEM

CHAPTER 1

HOW DO OUR CHILDREN GET SICK?

The question of how far early experiences have long-term effects extending into later childhood or even adult life has proved remarkably difficult to answer. However, it is clear that the links between infancy and adulthood are complex, indirect, and uncertain.

—Michael Rutter
*Stress, Coping and Development
in Children* (1983)

THE FIRST VOICE I HEARD BELONGED to Jonathan Wheeler, a colleague I'd known for some years. When we talked, it was usually shop, but I'd picked up, in bits and pieces, that he had a "troubled" son, the youngest of four children; I'd met Jonathan's wife, Louise, only a couple of times. Before seeing any therapists who worked with children, I wanted to set the tone by listening to a parent, so I called Jonathan immediately.

Here was this assignment, I said. Would he tell me about Carl?

Long silence. "Sure." He asked me to wait a minute, while he closed the office door and logged off the computer; perhaps he was also collecting himself. Then he began to speak, haltingly, as if trying to summon events he'd worked hard to put behind him. "Carl had been a nervous, excitable baby with digestive problems, so he always needed more attention than the others. Then when he was three, there was an episode that required intervention. While we were on vacation, Carl rolled in a clump of poison ivy. We didn't get to the brown soap soon enough, and he was covered with a nasty rash, which, of course, we kept smearing with calamine. On the pediatrician's advice, we even threw out all the clothes Carl was wearing that day.

3

"But weeks after we'd done all this, the rash persisted; it appeared every morning, and he scratched and scratched till his arms and legs were covered with open sores. The dermatologist could find no organic explanation. We finally took him to a child psychiatrist, who concluded it was psychosomatic: Carl had somehow internalized the original experience and was reproducing that rash overnight. After several months of therapy, the condition abated. We decided we'd gotten through the episode and hoped for better times."

When Carl started school, however, the Wheelers again saw odd patterns of behavior: he'd hide under tables and chairs, and the teachers found it stressful to keep tabs on him. "We knew we had a complicated child," Jonathan observed, but it was also pleasing to discover that Carl showed some musical talent and to start him on piano lessons, which he enjoyed from the first.

In fifth grade, however, the boy became very volatile. He punched two women teachers, and, Jonathan said, "the principal told us he couldn't stay unless he learned to control himself. So we sent him to a private school that specialized in dealing with problem children. The next year we put him in therapy with a psychologist, partly because he seemed resolutely unwilling to do any academic work, no matter how hard we and the school tried to engage him, even though by all tests he was in the top two or three percent of his class intellectually. He failed almost everything, and we hoped therapy might provide some answers."

Carl grudgingly agreed to go and stuck with it for three years: "I think he came to like the therapist, though he wouldn't admit it, but we saw no sign that he was learning much." At first the therapist wanted the family there too: then after a few months, the adults decided it should be mostly Carl's private time, and his parents didn't intrude with questions. But relations between father and son had become tense and angry.

In spite of this tension, Jonathan himself had found the family sessions quite worthwhile. He—ahead of his time—had grown up in a single-parent family, and he believed this affected the way he handled Carl. "I was perplexed about my responsibilities as a parent. I worried that if I became too tolerant of what I saw as Carl's irresponsibility to other people, I would fail to meet my obligations. In the therapy I was encouraged to see myself as the children might see me and to reconsider my rigidity and the weight of my anger. I came to realize I'd had no useful models of parenting in my own life. And perhaps it was helpful for him to hear me talking about the difficulty I had knowing how to be a father."

But by eighth grade the Wheelers had decided Carl himself wasn't benefiting emotionally or academically, and the therapist agreed there was no point going on. Carl was asked to leave the private school for problem children, with no alternative left but to sink or swim at the local suburban public high school, where the pattern of hostility and failure in everything but music began again. Gradually he got into smoking and drinking and pot, and he had two terrible years of deterioration, till he was stoned most of the time and even selling drugs out of his bedroom. "Having him in the house was almost intolerable," Jonathan told me, and "after several school conferences I suggested that Carl just leave school. A month later he was arrested for breaking and entering a Seven-Eleven and received a suspended sentence. This brought us to another therapist, whom he met with hostility. This one was a court-recommended specialist in drug abuse, who said Carl was certainly at risk but not yet addicted. Neither Carl nor I took to this therapist, but we stuck it out for eight sessions."

Then—at a point when Jonathan and Louise felt they had been around the therapeutic block several times and were feeling both cynical and desperate—an apparent miracle occurred. Carl, despite his resistance, had clearly been shocked by the conviction. Suddenly he agreed to study for general equivalency diploma exams with hopes of getting into the conservatory. He moved into an apartment, he studied, he took music courses, he practiced, he passed the GEDs easily, and he got into music school, where he was quickly recognized as someone with talent. "That first year he became a star," Jonathan remembered. "A couple of his pieces were performed, and he won a $2,500 prize. He began to work night and day and was allotted one of the premium studios—a perk for outstanding students.

"That's when things began to go down again. There were courtesy rules for using the studios—no food, no smoking, no pets—and Carl flouted them repeatedly. After many objections and offenses, the school finally told him he would have to leave, and the question of his returning was up in the air, until he could convince them he was ready to play ball. He did seek readmission a year later and was turned down; they said he wasn't truly penitent. Meanwhile he was moving from apartment to apartment because of quarrels with his roommates. Over the past year he's settled down a bit, although he practices only sporadically. He clerks in a shop that sells forties memorabilia and has become something of an expert on baseball cards. He's actually been called in to appraise some collections. Both Carl and I are pleased about that, but his music is at a standstill, and he's declined further therapy." I learned that the Wheelers, after some years of marital difficulties, had recently been divorced. Carl was now twenty-three, and Jonathan, while reconciled to the probability of chronic problems with his son, still hoped the young man would at least stabilize with maturity.

Over the next several years, as I researched first the article and then this book, I thought often of Jonathan Wheeler, who had, in a sense, given me marching orders. However valiantly he strained to be objective, to marshal the professional skills—composure, detachment, analytical ability, articulateness—to describe his experience for me, the anguish in his voice was palpable. The feelings that pervaded his account—bewilderment, self-doubt, vulnerability—were, I found, typical of parents, however competent and well-educated, who must make decisions while they and their children are suffering and who feel at a loss even to monitor the treatment—the least they might do with a physical disorder. And if in general the fathers seemed to take less of the heat than the mothers, they felt the special tension that comes from being culturally forbidden to let down the side.

What Jonathan told me had also laid out the puzzle, because Carl's case raises many of the questions that baffle parents and stir debate among professionals in the field of child psychotherapy. What combination of biology, temperament, environment, and experience caused this child's problems? How, if at all, were the symptoms he showed at different ages connected? What part did changes in the family dynamics play? Can therapists take credit for his short periods of success, or should they be blamed for not fixing him once and for all? Would medicine have helped?

These questions, moreover, reach beyond the domain of parents and therapists: they are the concern of teachers and school officials who must deal with troubled families; of the pediatricians, family practitioners, gynecologists, and allergists who are often called upon to advise whether a child or teenager needs therapy—and who should provide it; of policymakers who must decide what sort of mental health care is prudent for taxpayers to endow; and of the ultimate arbiters, the taxpayers themselves.

Discoveries in genetics and neuroscience have taught us much more about psychopathology than we knew even ten years ago; without doubt these developments, which further encourage the shift from analytic to biological (and consequently, pharmacological) approaches to treating mental disturbances, have shaken the psychotherapeutic tree. No serious clinician would now attribute a child's problems exclusively to poor parenting or a single traumatic event. There is accumulating evidence of what many of us, professionals and lay people alike, have always suspected—if with mixed feelings: that the child must bring something to the party. How often, for example, have we seen two children in the same troubled or peaceful family, one of whom is barely functioning while the other looks just fine? How many life stories of both criminals and captains of industry credit their denouements to poverty, youthful illness, and parental abandonment?

At the same time it often seems to nonprofessionals—reading the newspapers, talking to friends—that childhood mental disorders are rampant, whether our own turn of mind blames that phenomenon on social chaos, parental self-indulgence, or the marketing skills of mental health professionals. How accurate are our hunches? Are more children sick and troubled today, or do we just notice it more? Have we—collectively, as a society—pathologized ordinary obnoxious behavior, claiming that children are acting out when they're merely acting up, depositing our own failures in nurturance or discipline (depending, again, on how we choose to look at it) on the clinical doorstep? What then about the personal *we*— you, Dad, and me, Mom—for whom these questions are more painfully immediate? What does a mentally ill child look like? (Does he look, for example, like Carl Wheeler?) And how did he or she get that way?

For the past twenty years, research estimates of the number of children eighteen and under who suffer from diagnosable mental disorders have hovered around 12 percent of the population. But recent community epidemiological studies pursued in several countries suggest that the figure may actually be as high as 17 to 22 percent—11 to 14 million American children—an increase credited chiefly to sharper methods of diagnosis and classification, not some new *mal du siècle*. To put these figures into perspective, only 250,000 American children have muscular dystrophy and one in 600 has diabetes.

Moreover, it appears that many children with mental disorders are not getting treated. In 1988, a team headed by Dr. Elizabeth J. Costello, a psychologist in the psychiatry department at Duke University, interviewed 300 children and their parents who visited two branches of a health maintenance organization in Pittsburgh—one in a rich suburb, the other in a poor urban neighborhood—for routine childhood ailments.

Using the Diagnostic Interview Schedule for Children, a questionnaire developed by the National Institute of Mental Health that covers both feelings and behavior, and scoring it to detect "significant impairment and need for treatment," they found that according to either the child or the parent, 22 percent of the children qualified. There were, however, discrepancies between the parents' and children's scores that reflect two recurring themes in child psychotherapy: first that it's difficult to get diagnostic agreement between children and the adults in their lives, and second that, as the authors noted, "On the basis of parental reports three quarters of the children with behavioral problems, but fewer than half of those with emotional problems, would have been identified." Childhood psychiatric care is, then, a sad example of the adage that the squeaky wheel gets the oil: the child who disrupts the classroom will be seen to by the adults, but when a child aches silently, the adults will not notice—or will look away. Finally the *pediatricians* at the HMO did very poorly: they picked out less than six percent of the children as needing treatment for mental illness and actually referred less than four percent of them.

Still, while part of the spurt in psychiatric disorders may be credited to vigorous epidemiology, in almost everyone's estimation the times seem to be especially difficult for children. The suicide rate for adolescents aged fifteen to nineteen quadrupled between 1950 and 1988. (This frightening figure, versions of which appear everywhere, is, as we'll see shortly, more complicated than it looks.) According to the most recent census figures, 38 percent of all American children will have been involved in a divorce by the time they reach eighteen; divorce is what professionals in mental health call a "stressful" or "transitional" life event, one of those that put children at risk for developing mental disorders. "Divorce," says Richard Chasin, M.D., a family therapist in Cambridge, Massachusetts, "is the bread-and-butter of child psychotherapy."

The suspicion that today's children and teenagers are more troubled than were their older cousins finds some confirmation in a recent study done by Thomas M. Achenbach, a psychologist at the University of

Vermont, and a colleague, Catherine T. Howell. Achenbach is well known as the designer of the Child Behavior Check List, a widely used questionnaire for parents reporting on their children's problems (behavior classified as anxious, depressed, inattentive, delinquent, and so forth) and skills (in jobs and chores, friendships, social relations, and schoolwork). In 1976 he had administered that test to a large and diverse sample of parents. In 1989 he and Howell ran it by a similar sample and this time found that the parents identified nearly twice as many of their kids as showing problems worthy of clinical attention; the 1989 children's competence scores were lower too. Since the same test was used in both studies, the differences could not be credited to new ways of defining the problems.

While I was doing the research for this book, I was also circulating in the lay world—living a normal life, that is—and encountering the almost universal fondness of nonprofessionals for global statements about causes and cures. Besides the sweeping "It's biological" and "It's environmental," I heard innumerable sentences that began with "What these kids need is . . . ," "The parents today . . . ," or simply the words *They* and *It*. These sentences often seemed, on further examination, to stem from either political or personal convenience—the understandable need to feel more comfortable about some relative's problems by generalizing them to all children. One of the goals of this book is to establish for lay readers why such statements, as framed, are dangerous and to describe the intricate chains of circumstances that lead various children to display symptoms of psychological disorder.

The past decade has been a vibrant period for research in all psychotherapeutic orientations. New developments in therapy will be covered in later chapters, but it is useful to start here by sampling some different types of research to illustrate what each approach can and cannot tell us. I will also report on what some researchers have discovered about factors that place children at risk for developing psychological disorders. Before proceeding, I must emphasize the cherry-picking nature of the explanation that follows and its primary goal of sketching out how researchers work: one study is almost never sufficient to prove a hypothesis, and this chapter is an introduction, not a conclusion. At the same time it makes sense to choose examples that shed some light on issues that readers outside the field of mental health find compelling.

To understand more about psychological disorders, as I discovered, we must learn simultaneously to think with more precision and to tolerate considerable ambiguity. It is acquiring the first skill that affords us the second, and along the way we will likely be irritated, frustrated, and tantalized.

In 1989 a special section on child psychiatric epidemiology ran in the *Journal of the American Academy of Child and Adolescent Psychiatry.* As Dr. Elizabeth J. Costello, the Duke University psychologist already cited, explained it, epidemiology is "the classic 'counting' strategy: describe the pattern of disease occurrence in society; identify the high-risk group; categorize risk factors; isolate a common cause; establish an agent-host-environment relationship; intervene to break the causal chain. By the use of this strategy the current generation of children has been preserved from smallpox, and in the industrialized world from a host of other scourges." Over the past two and a half decades, interest in applying the counting strategy to psychiatric disorders has grown substantially: it parallels the ascent of medical approaches to mental health problems and has been reinforced by efforts to sharpen diagnosis. Thus if you want to find out whether adolescent girls in single-parent families are especially prone to depression, you have to start by agreeing on what depression is.

A good example of the epidemiological approach is an article on teenage suicide written by David Shaffer, a psychiatrist at Columbia University's New York State Psychiatric Institute, and four colleagues, and published in the *AACAP Journal* in 1988. Suicide is surely the terrifying subtext of all discussions of childhood mental illness; it may, perhaps, be the epidemiologists' white whale. The authors started by pointing out that teenage suicide—despite its alarming increase—is actually quite rare: in 1984 only nine out of 100,000 fifteen-to-nineteen-year-olds died by their own hand. What this means, therefore, is that scattershot school prevention programs are inefficient. They are also ineffective, the authors believe. In an earlier project Shaffer and some colleagues studied a thousand teenagers who had been exposed to a variety of these high school programs. The majority of the students, it turned out, didn't seem to need them. They started out with intelligent views and some knowledge about suicide—the warning signals, the value of professional help, and the importance of taking threats seriously, consulting adults, and sharing one's own suicidal preoccupations.

But up to a fifth of the students "expressed views that would generally be regarded as inappropriate"—and these views were not changed by the programs: that is, the students continued to romanticize suicide, considered it a reasonable solution to some problems, and believed in protecting the suicidal secrets of friends. The authors found that "relatively few students believed either before or after exposure to a program that suicide was a feature of mental illness," and they suggested that prevention programs run the risk of encouraging imitations unless suicide is clearly "depicted as a deviant act by someone with a mental disturbance." The researchers did believe that high school students might benefit from more education about mental health and the value of counseling, and that teenagers like the three percent who said they were now troubled or suicidal and wanted professional help would be better served by school screening programs (those aimed at picking out the children who need help, not generalized prevention programs) and individual therapy.

The authors also summed up the literature on factors that put teenagers at risk for suicide: boys, for example, are nearly five times more likely to commit suicide than girls, although sex differences are less prominent among Hispanics and blacks; whites commit suicide more often than blacks; and native Americans vary widely among tribal cultures. While drug overdose is the most frequent mode of suicide in the general population, teenagers of both sexes most commonly use a gun, and those who shoot themselves are likely to be substance abusers. (Hanging is the second most common method among boys; jumping is second among girls.) The phenomenon of imitative suicide after the appearance of news stories, television programs, films, and books has been sufficiently documented to be cause for alarm.

Among the risk factors for individual adolescents are, not surprisingly, a history of previous attempts and severe depression—although many teenagers with these risk factors don't go on to kill themselves. A couple of markers have been isolated, however, that might seem novel to nonprofessionals: "an excess of obstetric complications" in the birth histories of teenage victims and, in several small studies of adults, "low concentrations of the serotonin metabolite 5-HIAA in the cerebrospinal fluid of suicide attempters and completers."

The second factor illustrates an important new direction in epidemiological research that I will cover more extensively in Part V: studies aimed at finding the correlation between various biological factors and mental illness. The first, the "excess of obstetric complications," as described by the authors, illustrates the caution about hypothesis that characterizes contemporary psychological research. In the paragraph about birth history, the authors gingerly volunteered some possible explanations: "Along with having complicated obstetric histories, the mothers of the potential suicides received less prenatal care and were more likely to have smoked and taken alcohol during pregnancy. The excess of suicide in their offspring could reflect such associated factors as the central nervous system consequences of birth complications, exposure to some teratogen during pregnancy, the heritability of psychopathology, or the effects of inappropriate parenting by deviant mothers."

Several things are noteworthy about this extensive report, which is too long to cover completely here. The first is that in every paragraph it intentionally raises as many questions as it answers. Hypotheses are clearly marked. Like other surveys of its kind, it moves a step or two ahead of its predecessors and points the way for future research. And second, while it gives clinicians some guidance, it is the therapists, alone in their offices as the dusk lowers, who must put together innumerable tiny pieces of the puzzle, bits of history, and nuances of expression and character analysis, all of them barely hinted at by the researchers, to decide how imminent the possibility is that Ethan will take action. It is most dramatic for anyone who has read the basic psychiatric literature— Freud, Melanie Klein, D. W. Winnicott, and others—to contrast the ease with which those early writers, on the basis of just a few cases, constructed elaborate theories, with the restraint and humility of current writers. But cautious, quantitatively based research may not be the only useful means of illumination.

The single most compelling piece of research I encountered in preparing this book was the New York Longitudinal Study (NYLS), pursued between 1956 and 1981 by Stella Chess, M.D., professor of child psychiatry, and Alexander Thomas, M.D., professor of psychiatry at New York University Medical Center. Chess and Thomas are a wife and husband born in 1914 who followed 133 children (and thus their families) from infancy into early adulthood. The children in the main study came from middle- or upper-middle-class families on the Upper East Side of New York City and in one of its suburbs; Chess and Thomas intentionally chose a socioculturally homogeneous sample to minimize the effect of this variable on their findings, and they balanced it with control groups of 98 working-class Puerto Rican children from a neighborhood nearby, 52 mildly retarded children, and 243 children with congenital rubella, all studied (for financial reasons) for shorter periods of time. The NYLS is generally considered a landmark study, and it has strongly influenced my views.

I will talk more about Chess and Thomas's findings shortly; what is pertinent here is their comments on quantitative and qualitative research. (They opted to do some of each.)

As practitioners who came to maturity in the golden age of American psychoanalysis, the authors write that they were greatly enriched by "the research studies of Kraepelin, Freud, Bleuler, Meyer, Levy and Kanner . . . based on careful clinical studies and creative, systematic generalization from the data they had accumulated. These pioneers in no way felt restricted and frustrated by their inability to utilize various statistical strategies, such as correlation coefficients, analysis of variance, or factor analysis." They point out that in other branches of science, Darwin, Pasteur, and Piaget pursued the qualitative approach, "the derivation of scientific generalizations from the intensive qualitative study of clinical data . . ."

At the same time, during their clinical careers Chess and Thomas became increasingly "uneasy at the broad sweeping generalizations that were being drawn from a small series of cases . . . other interpretations were possible, and . . . the clinical studies as such did not allow for a judgment of the relative validity of the competing ideas. Frequently, recourse was made to 'my clinical experience' as a presumably decisive argument, when all too often this simply amounted to making the same mistakes for 20 to 30 years."

The authors realized that their own clinical observations could not be unbiased, that they needed "a scheme of objective quantitative ratings . . . to trace effectively the consistencies and changes in any child's characteristics over time," and they signed up a behavioral scientist to organize their data into scorable categories. In addition to the breadth and rigor that quantitative analysis brought to their study, it permitted a powerful new type of qualitative analysis: after discovering trends, Chess and Thomas could pick out individual cases that ran against type and analyze them in depth.

But as they observe, the quantitative approach has limits too, and today, when it has largely superseded qualitative methods, it is important for lay readers to hear and remember their reservations.

"Quantitative analyses," Chess and Thomas write, "are the product of routine methods involving a minimum of judgment and evaluation." Once you've decided on procedures and criteria, your work is routine; to ensure rigor, you aim to eliminate as many variables—and thus subtleties—as possible. "The mathematical precision of statistical methods in behavioral studies all too often confers an aura of authority and certainty on the results of the analyses which may be misleading." In real life, data do not fall so neatly into precise categories, and this "make[s] for fallibility." Finally they point out, "It is all too easy for the behavioral researcher to slip into the 'ivory tower' attitude which cherishes the 'good' measure of reliability above the 'right' measure of validity." They quote, approvingly, a 1981 psychological article by C. H. Kraemer: " 'When the right thing can only be measured poorly, it tends to cause the wrong thing to be measured, only because it can be measured well.' "

The reader who approaches quantitatively based psychiatric literature unburdened by professional tribal bias will likely, as I did, find it informative, persuasive, impressive—and sterile. The human texture of psychological illness—a significant dimension—has been carefully left out. For this texture one must go to the qualitative literature, in which sick children speak to us in idiosyncratic, compelling voices that cause three or five or seven decades to melt away. The early therapists—arrogance and quaint language notwithstanding—offer us the perceptions of the intelligent trained observer, the insight of the novelist, and the educative skill of the clinician. In dismissing these gifts we have much to lose.

With caveats established it makes sense to sample the flavor of some recent epidemiological research. The reason for doing this, as noted earlier, is to introduce lay readers to the kinds of questions professionals are asking nowadays. All of the papers described here were mentioned to me by clinicians during interviews; therefore one may assume that this research is influencing the way some practitioners do their daily work.

For most of this century both lay people and professionals in various fields that deal with youth have accepted the truism that adolescence is a painful time—more miserable, perhaps, for some teenagers than for others, but surely a territory fraught with *sturm und drang*. This belief, indeed, may prompt parents and teachers to "wait out" signs of turbulence they observe in a young person. A team of researchers in Chicago has for some time been studying adolescent disturbances, and their conclusions must give us pause. The principal investigator is Daniel

Offer, M.D., a professor of psychiatry at Northwestern University. Kenneth I. Howard, a psychology and psychiatry professor at Northwestern, continues to work with Offer, and Eric Ostrov, a forensic psychologist formerly at Rush Presbyterian St. Luke's Medical Center in Chicago and now in private practice, participated in the team's earlier studies.

Epidemiological papers usually begin with summaries of previous work in the field. In a 1989 *AACAP Journal* paper on gender differences, the authors start by expressing a view for which Offer is well known: "that, on the whole, most teenagers enjoy life and are happy with themselves. Pride in their physical development, endorsement of parents' values, comfort with sexuality, and confidence about the future prevail among most teenagers. The data indicate that the vast majority of teenagers have positive feelings toward their parents and are not continually rebelling or in a state of antagonism toward them. These empirical studies have been converging toward the conclusion that about 80% of teenagers function normally; that is, they do not present significant psychiatric symptomatology or experience marked or persistent stress or turmoil." Here the authors are not reporting data from one single study but are noting the convergence of figures from various countries published over a fifteen-year period.

What are we to make of this apparently good news? Earlier in this chapter I cited, in the alarmed tone that generally accompanies these figures, studies suggesting that more children and teenagers than we dreamed of have clinical symptoms and reporting the new numbers as 17 to 22 percent—right in the Chicago ball park. (Thus the figures on psychiatric symptomatology among teenagers approximate those for the larger population group of children *and* adolescents.) We are now encountering the half-full-half-empty question that has come to fascinate epidemiologists: Why do so many kids, even in the most horrendous of circumstances, *not* get sick? Can we solve the mystery of illness by studying the puzzle of health? In fact, the point the Chicago team wishes to make is that fully one-fifth of adolescents "present notable psychiatric symptomatology" and that "the belief in normal adolescent turmoil and symptomatology may have led professionals working with teenagers to minimize the importance of psychiatric symptomatology."

The authors studied 497 teenagers—half boys, half girls—in three local high schools, one in a rich, mostly white suburb, a second in a middle-class, mixed-race suburb, and a third in a black inner-city neighborhood. The students answered a battery of standard questionnaires, which the researchers had modified to suit the needs of the project.

The Chicago study—which did not report differences in results among the three high schools—corroborated others that reflect greater disturbance among teenage girls than boys, especially in the categories of emotional tone and body image. Many more girls than boys said they frequently felt sad and unattractive. More than twice as many girls as boys said they felt confused most of the time and had been easily upset and annoyed during the previous year. On the other hand, the boys led the girls in behavior problems: more than twice as many boys reported having damaged property, and almost twice as many said they'd been stopped by the police during the previous year. "These results," say the authors, "are consistent with the hypothesis that a teenage boy who is disturbed is likely to express that disturbance through acting-out behavior such as theft, running away, or substance abuse. A teenage girl who is disturbed may express that disturbance through inwardly turned symptomatology, such as depression and anxiety."

The reason for these differences is unclear, but there are several hypotheses: "Cultural factors emphasizing the desirability of girls being open to affective and interpersonal experience, and boys being prepared for action or oriented to problem solving, may be involved. In addition, fundamental biological differences may be operating . . . results presented here are also consistent with culturally based differential willingness (or ability) of boys and girls to attest to certain symptoms." In view of these findings, the authors suggest that clinicians might be particularly alarmed when a teenager's symptoms run counter to the gender norm: that is, a boy who is depressed and a girl who acts out may be more disturbed than a boy who acts out and a girl who is depressed. (Before proceeding with other studies, I should point out that while girls lead boys in psychopathology after puberty, the psychiatric patient in childhood is much more frequently a boy.)

The Chicago team took off from the discovery that most teenagers take adolescence in stride, then studied those who don't. Another variation on the theme of resilience-versus-vulnerability appears in the work of a psychologist named Cathy Spatz Widom, whose professional focus is on the consequences of child abuse and neglect: Widom's research illustrates, once again, how good quantitative studies can squeeze new juice out of old clichés. It has become an article of faith among both scholars and laymen that violence begets violence, that abused children and neglected children grow up to mistreat their own kids—despite a surpris-' ing lack of sound empirical studies of this proposition. In an article in the April 1989 issue of *Science,* Widom, then in the Departments of Criminal Justice and Psychology at Indiana University, deplored the "small sample sizes, weak sampling techniques, questionable accuracy of information, and lack of appropriate comparison groups" in earlier reports. Widom— whose institutional connection would explain her commencing with the roots of delinquency, rather than with other psychological consequences of abuse and neglect—undertook a two-year research project designed to overcome the defects of the previous work. The solution was "to identify a large sample of substantiated and validated cases of child abuse from approximately 20 years ago, to establish a matched control group of nonabused children, and to determine the extent to which these individuals and the matched control group subsequently engaged in delinquent and adult violent criminal behavior."

Widom took the court records of all cases of physical and sexual abuse and neglect processed and validated between 1967 and 1971 in the courts of one county in the Midwest—some 900 of them—in which the victim was aged eleven or younger. She found a control group of the children's schoolmates and neighbors matched by age, sex, and race; any whiff of evidence that a control child had been abused or neglected was grounds for exclusion. Then she combed the local, state, and federal law enforcement records to find which children got into trouble with the law in later life.

The first discovery Widom made was that "in comparison to controls, abused and neglected children as a group have a larger mean number of offenses . . . an earlier mean age at first offense . . . and a higher proportion of chronic offenders, that is, those charged with five or more offenses." Beyond this general statement, however, were various differences within demographic groups. Therefore, Widom says, "the type of abuse or neglect is not as powerful a predictor of violent criminal behavior as the demographic characteristics of sex, race, and age."

Widom's study has the requisite section of caveats, the most important being that poor and minority families are overrepresented in court records because cases of abuse and neglect among the upper classes are often hushed up (although, Widom says, studies of family violence have found that "those with the lowest income are more likely to abuse their children"). Also, some researchers have pointed out that charges of abuse and neglect against a family member start a long court procedure and bring on other events that in themselves may be traumatizing.

All of these findings are sad but not surprising. The most interesting of Widom's observations for our purposes, however, are these: "Twenty-six percent of child abuse and neglect victims had juvenile offenses; 74% did not. Eleven percent had an arrest for a violent criminal act, whereas almost 90% did not."

Criminality is not, of course, the only possible result of childhood abuse: Widom suggests that among other topics, researchers now study the incidence of depression, withdrawal, suicide, and early death among the victims, and in a book chapter written later she discusses the paucity of epidemiological studies that illustrate precisely and rigorously how abuse and neglect interact with other factors in children's lives to produce a variety of mental disorders—information we would surely love to have here. *Clinical* studies, as Widom agreed in conversation with me, abound; but this approach begins with the problem (suicide, depression, post-traumatic stress disorder, or indeed, juvenile delinquency) and looks backward for its possible cause, studying only those children who are already symptomatic. An epidemiologist like Widom—practicing a discipline that is still, unfortunately, in its infancy with regard to child and adolescent mental health issues—starts with the abuse and looks forward for its effects on a general population, and that is very different. (Now at the School of Criminal Justice at the State University of New York at Albany, she is currently pursuing the studies she recommended.)

Widom's observations evoke a simple medical comparison that helps illuminate what professionals do and don't understand about how children become psychologically disturbed. Suppose John and Mary go out to dinner and eat contaminated swordfish; John gets violent diarrhea and Mary vomits all night. A salmonella bacillus or, more loosely, the contaminated fish is the *etiology*—the medical term for the cause—of the food poisoning they both experience. But for a variety of reasons, once the bacillus enters John's and Mary's gastrointestinal systems, it attacks different organs in each.

The term for the process by which an etiology produces a symptom is *pathogenesis*. The correlation between a particular etiology and a given symptom is not inevitable. Widom is suggesting that the bacillus in this case—abuse—might be the etiology for other symptoms too. In another example, a mother might be, for a variety of reasons, so anxious about her children's physical safety that she overprotects them. As a result of this, one son develops phobias of everything from crossing the street to playing baseball, and his brother becomes counterphobic and goes skateboarding on the highway. A somewhat opposite example would be anorexia nervosa, which produces a well-understood, characteristic set of symptoms once the patient has started starving herself, but which has what psychiatrists would call a multidetermined (and still controversial) etiology. While nonprofessionals generally understand physical diseases as the result of a complex process, they may not realize that mental illnesses develop in similar fashion. It's useful to keep this in mind, particularly in reading Chapter 2, which talks about diagnosis, and later on, where this process bears on how different types of therapists define a problem.

Both Widom's results and the studies of adolescents in Chicago illustrate the direction of much important research over the past two decades. During the academic year 1979–80, for example, a group of distinguished child psychologists and psychiatrists gathered at the Center for Advanced Study in the Behavioral Sciences at Stanford to discuss what they knew about how stress affects children. The result of the seminar was *Stress, Coping, and Development in Children,* a book of twelve chapters by different participants edited by Norman Garmezy, a psychologist at the University of Minnesota, and Michael Rutter, a British psychiatrist. The papers explore biological and sociological as well as psychological views, and the basic questions asked in the seminar, as reported by Rutter, go to the essence of children's mental health. They should remain in our minds as we look at the way clinicians work with children.

In his introductory chapter Rutter notes "an increasing interest in the phenomenon of resilience, as shown by the young people who 'do well' in some sense in spite of having experienced a form of stress which in the population as a whole is known to carry a substantial risk of an adverse outcome." He asks "whether the processes involved in stress and coping differ according to the child's stage of development" and "whether adverse experiences or happenings in early life alter the course of subsequent development or influence the ways in which an individual responds to much later stress events." He asks, "Do stressful events *cause* psychiatric disorder or, conversely, does the presence of disorder (or its precursors in the form of personality or lifestyle variables) increase the likelihood of *having* stressful experiences? Or . . . are both stress and disorder due to some third set of variables with the interrelation between the first two purely artifactual?" Both researchers and clinicians are still asking these questions, often disagreeing and in fact changing their minds on the answers, and certainly acknowledging that those answers are always murky and always different in each individual case.

Garmezy's chapter, for example, examines the phenomenon of stress. It is now widely accepted, he notes, that individuals have different vulnerability to different stressors, but we can only guess why (that's pathogenesis again). Will we ever be able to predict how stress-prone a particular child will be? To do so, we would need research that considers "individual predispositional biogenetic and constitutional factors, patterns of family structure and interaction, rearing practices of parents, characteristic personality attributes of the individual and careful analyses of stressful situations and events, modes of coping and outcome, and potentiating and protective factors in the environment."

While children have been mistreated since the dawn of time, the effort to study how they react to stress is relatively modern. From the late nineteenth century through the thirties, Garmezy reports, pediatricians began noticing the high death rate and developmental retardation of children who lived in orphanages and hospitals; the solution was thought to lie in better hygiene and more attractive surroundings. Then during World War II large numbers of children experienced desertion, displacement, starvation, torture, imprisonment, and loss; researchers began to anatomize the immediate and long-term effects of this suffering. At first the studies described "hospitalism," "maternal deprivation," and "the affectionless character"; but later research suggested that "many children in institutions more than survived, and were not foreordained victims of developmental, intellectual, and characterological disabilities . . . only a minority of children were so affected." The initial reactions to the later reports were again to improve the institutions, this time in more sophisticated ways; the current path is to study the children.

While the conclusions of earlier studies on parental deprivation have been modified, the strongest theme of literature on stressors is still that "fear of loss and separation from loved ones will demonstrate marked staying power through the years of infancy, childhood, and adolescence." This fear lies at the core of many of children's psychological disorders.

Accordingly, researchers study the nature and length of the separation, the age of the child, the conditions in which the child is placed, and the relationships he had before. For example, children between six months and four years of age show marked distress after a stay in the hospital, but they are more disturbed if there's conflict in the family.

What emerges from much of the literature Garmezy cites is that as in the hospital studies, one stressful experience in itself is seldom sufficient to produce long-term psychic damage; repeated experiences, or experiences with a combination of stressors, can cause considerable harm. For example, "Multiple foster home and institutional placements in early childhood can contribute significantly to the development of later psychopathic and antisocial behavior," Garmezy writes.

The context of a child's life is crucial, most notably the relationships he has with significant adults before and after the experience. During World War II, for example, when England's cities were suffering savage air attacks, children were evacuated to rural areas for their protection (and thus taken away from their parents, who remained at home). This episode, Garmezy reports, produced among the children an estimated prevalence rate of "neurotic symptoms"—these are not spelled out here, but the term refers to anxiety, hysteria, phobias, obsessions, and compulsions—ranging from 25 to 50 percent. "Those who remained in the cities close to their families during the Blitz showed relatively few such neurotic behaviors, suggesting that the security engendered by parents compensated for the traumatic effects of air raids." At the same time most of the children showed some ability to adapt: the effects of the disruption depended on the children's age and how they got along with their own parents and with the families that boarded them.

Concentration camp children, however, whose experiences were more terrifying than those of the children who went through the Blitz, showed serious behavior disturbances: "They stole, cheated, formed gangs, engaged in varied forms of anti-social behavior. But mental disorders were an infrequent occurrence, and even neurotic symptoms, which a child had shown previously, disappeared. But the longer term effects remained—hostility, anxiety, a desire for vengeance. In some cases, these sometimes came to dominate the children's development."

Among the most moving descriptions in psychiatric literature—liberally excerpted by Garmezy—is the account of six children, survivors of the Terezin camp, whose parents had died in the gas chambers when the children were infants. After the war they were sent for treatment to Anna Freud's Hampstead Nursery. Freud and her colleagues reported:

> It was evident that they cared greatly for each other and not at all for anybody or anything else. . . . The children's unusual emotional dependence on each other was borne out further by the almost complete absence of jealousy, rivalry and competition, such as normally develop between brothers and sisters or in a group of contemporaries who come from normal families. . . . Since the adults played no part in their emotional lives at the time, they did not compete with each other for favors or for recognition . . . they stood up for each other automatically whenever they felt that a member of the group was unjustly treated or otherwise threatened by an outsider. . . . They did not grudge each other their possessions . . . on the contrary lending them to each other with pleasure . . . they were concerned for each other's safety in traffic, looked after children who lagged behind. . . . The children were hypersensitive, restless, aggressive, difficult to handle. They showed a heightened autoerotism and some of them the beginning of neurotic symptoms. But they were neither deficient, delinquent nor psychotic. . . . That they were able to acquire a new language in the midst of their upheavals, bears witness to a basically unharmed contact with their environment.

Another study of children who survived Terezin reports that 60 percent "showed no frank symptoms of mental disorder" but almost all "were scarred in certain ways by their great suffering; this was reflected mainly in their increased vulnerability and mental instability and in the fact that minor changes in their life situations tended to produce breakdowns."

Today there is no shortage of war-torn countries for child psychologists to study: Israel and Northern Ireland, for example, have been virtual petri dishes, and psychiatric reports from the former Yugoslavia appeared soon after its devastation began to dominate the evening news.

"In general," Garmezy says, "there would appear to be greater plasticity than had been anticipated in the adaptive capacities of children who have known separation experiences." Once we know that some children are resilient, of course, we've only begun to think in the right direction; the next question is which children, and why. Reports on high-achieving black children in urban ghettos, a famous longitudinal study of poor children from unstable families on the island of Kauai in Hawaii, and Michael Rutter's own work on the Isle of Wight all yield essentially the same three protective factors: temperamental qualities in the child, including social and cognitive skills; "family cohesion and warmth," which did not necessarily mean the presence of the father but did have much to do with how the mother coped in his absence; and supportive adults and peers outside the family. What is most significant in these studies, as Garmezy points out, is "the variation in adaptation in children exposed to similar traumatic circumstances." That is, the same stressor affects individual children quite differently.

The stress researchers study the variety of reactions among children exposed to extreme conditions—but most of us are shaped through the more prosaic struggles and rewards of daily life. Stella Chess and Alexander Thomas spent nearly thirty years illuminating how character develops and are even now finding questions to explore in the data they assembled. ("I'm not emeritus," says Chess, a tall, thin woman who wears her gray hair in a bun, favors T-shirts, sweat pants, and running shoes, and still gives the occasional touch-up session to some old patients. "We've kept our titles, although our salaries retired quite some time ago.")

When Chess and Thomas, both psychoanalytically trained, began practicing in the early forties, the psychiatric pendulum had swung far over toward environmental explanations of emotional and behavioral problems. "Whether the concepts came from psychoanalysis, learning theory, or behaviorism, the young infant was considered a *tabula rasa*," they have written. While many psychoanalytic theories did involve biological processes, they did not see individual differences as rooted in biology. Theories that recognized both heredity and environment "presumed that the contribution of each category could be parceled out—so much for heredity and so much for environment, so much for biology and so much for culture."

Both the research literature and the experiences of their clinical practice—his with adults, hers with children—seemed to negate these ideas. Chess found it extremely difficult to get useful information from parents who, abashed by what she later called "*mal de mère* ideology," dwelled on how they had traumatized their child; out of these stories she would pick up cues to the child's individuality and pursue the questioning in that direction. In addition to the matters of motivation that so preoccupied psychoanalysts, both Chess and Thomas—who, of course, compared notes at the end of the day—were intrigued by what they have called "a style of reacting or behaving." Moreover, Chess saw "that there were some parents who seemed to be reasonably good who had children with noticeable problems. Other parents who seemed to be quite rotten had children who were sailing through life without any trouble." The Thomases themselves had four children of their own, two biological and two adopted, who reacted differently from birth.

Finally the after-hours conversations yielded a hypothesis, which they called "goodness of fit." According to this formulation, "When the organism's capacities, motivations and style of behaving and the demands and expectations of the environment are in accord, then goodness of fit results. Such consonance between organism and environment potentiates optimal positive development. Should there be dissonance between the capacities and characteristics of the organism . . . and the environmental opportunities and demands . . . there is poorness of fit, which leads to maladaptive functioning and distorted development." Notions of dissonance and consonance, Chess and Thomas write, "have meaning only in terms of the values and demands of a given socioeconomic group or culture." Finally, development is not linear but a "continually evolving reciprocal" process.

To the contemporary ear, the general hypothesis sounds less than novel, testimony to the acceptance and corroboration of the authors' work over time. But the way in which the hypothesis was played out in their longitudinal study is still a revelation, especially for lay readers.

Starting with friends and friends-of-friends who had infants, Chess interviewed ten families at length about the minutiae of daily life with their children. Then they brought in a psychologist trained in quantitative research, and some independent observers to verify Chess's interview data. The psychologist analyzed this and came up with nine scorable attributes of temperament. To any parent, they should ring a number of bells:

Activity Level (how much the child moves around and how long his quiet periods last)

Rhythmicity (how predictable are her bodily functions)

Approach or Withdrawal (does the child embrace or shrink from new stimuli, whether they are people, toys, foods, or places?)

Adaptability (response to change; "one is not concerned with the nature of the initial responses, but with the ease with which they are modified in desired directions")

Threshold of Responsiveness (how hard you have to work to get a reaction from the child, whatever the reaction might be)

Intensity of Reaction

Quality of Mood (whether the child tends to be good-natured or grouchy)

Distractibility

Attention Span and Persistence (how long the child is willing to stick with an activity, and how determined she is to keep it up no matter who or what gets in her way)

These characteristics last throughout our lives. As Chess and Thomas point out, "it is often empirically useful to conceptualize behavior in terms of abilities ... motivations ... and temperament." Prevailing psychological theories, they believed, focused on the first two and ignored the third.

The notion of "goodness of fit" becomes far more complex when considered in terms of nine temperamental factors, and Chess further discovered that for some of the infants, temperamental attributes were clustered in three different patterns. "One group of parents, a small minority, reported graphically the difficulties they were having. Their baby cried loud and often, sometimes without apparent cause, reacted negatively and vigorously to new foods or most other new experiences, and then adapted only slowly. Sleep and hunger cycles were irregular, further increasing the difficulties of child care for the parents." These children, who numbered 10 percent of the sample, she termed "difficult." The "easy" children, 40 percent of the group, followed an exactly opposite pattern. Finally a third cluster, 15 percent, were called "slow-to-warm-up": they showed "a combination of negative responses of mild intensity to new stimuli with slow adaptability after repeated contact. . . . If given the opportunity to reexperience such new situations over time and without pressure, such a child gradually comes to show quiet and positive interest and involvement." The remaining children's attributes didn't cluster.

It is essential to understand that no single attribute or pattern in itself either doomed or protected a child: it was the confluence of temperament with family, school, society, and innumerable other fortuitous circumstances that shaped the child's future. "In the cases of poorness of fit between early childhood difficult temperament and dissonant parental handling, the temperamental characteristics preceded the negative parental attitudes. Furthermore, there was no consistent parental pattern that could be identified in these cases. Parental attitudes ranged from blaming the child to blaming themselves, from vacillation to extreme rigidity, and from excessive demands to appeasement. Also, many of these parents functioned quite differently with their other children who did not show this difficult temperamental constellation."

Chess and Thomas point out that the notions of "easy" and "difficult" temperament are themselves a cultural artifact; one of the many studies by other researchers amplifying the NYLS showed that "difficult" temperament enabled some Masai babies to survive a drought that killed off most of the "easy" babies in their tribe. The psychiatrically savvy parents in the NYLS group were laid back about irregular feeding, toilet training, and masturbation, and so few problems developed in these areas. On the other hand, "symptoms in the areas of sleep, discipline, speech, peer relationships, and learning, were prominent." The children's choice of symptoms dovetailed almost perfectly with the values of their upper-middle-class urban families, a population in which "an IQ score below 120 was considered to be 'below normal.' " Chess and Thomas offered guidance to the parents of four boys with low persistence and high distractibility, but the fathers thought lack of "stick-to-it-iveness" was a character flaw and balked at the simple suggestions for getting around it. In this case the parents stubbornly persisted in judging their children's behavior according to rigid cultural norms. This was the authors' most notable therapeutic failure.

Middle-class parents devoted to their children before bedtime were notably intolerant of evening and nighttime interruptions: the evening was their personal time, and then they needed a good night's sleep for demanding jobs the next day. The working-class Puerto Rican (WCPR) parents, on the other hand, didn't much care about enforcing regular bedtime and sleep habits for their preschool children. Only one child developed a sleep problem until the kids started school, a point at which parents laid down the law and bedtime tantrums became an issue for five of the children in the study. Most dramatically, "half of the WCPR clinical cases under nine years of age presented symptoms of excessive and uncontrollable motor activity, whereas only one NYLS youngster displayed this symptom." The Puerto Rican children came from large families jammed into tiny apartments in unsafe neighborhoods where their parents were understandably protective, and those with a high activity level and certain other temperamental qualities exploded.

The authors studied the NYLS sample of 133 Upper East Side children through IQ tests, psychological questionnaires, and interviews with parents and children at regular intervals from infancy to early adulthood. In exchange for their cooperation, the parents got whatever free consultations they needed; children who required therapy were either referred out or treated by Chess (or Thomas, in the case of young adults). Financial restrictions limited the length of time the team could study the different control samples, but they were followed to some point in elementary school.

After the children underwent their final interviews, Chess and Thomas analyzed the group data for factors that predicted problems, finding that "the combination of difficult temperament and parental conflict in a preschool child does create a higher risk for poorer than average functioning in early adult life, at least for a population with the sociocultural characteristics of the NYLS." In this high-risk group 80 percent developed behavior disorders, and they came down with them earlier than the sample as a whole, in which less than half showed behavior disorders, many of which were relatively mild. Oddly enough, the low-end risk group (easy temperament, low parental conflict) also had slightly more behavior disorders than the sample overall. In agreement with other studies, the NYLS found preadolescent boys—easy or difficult—more vulnerable to parental conflict than girls, and in general more likely to develop behavior disorders.

Which children recovered in later life? Interestingly, all those in the extreme high- and low-risk groups outgrew their problems; the worst outcome prevailed in one of the middle groups—with easy temperament and severe parental conflict—in which two out of three cases continued to show serious disorder as adults.

What Chess and Thomas did next—and perhaps the most intriguing part of their study—was to focus in-depth on the children who went against type. Each of these cases is a miniature novel, showing the interaction of character and circumstance. There was, for example, Bernice, rated a child with easy temperament and low parental conflict but "occasional quick intense and even impulsive behavior with resulting mild difficulties" (the kind of erratic child that quantitative studies tend to miss). Working as a team, her parents handled her well, and the problems disappeared. But when Bernice was thirteen and just beginning to face the demands of puberty, her father, a strong and stabilizing figure, died suddenly. Her mother, stretched to the limit by four children and a demanding job, couldn't cope. Bernice developed "a severe sociopathic behavior disorder, including truancy, sexual promiscuity, stealing and lying." Psychotherapy failed to reach her.

By the time Bernice turned eighteen, her mother and three sisters were totally demoralized by her violent tantrums, which threatened to split up the family. Finally Thomas "pointed out to the mother that she could order Bernice out of the house . . . and, given their complete alienation from each other, this might be the only solution, however regrettable."

The expulsion was a gamble that happened to work. It turned out Bernice could manage when she had to. She discovered a career in which she had talent and did well, became self-supporting, and made friends. In her final interview at age twenty-two, she turned out to be thoughtful, articulate, and friendly, able to analyze her temperament and its role in her life. The Thomases felt she was not out of the woods: she would prosper if her career and love life went well, but it was "a toss-up" whether she could handle bad luck.

The most successful child in the sample was a combination of that same resilience that, as we've seen, so intrigues contemporary researchers, and old-fashioned privilege. Barbara's parents were divorced when she was two, and both remarried later. "She had clearly been able to use four parents, instead of two, as sources of strength and support, and to identify and compare different styles of coping in the two households, taking what was best from each." It didn't hurt that Barbara's working mother had a full-time housekeeper or that Barbara herself had an IQ of 164. But Stella Chess gave me an amazed, amused description of her final interview with Barbara: "I called her and she said, 'I think I have the ideal time to meet with you. We're moving to a new house and we're having the closing. I'm pregnant. I developed diabetes in pregnancy, and when I deliver, that will be over. It's going to be an induced delivery, so that by three weeks after we'll be in the new house even though it won't be unpacked, and I'll still be on maternity leave.'

"So I come to the house," Chess continued. "She had an adopted child, a Korean baby, and then they discovered she was pregnant. So this little girl was there with Barbara's stepmother who had come to help her, a lovely woman whom I had seen in therapy—not her mother but her stepmother—and Barbara was nursing the baby all through the interview. Then she said, 'I'll drive you to the airport,' and I said, 'That's not necessary, I'll take a cab.' But she had promised the other child a ride to the airport, so she drove me. After Barbara's parents broke up, the mother remarried and later divorced her second husband. And while Barbara respected and liked her stepmother, she never got very close to her. She really got her nurturance from her friends, and her relationship with her husband was obviously very close. She's close to her two children. She was a winner from the word go."

In drawing conclusions from their study, Chess and Thomas point out that "a number of our NYLS subjects were 'defiers of negative prediction." These were the children who underwent "dramatic reversals in their developmental course." Two protective factors that emerged from Chess and Thomas's distinctive mixture of quantitative and qualitative data analysis were "the therapeutic value of a firm commitment to a specific career direction . . . and/or the ability of the youngster to achieve emotional distancing from a pressuring and intrusive parent."

Not surprisingly, there is good news and bad. Among the children in the New York Longitudinal Study who developed disorders, "a significant number of cases did not improve or even grew worse in adolescent and early adult life, and it was frequently not possible in childhood to predict negative outcome. Hence, we would recommend parent guidance and other appropriate therapeutic intervention in all cases." The Thomases attest that "the emotionally traumatized child is not doomed, the parents' early mistakes are not irrevocable, and our preventative and therapeutic intervention can make a difference at all age periods."

In the chapters that follow, I will describe the ways different types of therapists provide that intervention and what assumptions underlie their work. But it is important for lay readers to keep in mind that etiology and pathogenesis are processes of almost unimaginable complexity, that in these phenomena the insights of the novelist are often as acute as the conclusions of the statistician, and that—while we know many things today that we did not know even ten years ago—it is still quite impossible to unscramble the egg.

Because children present special complications to clinicians and researchers, child psychotherapy lags a good ten years behind the treatment of adult mental disorders and way behind physical medicine. In child therapy the patient is not the customer, a circumstance that raises difficulties for the parent, the child, and the therapist; it is usually not children who come in saying, "The pain is intolerable, give me relief," but some adults who have made the decision for them (and possibly hauled them in by the hair). That is one of three special characteristics of child work that professionals have long noted; the others are that the child's verbal and conceptual abilities, the entry points for psychotherapy, are limited, and that in every area of development the child is a moving target. Finally research in pediatric psychopharmacology has moved slowly because of caution about side effects.

Unless a child is clearly psychotic, the idea of therapy troubles and perplexes most parents. Since many laymen haven't caught up with research on the complex origins of mental disorders, the assumption of parental guilt, however wrong-headed, is bound to creep in, still subtly or overtly encouraged by popular literature and by some school officials and mental health professionals. So perhaps the child is just *really* terrible two, or having a *very* difficult adolescence. Indeed, while Carl Wheeler's ups and downs are ambiguous, there's evidence that some problems do go away without treatment. (In his book *Child Psychotherapy: Developing and Identifying Effective Treatments*, Alan E. Kazdin, a professor of child psychology at Yale, cites fighting, stuttering, and enuresis as behaviors that sometimes emerge and disappear.) Some problems don't, however. "Children who show early signs of dysfunction such as unmanageability, aggression, social withdrawal, speech and language problems are at risk for subsequent psychiatric disorders," Kazdin writes, noting a need for "intervening in response to early signs . . . to prevent them from becoming worse." Particularly when symptoms are mild, parents may wonder—and even disagree—whether therapy is a useful emotional vaccination or a fashionable indulgence. (One of the goals of this book, of course, is to help the parents work out an answer to this question in relation to their own child.)

Those who believe in informed decision-making may be daunted by the choices: Kazdin identifies 230 different types of therapy available to children, from "activity-interview group" to "Z-process." (Perhaps he's stretching it to make a point, but the point is telling.) Different approaches, not to mention different practitioners, relate to parents in different ways, and this affects the parents' own comfort.

Most important, the different approaches are vastly divergent in time and therefore in cost. As this is written, the manner of payment for psychotherapy, like that for all health care in the United States, is in flux and is not likely to be firm for some years. What is sure, however, is that the mental health care system is increasingly cost-driven, and even appropriate economic concerns, if they enter the picture at the wrong time, can blur the clinical assessment of what is the best treatment for a particular disorder—or a particular child—at a particular time. How narrowly, for example, should we focus on the symptom? Does the child need several kinds of brief therapy, longer treatment, residential care? What trade-offs and compromises are safe? What, if anything, constitutes false economy in this child's case? How do we decide if a particular kind of therapy is working, and what does "working" mean? What is measurable, what is not, and what do current techniques of measurement tell us—or not tell us—about the effectiveness of a therapy?

While most clinicians would agree with the late British psychoanalyst D. W. Winnicott that the purpose of therapy is to "let the developmental processes simply take over as the analysis begins to succeed," each therapeutic approach meets—and even describes—the challenge differently. (The word *analysis,* of course, is anathema to some kinds of therapists, but as I discovered, there is no language but bureaucratese that's acceptable to all professionals, and that language is uncongenial to me. So the professionals will have to put up with the strictures of plain English.) In July 1982 *American Psychologist* published a survey of 415 members of the American Psychological Association in clinical practice, asking them, as it were, to label themselves. The largest percentage, 41.20, said they were "eclectic"; 10.84 percent called themselves "cognitive-behavioral"; 8.67 were "client-centered"; 6.75 "behavioral"; 2.65 "family therapists"; smaller percentages were "Adlerian," "reality," "Gestalt," "existential," "rational-emotive," and "transactional"; and with all these tags available, 9.16 percent still called themselves "other." While the field still seems hopelessly splintered, it's reasonable to subsume these approaches into three broad categories; each takes a distinctive view of its own task and of the patient. All these therapies may be used in conjunction with pharmacotherapy (treatment with medicines that affect thought, feeling, and behavior), which is discussed in Part V.

Psychodynamic therapy (covered in Part II) looks inward: it aims at helping the child understand his emotions. To do this, the therapist must find the origins of the problems; dynamic therapists tend to view the patient as a text to be explicated, with clues often presented in symbolic form. Classical psychoanalysis—which generally requires four sessions a week—is only one form of dynamic therapy, and while it's the form best known to laymen, it is so expensive and time-consuming that it is seldom used on children. Dynamic therapy (with one or two weekly sessions) is, however, the type most likely to take several years.

Cognitive-behavioral therapy, on the other hand, looks outward (see Part III). It trains the child to see the world differently and to change her behavioral patterns. It has its roots in experimental psychology and is dedicated to rigorous data-gathering and measurement of results, the practices that prevail in laboratories. Cognitive-behaviorists, who prefer the term *client* to *patient,* tend to look at the client as a machine with a broken part that needs fixing. Aimed at alleviating a particular group of symptoms, cognitive-behavioral therapy usually lasts between four months and a year.

Family systems therapy (see Part IV) holds that problems are not individual but reflect a malfunction in the family unit, although rapid evolution in this young field is moving many of its practitioners away from any notions like "malfunction" that might appear to be judgmental to the most sensitive observer. The family systems view—in which a symptomatic child is called the "identified patient"—has traditionally drawn on cybernetic theories of feedback and on cultural anthropology. It uses both psychodynamic and cognitive-behavioral techniques. Family systems therapy can range from one or two sessions to several years in length.

Without question, all child psychotherapy has become more eclectic in recent years, because most good clinicians agree that doctrinal purity doesn't get the job done. Edward M. Hallowell, a psychiatrist who practices in Cambridge, Massachusetts, offers an illustrative case. "A high school senior, the youngest member of a family of three children, has a sudden onset of panic attacks. Her heart starts beating, she gets light-headed, she starts sweating and trembling and becomes immobilized—she's afraid to leave the house. She then begins to have intrusive thoughts she can't control that tear down all her achievements, that say life is meaningless and all she's grown up to believe in is just a put-up job.

"The panic attacks recur so frequently that she's afraid to go out with people, afraid she'll have an attack in the middle of a date or right on the hockey field. So she gives up hockey, she gives up dating, she considers dropping out of school. At that point she comes to see me. After interviewing her, I ask to get more information and to see her mother, who comes in and tells me about the family. It turns out the father had been drinking for a number of years while the kids were growing up, and while it didn't interfere overtly with any of their lives—he continued to make a living and they all went on vacations together—it did undermine the parents' relationship, and she thinks it might have influenced the children.

"My treatment plan was threefold. I prescribed a tricyclic antidepressant to reduce the panic attacks, and within a week they had stopped. But I also felt the cause had to do with what was going on in the family, so I arranged to start family therapy with the mother, the father, and the three children. Sure enough, by the second session, the mother and father began to tell of their resentments for each other over the years. My patient said, as she listened to it, 'I've never felt such a relief—this is the secret I've been growing up with.' Rather than feeling anxious, she felt relieved. The third part of the treatment was individual therapy with her because she needed to resolve dynamic issues of her own.

"She had to bear the message before she went off to college that something was amiss. The panic attacks got attention. That was unconscious, so in that sense psychodynamic, but this is what the symptom achieved, and she wouldn't have achieved it if she hadn't come to see someone who believed in family therapy. But I don't think family therapy alone would have taken care of the attacks: she needed medicine for those right away. Family therapy wouldn't have taken care of her individual issues either."

But however flexible and savvy a particular therapist may be, he or she was trained somewhere, is a member of certain professional organizations, keeps up with particular journals, and attends specific conferences where papers are presented; in other words, tribal affiliation narrows the focus and can't help affecting the bent of the therapy. I often found clinicians unaware of important work done by practitioners with different orientations. Inhabitants of some metaphorical archipelago, they seemed distressingly insular: the Bugis didn't know what the Toraja were doing, and their view of the Toraja, learned long ago in graduate school or even in college, was oversimplified and outdated. This is understandable: the volume of psychotherapeutic literature is so enormous that a practicing clinician is hard put to keep up with developments in his or her own area, let alone others. But it highlights a serious defect in the treatment that children may receive.

It is also noteworthy that patients have changed since many practitioners received their training: as America looks increasingly varied, researchers are becoming more aware of cultural differences among ethnic groups and the way they affect a child's and a family's behavior, not to mention clinical notions of normalcy. And as the psychologist Judith Wallerstein, a specialist in the problems of divorced families, has pointed out, the basic theories underlying psychotherapy were all constructed assuming an intact two-parent family, one that is far less common than it used to be. Insofar as practitioners are mindful of these differences, therapy is much more sophisticated than it used to be.

The breadth of the individual clinician's knowledge varies; some are defensive about what they don't know. The fragmentation of the mental health care system is an important subject for policymakers to address, but until they do, it behooves lay people making decisions about child therapy to inform themselves. Practicing psychotherapy is a skill that deserves respect, not a black art that requires reverence; with certain exceptions, most of what the clinician can read and understand the nonprofessional can digest equally well. (That has been my premise in writing this book.)

Lay people are often confused by the different types of practitioners in the field. Whether a therapist is a psychiatrist, a psychologist, or a social worker, that person ought to have special training and experience in treating children and adolescents.

A psychiatrist is an M.D. who has had four years of medical school, one year of internship, at least two years of approved residency training in general psychiatry with adults, and a two-year residency in child and adolescent psychiatry, which includes supervised experience in a range of therapies and settings. All certified psychiatrists have passed an examination in general psychiatry given by the American Board of Psychiatry and Neurology; after completing the second residency, child and adolescent psychiatrists are eligible to take another test for certification in their subspecialty.

A child analyst may or may not be a psychiatrist or have a medical degree: he or she has been trained at a psychoanalytic institute, which studies the influence of early life experiences on mental illness. Psychoanalytic training alone does not qualify a practitioner to prescribe drugs (which can be done only by a physician), diagnose physical symptoms, or offer behavioral or family therapy.

A clinical psychologist in private practice is a Ph.D., a Psy.D., or an Ed.D. who has had about five years of graduate training, including a year of internship and several half-year practica, which are programs of supervised clinical experience that graduate students take along with their courses. Some states also require postdoctoral practica for licensing. Psychologists who work for state institutions may, in some cases, have a master's degree instead of a doctorate.

A clinical social worker should have an M.S.W., the result of a two-year graduate program of classes, internship, and fieldwork; several years of postgraduate experience may be required for a state license, which entitles practitioners to use the letters CSW or LCSW or some other state variation after their names. Members of the National Association of Social Workers who meet prescribed educational requirements, pass an examination, and submit professional references may join the Academy of Certified Social Workers and use the letters ACSW after their names.

Some thirty-two states now certify or license marriage and family therapists, who are then entitled to use the letters L.M.F.T. after their names. As with other practitioners, state requirements vary but are generally similar to those for clinical membership in the American Association of Marriage and Family Therapists: a master's degree in marriage and family therapy or a related mental health field from a regionally accredited institution, including certain required courses; a three-hundred-hour clinical practicum; and a specific number of "client contact hours," some of which are under supervision of an AAMFT-approved supervisor.

Psychiatrists (not individually but as a group) look down on nonmedical practitioners. Psychologists (whose private practice fees are often just as expensive as those of psychiatrists) respond that they refer patients to M.D.s for physical diagnosis and prescription and point out that neither

Anna Freud nor Erik H. Erikson nor Bruno Bettelheim, among other distinguished theorists, was an M.D.

Some psychologists may condescend to social workers, but certain aspects of social work training (women's issues, ethnic and cultural studies) are unique and may have particular value to some clients. "A good social work clinician should be able to relate a child's problems to something in the home or school environment," says Carol H. Meyer, a professor at the Columbia University School of Social Work. "Whether the kids are rich or poor, nobody else wants to get their hands dirty in the environment. When a psychiatrist who has a patient on psychotropic drugs sends that patient out into the community, the social worker deals with how he'll manage. When a psychiatrist says 'this child is abused, take her away from her mother,' the social worker deals with the mother and child."

To compare the numbers of psychiatrists, psychologists, and social workers who deal with children is difficult because analogous figures don't exist, but the following numbers (the most recent available for each profession) ought to give some sense of the demographics of therapy. In 1994 some 7,500 child psychiatrists were practicing in the United States. In 1989 there were 56,530 clinically active psychologists, although only a few thousand of these were "child clinical" specialists; that same year there were 81,737 clinically active social workers, most of whom work with children at least part of the time. Thus nonmedical practitioners are engulfing the psychiatrists, putting them on the defensive. Moreover, to be fair, it is important to note that there are enough "therapists" hanging out shingles without adequate credentials of any kind to invoke wariness in the consumer.

The type of practitioner a patient encounters depends somewhat on the therapy chosen. Psychiatrists tend to concentrate either in psychopharmacology or in traditional psychodynamic therapy, with a few Turks in family systems. (A social worker who practices at a prestigious family therapy institute may be as expensive as a psychiatrist; clinics have their own fee structures; and private practitioners are, so to speak, free agents.) The cognitive-behavioral field, derived from psychological research, is mostly Ph.D.s. There are, however, both psychologists and social workers doing dynamic therapy. Fees are more a matter of the setting than the therapist's academic credentials, although insurance companies may not reimburse for all therapists equally unless required to do so by state law.

Private patients, whatever the practitioner's training, are charged what the local market will bear. Clinic patients will pay lower fees in exchange for using supervised student therapists; they might also barter the right to be observed or taped for research purposes. What all this boils down to is a vigorous marketplace competition in addition to religious war.

Let us, then, watch some clinicians at work.

CHAPTER 2

FINDING THE LESION

A child's loves and hates cannot be evaluated without an inquiry into the loves and hates of those around her.

> —Erik H. Erikson,
> *Childhood and Society* (1950)

In classification of a series of cases one can use a scale: at the normal end of the scale there is play, which is a simple and enjoyable dramatization of inner world life; at the abnormal end of the scale there is play which contains a denial of the inner world, the play being in that case always compulsive, excited, anxiety-driven, and more sense-exploiting than happy.

> —D. W. Winnicott,
> "Appetite and Emotional
> Disorder" (1936)

"IF YOU COME ON TUESDAY, YOU'LL SEE a little boy who thinks he's a dinosaur," says Gabrielle A. Carlson, M.D., a small, animated woman with short curly brown hair. Carlson is director of the Division of Child Psychiatry at the State University of New York at Stony Brook. The tone of her invitation (though certainly not the idiom) is, "Come along, Watson, the game's afoot!"; while she has published many articles on affective disorders, it is the complexity of all psychiatric diagnosis that clearly seizes her.

A few days later we are sitting in the cafeteria of University Medical Center being briefed for the case conference that is about to take place. The boy has been in the hospital for observation over the last two weeks;

Carlson met him the day he was admitted. Now she is returning for a second look, to hear what the staff has learned, and to help diagnose his problem and arrive at a plan for treatment.

"His name is Hector Lopez, and he's seven years old," says Silvana Fennig, the postdoctoral fellow who's in charge of the case; she speaks in a heavy Italian accent. "He lives with his biological mother, and he attends first grade special education classes. Special education is not for learning disability in his case. He is classified [by the school committee that evaluates children for special ed] as emotionally disabled. He needs to attend small classes, with eight students, one teacher, and one aide."

Carlson is punctuating the narrative with explanatory comments. "With that small a classroom environment," she tells me, "that means he's been in deep trouble already."

"I'm going to begin with what was the reason for his admission," Fennig says. "After this I will come back to the story. The reason for the admission was increasing disruptive, aggressive behavior. The second point was accident-prone behavior—he was running into the street without any specific reason, but he explained this as 'I don't know, I don't care, it doesn't matter.' "

" 'I don't care what happens to me' was the point," Carlson says.

"The third reason," continues Fennig, "was increasing fantasy involvement. He was always playing as a dinosaur or another animal, I think you say for ten hours a day. The mother reports that he was hearing voices that said, 'Do bad things,' like running into the street or hurting people. He doesn't want to do things at home, he was fighting with other kids, and he was all the time jumping and running from one place to another with a reduced attention span, high distractibility, not able to wait or play with other people in games, and very impulsive behavior."

"What's important to listen to is we have a young kid, only seven, who is classified by first grade," Carlson tells me. "It means that whatever he's got, he's probably got it severely and has had it for a while. Most of the symptoms aren't all that unusual. They're garden variety—hyperactive, impulsive, aggressive behavior. But playing you're a monster or dinosaur ten hours a day is fairly unusual, and putting yourself into life-threatening situations and not caring what happens to yourself is very unusual, and supposedly hearing voices is certainly unusual."

Fennig reports that Hector had had no birth complications and his earliest abnormality was speech delay: his speech is fine now. At age two he had gone to a Head Start–type program where he was considered highly aggressive and inattentive, but despite his placement in special ed, he had never been given any medication or treatment for this behavior. "It is a very important question, what happened with this family," Fennig says. "It seems this behavior can be related to family traumatic experience from the beginning.

"The mother has a long history of affective pathology that we don't know in detail, but in early adolescence she was hospitalized more than once because of suicide attempts. When Hector was born, she continued to be depressed and was practically unable to take care of him. She also described some high periods, but we don't know exactly if they are manic episodes. She's aware that she is physically abusive to the kid when she is irritated. Three months ago she was hospitalized for a suicide attempt, which seemed to be tied to some disappointment in her gay relationship with her girlfriend.

"Now we come back to Father. Father was described also as having a long history of psychopathology. It seems that from early childhood he was always very suspicious and jealous, and he has also been hospitalized because of inability to function. The mother and father were divorced when Hector was two years old, and the father became involved in a new triangular relationship with the best girlfriend of the mother.

"Hector was always exposed to aggression and violence. The father was jealous of the mother and her girlfriend. The end of this situation was a few months ago, when the father killed this woman. He explained it as accidentally."

"Manslaughter, not malice aforethought," notes Carlson.

"Hector saw a videotape of the father with the handcuffs," Fennig says. "I think the mother videotaped the news, and when Hector didn't believe her and accused that she wanted to separate him from his father, she showed him the videotape."

It's time for the case conference. We bus our trays, and as we're walking upstairs, Carlson describes the diagnostic issues. "You collect your information with the idea of hypothesis-testing," she says. "Am I dealing with a hyperactive kid? Am I dealing with a retarded kid? An emotionally disturbed child who is anxious or depressed? A psychotic youngster who has been so traumatized by events in his life that he just can't see straight? Is it all of this or much of this? It needn't be just one thing. So you collect all this information and start lining it up under different diagnostic possibilities."

The diagnostic team is beginning to gather in a small sitting room. It includes Joe Gartner, the medical director of the children's inpatient unit; Shel Weintraub, the clinical psychologist on the unit; Rick Schwabish, a school psychologist who consults on the unit; Debbie Lane, the boy's teacher at the in-house school he's been attending during his hospital stay; and Corinna Walsh, one of the nurses. Gartner, who is in his thirties and has curly brown hair and glasses, asks Fennig to review the history, which she does briefly. "What was our differential diagnosis at the entry point?" Carlson wants to know.

Fennig's answer throws the book at Hector, so to speak: she appears to be reading the table of contents of the DSM-III-R—the American Psychiatric Association's *Diagnostic and Statistical Manual of Mental Disorders,* third edition–revised. "We talked about Attention Deficit Disorder, Oppositional Defiant Disorder, Conduct Disorder, some kinds of psychosis. Also, his environmental history was Posttraumatic Stress Disorder because of the episode of the murder, and all his life was another trauma and another trauma, and maybe some of the fantasy behavior was related to that. We need to also realize some learning problems at school." All these are mental disorders spelled out in the manual.

While lay people tend to describe children's behavior (or misbehavior) in cosmic terms, clinical diagnosis is highly precise: nuances make a world of difference in what treatment the patient eventually receives. In brief, according to the edition of the DSM in use at the time of this case conference, the patterns of behavior associated with Attention Deficit Disorder were inattentive, hyperactive, and/or impulsive to a developmentally inappropriate degree; the patterns of behavior tied to Oppositional Defiant Disorder were negativistic, hostile, and logically enough, defiant; and the more serious Conduct Disorder, according to the manual, embraced "a persistent pattern of conduct in which the basic rights of others or major age-appropriate social norms or rules are violated . . . at home, at school, with peers, and in the community." (While current definitions of psychosis vary with the particular illness, the diagnosis always requires that there be some sort of delusions and impairment in what professionals call "reality testing," which means the ability to distinguish inner experience from experience of the outer world. Posttraumatic Stress Disorder in children involves disorganized or agitated behavior and a host of other symptoms that follow exposure to actual or threatened death or serious injury to oneself or people one is close to.) The manual represents an effort—sometimes successful, sometimes less so—to grab hold of these nuances, and it has left its authors open to both intelligent disagreement and frivolous ridicule. The changes in the criteria for each of these disorders that were made in the revised edition of the manual—DSM-IV—published in May 1994, a year after this case conference, would seem to a nonprofessional eye to be minor.

Carlson asks Fennig to describe how Hector's mental status (what lay people would call his demeanor—the outward expression of whatever might be troubling him and the first evidence the clinical observer can draw on) relates to the various diagnostic possibilities.

"I think the mental status I describe now is also observed by the unit. He is a small cute boy, Hispanic, who tends to be a little young for his stated age—he seems like a five-year-old. It was difficult to have communication and also make eye contact with him because he was jumping all over the place. He was acting like an animal during the interview and, most of the time, making faces and jumping on the furniture like a monkey, like a dinosaur, like a cat. Most of the time he was unable to focus in a conversation, but at times, both in the interview and when he stayed here in the unit, he could talk and relate with people and have good eye contact and talk about regular things in a normal way—not crazy, bizarre things. He was able to sit with a book and tell you the story without a problem."

"He was in touch with reality, then," Carlson says. "He wasn't sitting off on some other planet, totally consumed by the fact that he was a dinosaur."

"During this week of observation," Fennig answers, "we looked at his bizarre behavior and said, 'Stop with this. We want to work with you as a boy.' And he was able to talk like a boy. With commands and requests his behavior was under control. Most of the time I think he had an angry affect. He was not sad, he was not happy, but he was irritated and angry." (The term *affect* refers to both feelings and their manifestations, which would be cognitive, behavioral, and physiological.)

Gartner, the medical director of the unit, chimes in. "At times he would persist in acting like a dinosaur, but with very firm limits you could get him to stop that, and at some point you could engage him. You wouldn't know from the conversation alone—except that he moved around too much and was more easily distractible—you couldn't pick up that he was psychotic. He was cogent, logical, and developmentally appropriate."

Weintraub, the clinical psychologist, a slightly built man with white hair, says, "We were concerned about the report that he heard voices, so when I saw him the first day, I really talked to him about that. I was curious because he said he was hearing voices right then, but his affect and behavior were not consistent with someone hearing voices. Nevertheless, he described hearing voices at other times in the past, and it still had us quite concerned that there might be some psychotic disorder."

Gartner contends that "along with the genetic history, it is very clear that it's a psychotic disorder. It really makes us wonder if this is a kid who is developing the same problems that his parents had. So that was the most worrisome question—whether he was psychotic or whether his behavioral problem, including attention problems and oppositionality, was secondary to a primary psychotic disorder." Does Hector, that is, have two different disorders, each of which has a separate etiology and needs separate treatment, or is there one treatable disorder that has resulted in two sets of symptoms, one subordinate to the other?

Now Carlson asks, "Silvana was talking about how Mom was depressed and that she had mood swings. We had discussed whether this kid could be bipolar [the current term for manic depressive] or have a manic psychosis. Was he euphoric? Did he have any sleep problems particularly? Is there any diurnal variation in his behavior? Is he silly, infectious? Does he make you want to laugh because he looks like he's having such a good time?"

"He looks pretty much the same every day," Gartner says. "You don't see wild periodic swings from irritability to euphoria, at least not on a day-by-day or week-by-week basis. He doesn't have a clear-cut history of sleep or appetite problems. It's really a picture of disruptive behavior that is continuous, with a recent onset of more disorganized behavior. The irritability was one thing that might be suggestive of a mood disturbance, but there was no grandiosity. He does have an infectious quality, but that's more because he's so involved in his play, almost too far into fantasy but still on the normal spectrum. He'll smile at you when he's pacing back and forth on his bed as a dinosaur, so it's playful, not driven. But when he first came in, you had to redirect him over and over. It was like his behavior had taken on an autonomous quality where he wasn't responsive."

Schwabish has given Hector two projective tests to smoke out disordered thinking: the Rorschach and the TAT, or Thematic Apperception Test, in which the subject is shown a series of cards depicting scenes that might illuminate attitudes toward aggression, achievement, parents, siblings, and fears and is asked to make up stories about them. Hector, it turns out, performed very differently on each of these tests. "On the Rorschach he had difficulty processing stuff," Schwabish reports. "His perceptions violated the contours of the blots, which is not all that unusual for little children because they don't really follow the shape anyway. But what was interesting was, he would look at the shape quickly and come up with a picture and then go back and change it and change it and change it."

"Was this an impulsive response?" Carlson asks.

"He would stare at it for a while, but his response was very quick. He was like he hadn't really processed what he was looking at." Carlson presses Schwabish on this, because it doesn't sound like an actual thought disorder, just a problem in figuring out what the shape might be. The boy's answers, she is told, didn't have much to do with the form of the blot, but he stuck to his guns on what it looked like to him. Then "on the TAT he gave very, very good stories," Schwabish says. "Usually with small children you have to prompt them continually because you want all this information out of them. 'How do the characters feel? What are they thinking? How is the story going to turn out?' And he had no trouble. He gave half-page stories, and they were appropriate, they made sense, there was cause and effect. All of them had happy endings. Usually the character had a conflict that was somehow solved. There was one where he told a violent story, but it was a violent card. It all surprised me, considering how poor his Rorschach was."

Weintraub, who is doing a research project on high-risk children, has given Hector some tests from the project on something called "cognitive slippage, which is kind of a watered-down version of formal thought disorder, looking at the form of the disorder and not just the content. Violent and morbid thoughts certainly dominated his fantasy, but there was no disturbance in the *form* of his thought. He would have been in my study, as the offspring of psychotic parents." In other words, Hector didn't think dinosaurs—or even criminals—were pursuing him. Gartner asks if Weintraub found any grandiosity; Weintraub says, "He's small for his age and he still sees himself as the biggest child in the school—he could beat up any of the other kids. That could qualify as grandiose."

Hector's IQ is 90 full-scale, "at the low end of the average range,"

Schwabish says. "His verbal was ninety-eight and his performance was eighty-three, which means he is better able to process information using his auditory as opposed to visual-perceptual faculties. It is interesting that he was highest in Similarities—abstract reasoning—where he got a twelve. His lowest score was a four, on Picture Arrangement. He had some difficulty perceiving social situations accurately." (In general, the average score on each IQ subtest is 10, and scores between 7 and 13 are considered within the average. So Hector's highest score was a high-average, while his lowest, the 4 on the Picture Arrangement subtest, was two standard deviations below the mean—significantly low.)

Carlson asks how Hector organizes events in his life; Schwabish says that the Rorschach suggests a problem putting things in the right order, but the well-sequenced TAT stories dispute that.

Now it's Lane's turn to tell how Hector's doing in her classroom. He's a couple of months below grade level. Carlson says, "Considering his life, that's not bad." Otherwise, Lane's report has much in common with everyone else's: in the beginning he did a lot of playing dinosaur, but when you were very firm with him, he'd come back to reality. Lane finds him "very manipulative and very oppositional," which previously interfered with his schoolwork, but he's doing much better now.

"Do you think he's just more compliant now, or do you think he's paying better attention?" Carlson asks. It's both. Lane says he likes to make up plays with other kids, and when and how he does this is entirely *appropriate* (which I have learned, over the past couple of years, is one of the buzzwords in the world of mental health).

Walsh checks in with a similar picture, saying that Hector's dinosaur play alienated many of the other kids on the unit, but—except for the occasional growl or hiss—he's much better now. Weintraub explains to me: "When you're working with kids, you have to know something about the mental norms, and this kind of play, you know kids his age play with imagination, but it was the way he did it, and it set the other kids off."

Finally Carlson moves the discussion to Hector's relationship with his mother. Fennig says, "He is very aware of where his father is now, what happened with this woman that was with his mother, and what happened with his mother. But he loves his mother, and he needs his mother, and he wants to go back to her. At the beginning, when the mother came here for the first visit, she was very depressed, complaining that she felt detached from the child and depressed about her lack of self-control with him. We were very active with her because she needed treatment and she wasn't going to go get it. But now she's more in contact with the child and says he's better with her also, not always talking about fantasy and animals. The mother is involved in another new relationship with a woman who comes to live with her now. This woman is also very involved with Hector—she was here and was kissing Hector on his mouth. That is something we will need to talk about and the ability of the mother to take care of Hector."

Gartner's next comment evokes the interactive process described by Chess and Thomas. "The history of the mother, of course, is of having major ups and downs, being grossly impaired, being not available, and the kid reciprocally being progressively autonomous and not involved with the environment. His history is very long for that, with major periods of the mother being unavailable, impaired, hospitalized."

Fennig says Hector was always able to play animal games for hours, but now this is exaggerated; his mother is delighted by his rich fantasy life and his ability to amuse himself. This leads Carlson and Gartner to puzzle over his perseverance, which doesn't seem typical of a child with attention deficit disorder. Finally Carlson says, "Shall we have him come in now? How will he be with a roomful of people? Will it scare the crap out of him?" Gartner suspects he will be rowdy, which is fine with Carlson. "I don't want him to be quiet," she says.

As the others move chairs around, Carlson folds a piece of yellow paper into that familiar childhood open-and-close shape that fits over the fingers. "When I was a kid," I tell her, "we called that a cootie-catcher."

Now a small Latino boy with dark curly hair and glasses is brought in. His face is arranged in a flamboyant and charming pout. "I was making a toy for you, Hector," says Carlson. "Have a seat for a second. I'm trying to make a toy for you because I knew you'd be annoyed at coming in here. What color Easter eggs were you making?"

"They were real ones, blue and green."

Carlson is opening and shutting the cootie-catcher. "Do you want to put some eyes on it? Does anybody have a pen or something?" Lane hands over a Bic. "This is the mouth," she says, snapping the jaws, "so we'll put the eyes there. . . . Is it going to be a lady or a man?"

"A lady," Hector says.

"Do you want to put some lipstick on? Does the lady have a name? What we really need is a Magic Marker."

"That might explode," says Hector. "You might drop it."

"A pen that explodes when you drop it? You were showing me this morning the bombs on your Super Mario Brothers, and everything exploded. And that pen explodes too. What do you do with it when it explodes?"

Hector says, "I don't know. Throw it away," and he appears unresponsive to this line of questioning, so Carlson moves on. She and Hector are making a face on the cootie-catcher, and once again she asks him to name it. "Andrew," Hector volunteers.

"I thought you said it was a girl. I never heard of a girl called Andrew. You could make me Andrea. What's your mom's name?"

"Marta. How about Danielle?" Without missing a beat.

"Oh, that's a pretty name," says Carlson in a high, squeaky voice. "I like Danielle. What's your name?" she asks, walking Danielle under Hector's chin. Hector giggles.

Something has happened to this woman of usually impeccable professional demeanor. She has become a thoroughly dedicated puppeteer. The room is silent; no papers move. The onlookers are transfixed.

"I'll behave myself," squeaks Danielle. "What you have to do to make me behave is to ask. What do you want me to do?"

"Behave."

"What means behave?"

Hector is giggling. "Please be good." Danielle asks if he will take off points or put her in the time-out chair ("no") and if he'll still like her if she's good ("yes"). During all this Hector is intently drawing on Danielle, laughing and shrieking and appearing to have a wonderful time, and Danielle is asking questions in her squeaky, bantering tone. She elicits mainly that Hector has a friend on the unit named Michael.

"Somebody told me you liked to play games with animals, dinosaurs." The conversation is keyed-up and giggly on both sides. "What kind of dinosaurs do you like?" Danielle asks.

"Meat-eaters."

"They eat hamburgers?"

"They eat other dinosaurs."

"Dinosaur burgers." Danielle is growling, and they talk more about dinosaurs. Hector claims to have met a Tyrannosaurus rex. "I thought they were extinct. Do you know what extinct means?"

"They still live."

"You mean for real or in your head?"

"In my head. I saw a dinosaur with Michael."

"Are dinosaurs big and strong? Why do you like to pretend you're a dinosaur?"

"I like to make them growl."

"I bet dinosaurs are bigger and stronger than little boys, aren't they?"

"I wish I was a dinosaur." While this is the sort of exchange that would not be out of place in a child analyst's office—surprising, because Carlson hails from the world of biological psychiatry—it turns out to be a blind alley. Nothing substantive comes out of Hector, who proves to be an artful dodger despite some clever questioning. When Danielle, perhaps, is getting a bit too close to the bone ("Does your mom ever make you sad?"), Hector says to the puppet with irritation, "Stop opening your big fat mouth and shut up. Get back there!"

"You hurt my feelings."

"Please get back."

Hector, for all his rowdy giggles, appears in touch with reality, able to control the conversation, and focused on what he wants to do (draw teeth on Danielle).

They are wrapping up the interview. Carlson, herself again, offers Danielle to Hector, showing him how to work the puppet, and asks him to return the pen to Miss Lane. Then he is gone, and the tension in the room drops.

Shel Weintraub says, "Did you uncover anything, Gay, in that interaction that you were concerned about?"

Carlson answers slowly, "I think the fact that he felt more like a preschooler. I felt like I was playing with a four-year-old, not a seven-year-old."

"Immature, delayed, but not aberrant," says Gartner.

"Not deviant, no, and talking about what he wanted to talk about," Carlson goes on. "He seemed engaged and interactive and not entirely inappropriate. Sometimes he said things I didn't understand, but I still don't get Long Island accents. His mother's name was Maaah-ta? The ringer here, of course, is he's on Ritalin right now—so the sixty-four-dollar question is, What would we have seen had he not gotten . . ."

Ritalin is the drug of choice for attention-deficit/hyperactivity disorder. It's a ringer for the visitor: I hadn't been told.

In four long discussions I've had with Gabrielle Carlson over several years, she's been a fount of diagnostic puzzles like Hector. It was, indeed, these puzzles that got her into child psychiatry. "At Cornell Medical School I did an elective in psychiatry, which I hated," she says. "I talk a lot. I could never be a real psychoanalytic person: I couldn't keep my mouth shut. My supervisors would pull these interpretations out of the air, and I'd say, 'There's no way in hell I could come up with that kind of interpretation.' I had a wonderful internist supervisor, and I thought I would go into hematology.

"So I did a medicine internship at Washington University in St. Louis. By the end of October, I'd been in the emergency room numbers of times. And I am tired of waking up at three o'clock in the morning to treat yet another twenty-three-year-old female who comes into the ER with abdominal pain with no known etiology, and you figure there's something going on in this kid's life and it ain't her stomach.

"I figured I need to know more about psychiatry. Washington University has probably been the single most influential source in the nosology [classification] and formulation of diagnosis in psychiatry. I said, 'This I could do. I can't keep my mouth shut for hours at a time, but I can do this.' I'm a problem-solver."

Carlson became interested in children during her second year of residency. "I was treating a woman who came essentially because she had a little twelve-year-old who was a four-plus brat. Everybody decided there was something wrong with this mother, and I was supposed to treat her in therapy.

"She was a lovely woman, and after the two years I treated her, she was doing beautifully and her kid was still a brat. I remember thinking that if somebody comes to me with a stomachache, I know what to ask to find out whether they ate too much pizza, or I'd better get them to the surgeon, or it's just their ulcer acting up. I didn't know what to ask to see whether this is a relationship problem or whether the *kid* really needs an evaluation and treatment.

"Number two, I was always interested in depression and manic depressive illness. It's been known since practically Hippocrates that this runs in families—and yet people were saying it didn't occur in children and adolescents. I thought maybe I needed to know more about children and adolescents to understand why this disorder didn't occur. Of course, once you get into it, you realize it does occur—you just haven't been looking for it."

The medical approach to diagnosis—which starts by nailing down criteria that define a disorder—is favored by many psychiatrists trained in the past two or three decades: practitioners with Carlson's point of view are riding high these days. "There is a long heritage to this," she points out. "When physicians started looking at fevers, they studied the pattern of the fevers and found they weren't all the same. You have fevers that peak at four o'clock in the afternoon, and fevers that peak every three days, and fevers that are low and chronic, and maybe something different is causing each of those fevers, and by golly it is. Every three days is malaria. Tuberculosis peaks in the afternoon. Low and chronic is cancer. So there is some notion that if you look at the pathology and the etiology, there's a relationship.

"I was in medical school at just the time the CAT scan was developed," Carlson remembers. (She graduated from Cornell University Medical College in 1968.) "I can hear my neurology instructor saying this would change the way neurologists practice, because until you were able to get a cross-sectional picture of the brain, you had to do a very sensitive neurological exam, and you spent half your life trying to decide where the lesion was. Medical students these days are not trained to take a history anymore, not the way I was trained, nor are they trained to do a physical examination the way I was trained."

But neurology is not psychiatry, in which, as Carlson says, "you're still looking for where the lesion is. And the only way you can go about it is by taking a meticulous history and doing a very sensitive evaluation of the patient—how he thinks, how he feels, how he answers particular questions, how he interacts—and by putting that together, much as Osler did by the bedside in clinical medicine at the turn of the century, because that's all he could do."

Besides the case conference at Stony Brook, I watched Carlson at work diagnosing a schizophrenic thirteen-year-old boy in a special-ed public school and interviewing an upper-middle-class couple in advance of meeting their hemophiliac son; the parents hoped Carlson would "help Philip feel better about himself, help him deal with his problems, his very real frustrations." In all three situations and in the two conferences where she played the Eminent Authority consulting with colleagues of varying credentials, Carlson appeared to have interpersonal perfect pitch, even though "working with people" had not been her motive for choosing psychiatry. Her tribal affiliation is with biologically oriented practitioners, for whom pharmacotherapy is central: thus professionals in other branches of mental health call them "pill-pushers."

"At the moment," Carlson had said to me the first time we met, "the biological framework is very important, very compelling, because everybody hopes—and I hope too—that we will find the spirochete, the vitamin deficiency, the genetic mistake. . . . Ninety percent of what was in mental hospitals a hundred years ago was tertiary syphilis. Maybe we have a recrudescence now and then, and we have AIDS now, but the fact is, you don't have to worry about psychological treatment of general paresis because you don't have tertiary syphilis anymore. You don't have to worry about the dementia you get with vitamin B deficiency because basically, except for alcoholics, you don't have vitamin B deficiency. So the hope is that if you could find the quirk that makes people develop a panic disorder or that makes people schizophrenic or depressed, you could wipe those illnesses off the face of the earth or just give people what they need and take care of them.

"That's a wonderful thought, but it isn't going to happen next week or within the time I have to deal with Mr. and Mrs. Jones and George. What you have to deal with is what you've got in front of you, and you have to deal with it the best way you can."

Medically based diagnosis has been pursued wholeheartedly by practitioners in Carlson's tribe but is accepted more grudgingly by other groups of professionals, who balk at putting psychological problems in neatly labeled boxes. She finds it most useful because "somebody can say their child's impulsive, and you don't know what that means. I'll be thinking, here's a kid who sees a ladder out the window and his first impulse is to run up it and look off the roof. Somebody else means impulsive is a seven-year-old kid who sees his five-year-old sister with a toy he wants and he'll go grab it out of her hand. That's not a mental disorder in my book—that's a typical seven-year-old snatching a toy from his less competent sister. If that's what you mean by impulsive and you want to help that boy mediate those impulses so that he asks his sister for her toy, that's minimal to psychotherapy. So it's important that we understand what impulsive is and then decide what kinds of treatments are there."

Most of us, for example, get the blues from time to time, particularly if there's trouble in our lives; one would hardly expect a cheerful outlook in a boy with hemophilia. Sadness alone is not necessarily deemed pathological. Nonprofessionals who say, "God, I'm depressed today," are being clinically imprecise; clinicians would use the term *demoralization* to describe situational gloom and *dysphoria* to denote a sad mood. It's only when dysphoria is accompanied by certain other symptoms (forming a *syndrome*) and this clinical complex has "a specifiable course, duration, outcome, response to treatment, and potential familial, psychological, and biological correlates" that the patient has a disorder.

Children's mental disorders are particularly puzzling to define because some arise in childhood and recede in adulthood, others seem to begin in adolescence, and a third group shows symptoms that vary with age. For a long time, Carlson says, there were two views of childhood depression. "The psychoanalytic people said depression doesn't happen in children, they don't have the ego constructs, they don't have the moral concepts, they don't have self-esteem, let alone worrying about the loss of it. They can't think about the future." Depression, according to this point of view, requires a certain level of intellectual and emotional maturity.

"Another view said they do get depressed but not the way adults do. They run away, become aggressive, take drugs, stop eating, develop anorexia, get pregnant. This was the 'depressive equivalence' notion.

"What we have now evolved—I've written a paper about it—is that a substantial number of children have at least two separate problems. They have a behavior disorder or some other disorder that gets the clinician's attention first—usually what the parent complains about. 'Johnny's still wetting the bed.' 'Mary's defiant.' 'George is not doing well in school.' When you spend some time talking with Johnny or Mary or George, in fact you find they are quite depressed."

This means they exhibit certain "core symptoms" of depression that adults and children share: sadness, anhedonia (a most evocative dictionary definition of this is "incapacity for happiness"), low self-esteem, and difficulties with eating and sleeping. In addition, children and adults have a few separate depressive symptoms that are, so to speak, developmentally appropriate; for example, irritability is apparently a more common symptom among depressed children than depressed adults, because they are less able to identify and describe their moods.

"I think there is a definite familial aggregation of the disorder, and the more pervasive it is, the more validated you are in deciding that's what the kid's got," Carlson says. "There's good data to show the odds are much less without familial incidence, but that doesn't mean it won't occur. In general, what we call 'co-morbidity'—having more than one disorder at the same time—seems to be particularly common in children, attention deficit disorder plus depression, or conduct disorder plus depression, or anxiety disorder plus depression. When there's no family history of depression, the depressive symptoms might be secondary to the other disorder. If the family is riddled with different disorders, that complicates the diagnosis even further, and the more you've got wrong with you, the worse off you are."

The publication of DSM-IV in 1994—a year after I sat in on Hector's case conference—met with a slew of angry articles that seemed to reflect the same emotion aroused by developments in psychopharmacology: indeed, the ascendance of biological psychiatry has hit a raw nerve, not only among those mental health practitioners who are in a position to suffer from it but in the general public as well. The DSM, as we will see, is very much a work-in-progress and far from perfect, but the ferocity it provokes appears irrational. It is not the tool of evil drug companies but a logical step in a hundred-and-fifty-year-old effort to understand the kinds and dimensions of mental illness in the United States. This attempt began with the 1840 census, which recorded only one diagnostic category: "idiocy-insanity." The classification system had bloomed into seven categories by 1880, and by 1917, the Bureau of the Census was beginning to collaborate with the forerunner of the American Psychiatric Association to gather more scientifically accurate statistical data. Once the psychiatrists entered the picture, the project also aimed to produce a clinically useful document.

After World War II the need to develop workable diagnostic criteria for mental illness among veterans brought urgency to this effort. The World Health Organization published a section on mental disorders in its current *International Classification of Diseases,* and the APA's variant of this became DSM-I, which came out in 1952. Subsequent editions of the manual, reflecting contemporary diagnostic refinements, appeared over the years.

One source of the anger, maybe, is the growing use of the DSM as the bible of reimbursement by insurance companies and government agencies. It is true that biological psychiatrists, rather more than practitioners with other orientations, tend to describe cases in DSM-lingo (which is as much a jargon as the formulations of psychoanalysts), but it is fair to say that the Procrustean reverence for the manual's diagnostic categories— what doesn't appear in the DSM doesn't exist—is more the attitude of bureaucrats than psychotherapists.

Perhaps the most diagnostically controversial of children's disorders is what is now called attention-deficit/hyperactivity disorder (familiarly shortened to AD/HD or ADD), one of the possibilities in Hector's case. It's a source of contention because the diagnosis occurs so frequently and the treatment of choice is medication. Local schools often refer possible AD/HD cases to Carlson for assessment; for the most part, she says, children who come in via school are less troubled than those brought by their parents. "There may be any number of different reasons why the child is having problems paying attention, and the school can't make that distinction. I can sometimes make it with a bunch of different questions I ask. So you have: the kid isn't paying attention because he's bored out of his mind. He just doesn't understand what's going on, and it's hard for anybody to pay attention to something they're not interested in. The child's got a learning disability of one sort or another. Or he may have an ADD. Or he's misbehaving because he's very seriously depressed: one of the problems in depression is you can't concentrate, your mind wanders. So you've got several different phenomena with very different treatment approaches."

In 1989, Carlson and a psychologist at Stony Brook, Mark D. Rapport, published a paper that included a historical review of the diagnostic issues in AD/HD. The review retraced what seems a yeoman effort by researchers over nearly three-quarters of a century to nail jelly to a tree. The first link between known brain damage and hyperactivity was noted in 1902; some years later, children who had been stricken with encephalitis in the 1918 epidemic were found to be "motorically overactive, inattentive, aggressive, and suffering with impaired judgment" as well as learning disabilities. When other hyperactive children were observed to have neurological "soft signs" (such as clumsiness, left-right confusion, and perceptual-motor dyscoordination), clinicians began to use the term MBD, for "minimal brain dysfunction." It turned out, however, that soft signs and a history of birth difficulties were neither unique nor universal among children who were "squirmy, immature, disruptive," so MBD fell by the wayside.

But these children didn't go away. Researchers began to focus on defining hyperactivity, and they devised various rating scales and questionnaires for parents and teachers to fill out; some of these are still used. But this next batch of studies found "that there were no consistent psychologic, biologic, genetic, therapeutic, or prognostic implications that confirmed the utility of focusing on motoric hyperactivity and its various descriptors as the core of a disorder." Still, it was found that whatever elusive behavior problem this mysterious group of children had, many of them didn't outgrow it. They displayed, as adults, "a more subtle fidgetiness." Moreover, "the outcome of the disorder ranged widely from underachievement to academic failure and at times included moderate to severe delinquency."

In some children inability to pay attention stood out; in others the predominant symptom was noncompliance. At length, as the field of classification became more complex and sophisticated, the DSM-III-R identified a broad category called "Attention-Deficit Hyperactivity Disorder (ADHD)" characterized overall by "developmentally inappropriate degrees of inattention, impulsiveness, and hyperactivity. People with the disorder generally display some disturbance in each of these areas, but to varying degrees." Oppositional Defiant Disorder and Conduct Disorder (described earlier in connection with Fennig's assessment of Hector), while frequently coexisting with ADHD, were separately classified. There were differences between the groups of children with pure ADHD and those with pure conduct disorders.

The notion of co-morbidity, which Carlson discussed in relation to depression, is popular now: instead of finding a group of children with the same set of symptoms and no others, medical diagnosticians are much more likely to decide a particular child has several disorders, each of which must be dealt with in its turn. There is still a school of thought that holds that attentional dysfunction appears in so many other childhood psychiatric disorders that as an independent entity it doesn't exist at all. And the attempt to understand and treat AD/HD, as we'll see throughout this book, is certainly not yet complete.

Carlson was a member of the American Psychiatric Association's DSM-IV Child and Adolescence Work Group, the team of psychiatrists and psychologists who revised the criteria for children's mental disorders listed in the 1994 edition of the manual. A co-chairman of the group was David Shaffer, the British-born psychiatrist who now heads the pediatric psychiatry department at Babies Hospital at Columbia-Presbyterian Medical Center in New York and is also director of the Division of Child Psychiatry at New York State Psychiatric Institute. (One of Shaffer's papers on teenage suicide is discussed in Chapter 1.) I talked with Shaffer about the assumptions that underlie the DSMs and how the manuals have evolved since they first appeared in 1952. They are still tied to the World Health Organization's *International Classification of Diseases*; an obvious purpose of the successive DSM editions is to enable an American clinician or researcher to communicate with his counterparts in Japan or Finland or Portugal, and to allow psychologists and psychiatrists of different theoretical religions to converse with relative civility. But despite their clear practicality in this respect, the manuals do arise from a postulate that makes some practitioners grumble.

"For some time now we've known that you can describe a person on the basis of the behavior they show or the thoughts they have or the emotions they feel in a way that allows you to predict what's going to happen to them," Shaffer said. "Until quite recently in child psychiatry, there have been many people who have dismissed behaviors you could see as surface phenomena that really didn't tell you very much about the patient." Shaffer is talking about what psychodynamic therapists call symptom substitution: that if you clear up one symptom without getting to the underlying disorder, you are almost provoking another symptom to appear in its place. "I think now we've accumulated a lot of evidence that shows that's not true," he said.

"When we have a group of kids with what we call a conduct disorder— they consistently show aggressive behaviors or disregard of rules or the rights of others, for example—we know that their prognosis and their natural history and their response to treatment is going to be different from what happens with a group of kids who are anxious about being separated from their parents or about engaging in activities. So these 'surface phenomena' are actually terribly important and get at things beneath the surface. Once you accept that, you can actually describe people on the basis of what you can see.

"Traditional Freudian psychoanalysts would believe that unresolved conflicts may be seeking their way to the surface, and they would mainly be concerned with the satisfactory resolution of these struggles. It's a highly theoretical viewpoint, and there's absolutely no evidence that it's related to mental illness. There are other highly theoretical viewpoints—again, with very limited evidence of their relevance to psychiatric disease. So you end up with a classification system that is trying to avoid at all costs making reference to theory or cause, because if you take a roomful of psychiatrists, they'll all have different beliefs about how conditions come about. If you start writing any of those beliefs into your description of a disorder, some people will fight it.

"So the DSM system was a breakthrough in being 'behavioral-descriptive,' a description of usually obvious, observable phenomena, with no implication about the cause. But when it was first written for DSM-III in the late 1970s, a lot of behaviors that were described as characterizing a disorder were obtained not from research but just from the experience of clinicians who had seen a lot of kids or had done just a little research. This led to other people investigating whether the descriptions in DSM-III were true. It has produced an enormous volume of research over the past decade. The DSM was also revolutionary in trying to be very specific about how frequently and how long a behavior had to be present before you could call it significant, and nobody had ever dared to do that before."

DSM-IV is (as readers besides this one have noted) a veritable Chinese menu: in order to qualify for what is now called "Attention-Deficit/Hyperactivity Disorder"—punctuated to take into consideration the long history of disagreements described in Carlson and Rapport's paper—a child must have exhibited six out of nine symptoms of inattention or six out of nine symptoms of hyperactivity-impulsivity for "at least six months to a degree that is maladaptive and inconsistent with developmental level." The patient must have developed some symptoms by the age of seven and must show impairment from the symptoms in two or more situations (such as home and school or work). The disturbance must "cause clinically significant impairment in social, academic, or occupational functioning" (allusions to work reflect the fact that teenagers and adults are sometimes diagnosed as having had AD/HD for all these years without knowing it), and the symptoms "do not occur exclusively during the course of a Pervasive Developmental Disorder, Schizophrenia or other Psychotic Disorder, and are not better accounted for by a Mood Disorder, Anxiety Disorder, Dissociative Disorder, or a Personality Disorder."

The criteria for AD/HD have been revised to reflect the direction of current psychiatric thinking, but they also take note of the criticism, as Shaffer explains, "that we're really just talking about normally active, feisty, outspoken kids, and the medical profession is conspiring to put them in a chemical straitjacket. Everybody was very sensitive to that accusation, so the criteria were rewritten to make sure that these kids were really suffering, that as a result of their hyperactivity or inattention, their school progress was severely impaired, their ability to make friends was impaired, and they weren't just normal overactive kids."

The complaint that "we were trying to psychiatrize normality," as Shaffer puts it, seems to have been a running theme in the revisions drawn up for DSM-IV. Conduct disorder is a diagnosis applied to some of the children described in Carlson and Rapport's historical review. Shaffer says the criteria for this had been toughened in the previous edition of DSM—"you didn't need to be a serial killer to get it, but you had to be pretty bad or consistently doing a lot of bad things, and there was a plea from the profession to see whether we were setting the threshold too high. A lot of research had come out that suggested we weren't, and the net result was not to change that very much. It means that a high proportion of kids with conduct disorder will end up getting in trouble with the law, but also that conduct disorder is a serious diagnosis. It's not for kids who are a nuisance or don't do what you tell them to do.

"Oppositional defiant disorder symptoms are less severe, more common—you often see them as a precursor to conduct disorder, and there was a suggestion that the two be merged into a single disorder, but that was opposed successfully on the grounds that conduct disorder is so stigmatizing, we don't want to extend it more than we have to."

While the overdiagnosis of AD/HD and conduct disorders still worries many thoughtful professionals, the DSM-IV work group appears to have made a conscientious and respectable effort to winnow the disturbed wheat from the merely spunky chaff. But the attempt to resolve the various issues Shaffer describes produces another set of problems: the manual is, to some extent, a diagnostic camel designed by a committee.

Carlson herself expresses two reservations about the DSM, and it is well to keep them in mind. When we talked about Hector, she said, "You can say, 'Yes, this child meets the criteria for attention deficit disorder and oppositional defiant disorder.' But so do a million other kids, and that doesn't tell you anything about that child. It seems to me that when you give a diagnosis, it ought to speak about a particular kid. It says nothing about Hector's dinosaur preoccupation. There's no diagnostic hole that you can put his dinosaurs in, even though they may be a fairly salient feature. We don't have criteria that say, 'Obsession with peculiar play,' and he's not delusional; if he were, we have a slot for that. So you say, 'Okay, at the moment we don't have any way of explaining that.' "

Carlson's caveats about diagnosis by classification—which is, after all, her life's work—recall Chess and Thomas's comments on quantitative research. It is, she says, like saying, " 'I know a garden because it has pansies, petunias, tulips, and violets.' That's a garden, and so we have a structured interview for gardens, and we ask people, 'Do you have pansies, petunias, tulips, and violets?' If it turns out they have peas, squash, tomatoes, and eggplant, they don't have a garden. So you're stuck with the fact that you very narrowly define a garden. You don't have questions about what a tulip or a pansy or a petunia is. You have good reliability on what those flowers are, but we can't agree on what a vegetable is. Some people call a tomato a vegetable and some people call it a fruit. So that's an unreliable item, and we don't want unreliable items on our questionnaire because we can't get people to agree on them, and that's fine. But then you come to the conclusion that if it has tomatoes in it, it's not a garden, when you really just can't get enough agreement on what a tomato is. There are an awful lot of things we can't be precise about, like this little kid with his dinosaurs."

Her second concern is that "most of the people on the DSM committee are experts. They don't see patients, so they don't see the kids who fall between the cracks. They see the ones that fit their screening criteria and go over eight layers of hurdles to come into the system. They don't have the sense of the spectrum, and that can make you tunnel-visioned. If your only acquaintance with attention deficit disorder is what comes in on the in-patient service, you say, 'Oh, what an awful disorder.' I attend on the inpatient service because that's what I do—but I do school consultations to keep my sanity. In school consultations the kids are less severe. I consult at an honors program because I want to see kids who can function."

Perhaps the most conspicuously absent tomato in the DSM garden is a detailed developmental perspective beyond that convenient and ubiquitous phrase, "developmentally appropriate," and beyond descriptions of stable character features like mental retardation, learning disabilities, and "pervasive developmental disorders" (the term for varieties of autism). Carlson herself, in a book chapter written with Vanderbilt psychologist Judy Garber, called for studies that link developmental adaptation at each age level with subsequent disorders. Biological psychiatrists don't walk around quoting Anna Freud, but her work on assessment— despite a thicket of psychoanalytic language that ties it to the formulations in Part II of this book—is both highly relevant and illustrative of the need to break tribal boundaries.

Back in the sixties Anna Freud and her colleagues at the Hampstead Child-Therapy Course and Clinic in London evolved a Developmental Profile for use in the assessment of child patients; papers on this work appeared in *The Psychoanalytic Study of the Child*. This is the most classical of journals, and Anna Freud was approaching the very audience that Shaffer mentions as disparaging the importance of discrete symptoms. In the third of these papers, she writes:

> Analysts have always been proud of the distinction that theirs is a causal therapy, aiming directly at the conflicts and stresses which are hidden in the patients' personalities and underlie their symptomatology. Inevitably, with this approach they find themselves at cross-purposes ... with the parents of child patients who are concerned only with removing the disturbing manifestations in the child and completely disregard the pathological turn in the child's development which is revealed by the disturbances that trouble them.

The Developmental Profile was designed to serve psychoanalytic purposes, and Anna Freud certainly endorsed the psychodynamic view Shaffer mentions—that curing a symptom without getting at its root cause would only result in another symptom springing up in its place. One needn't agree with that view to accept the reasoning beneath the profile.

Anna Freud's first paper points out that children's symptoms are sometimes "transient appearances of stress which emerge whenever a particular phase of development makes specially high demands on a child's personality." After the child has adapted to that phase of development, they either go away or are replaced by others, leaving "no more than an area of heightened vulnerability." The lay term for this phenomenon, "outgrowing" the difficulty, is to Anna Freud "quite appropriate." Symptoms in themselves aren't infallible predictors of a child's future course. On the other hand, "there are no childhood alternatives to the adult's efficiency or failure in sex and work"—the markers of health or illness in adult psychiatry. The job of a child is to develop, and the failure to do so is the most significant indication of mental illness.

The Developmental Profile assesses disturbances by seeing "any given child against the background of a developmental norm." Because children's developmental progress is frequently skewed—at the simplest level, most parents remember their toddlers walked early and talked late or vice versa—the profile assesses progress along each of several developmental lines that lead

> from the infant's suckling and weaning experiences to the adult's rational attitude to food intake; from cleanliness training enforced on the child by environmental pressure to the adult's more or less ingrained and unshakable bladder and bowel control; from the child's sharing possession of his body with his mother to the adolescent's claim for independence and self-determination in body management; from the young child's egocentric view of the world and his fellow beings to empathy, mutuality, and companionship with his contemporaries; from the first erotic play on his own and his mother's body by way of the transitional objects to the toys, games, hobbies, and finally to work, etc.

While the detailed descriptions of what the child's problem is and how it came about are formulated in psychodynamic terms, a good assessment of an individual child by any sort of therapist will include questions of how the child is doing on the developmental continuum. As Anna Freud points out, the profile "is intended to draw the diagnostician's concentration away from the child's pathology and to return it instead to an assessment of his developmental status and the picture of his total personality." Especially when the child is not displaying dramatic symptoms but a nonprofessional has a sense that something isn't quite right, the developmental framework makes a most useful context for taking a closer look.

The assessment tools that go hand in hand with the medical model of diagnosis are rating scales and structured interviews. Parents and teachers are given a questionnaire on which they check off which symptoms are present, how frequently they appear, and how severe they are. The clinician scores these against some norm. Hector, for example, was rated against the norm of patients within the hospital's children's unit; this norm is measured against that of children who aren't hospitalized. When Hector came in, he seemed about as attentive as the hospital norm; a couple of weeks later, he was more than one standard deviation below that norm and two standard deviations below in oppositional behavior. The hospital started him on Ritalin, and his attention span improved to one standard deviation above the hospital norm, a significant increase. "There are tons of rating scales and they measure just about everything— anxiety, depression, tension," says Carlson. "The ones you use depend on what you're interested in. They're like a thermometer. They tell you whether something's there and maybe whether it's severe, but they don't tell you why it's there."

A structured interview is designed to get a patient's history; it is usually designed with DSM criteria in mind and aims to make sure that all the right questions are asked, whether the interviewer is in a clinic in Lower Squeedunk or a major teaching hospital, and even if Gabrielle Carlson is impossibly harried or coming down with the flu. If the parents have filled out a questionnaire, Carlson can use it as a guide to spend more time on the problems they check off and skip the areas that don't apply at all. In a research project the interviews are used with strict adherence by the graduate students who usually do the intake.

The trend toward precision and quantification in assessment has plunged projective tests—the tools so familiar to nonprofessionals who took Psych 101—into disfavor: the clinicians I encountered who were less rigid now tended to look on projectives, which are designed to tease out hidden thoughts and feelings, as "one more piece of information that can be useful." The most frequently used projective tests are the Rorschach, in which the child is shown ten inkblots and asked to say what each reminds him of; thematic cards such as the Children's Apperception Test (CAT), the Thematic Apperception Test (TAT), and the Tasks of Emotional Development (TED) test, all of which show pictures for which the child must make up a story that will reveal his attitudes toward issues like achievement, sibling rivalry, sexuality, and aggression; and drawing tests like the Draw-A-Person, the House-Tree-Person, and Kinetic Family Drawings.

In recent years efforts have been made to adapt the Rorschach to current modes. There is an elaborate scoring system that can be used with a computer to produce a comprehensive picture of the child's psychological makeup. Robert Brooks, a psychologist who is director of Child and Adolescent Psychology and Psychoeducation Training at the Hall-Mercer Center for Children and Adolescents at McLean Hospital near Boston, is something of a fan of projectives, but he doesn't use them either in that way or in the strictly psychodynamic style that once was popular. As Brooks wrote some years ago, at a time when the tests were particularly controversial, "Projectives are not simply instruments for obtaining a differential diagnosis (a practice that research calls into question) or for labeling a child; rather they can provide stimuli and strategies for understanding a child's cognitive and affective functioning in order to assist the child's development."

"I want to paint a portrait of the person I'm trying to evaluate," Brooks says, "some of the intricacies and the uniqueness of each individual. You can observe me giving the Rorschach and the symptomatic cards and doing a diagnostic interview, and you could observe four other psychologists interviewing the same person. There would be some overlap, but we all have our own way of looking at things. I'm interested in the concept of self-esteem as a guiding principle, so I'm always looking at, In what areas does this person feel more competent or less competent? In what ways does this person feel they have some personal control over their lives? Do they entertain any notion of hope? Because hope goes hand-in-glove with resiliency. I find projective tests a very useful measure of how people think, how they articulate feelings. Why is it that a person could make up a very rich story to one thematic card, but on the next card they can barely say anything? Under what conditions does a person have more difficulty expressing themselves or articulating how they feel? If they seem to be seeing something that almost no one else would see on some cards—and not on others—one would have to raise the question, What is it about this particular card that leads them to see things so differently?"

Projectives are a window for Brooks, a variation on the puppets that many child therapists (including Carlson with Hector) find useful. "Some kids can get more easily to the puppet, other kids do better with the Rorschach," Brooks says. "I remember one child who saw a picture on one of the Rorschach cards of a dog starving to death, but there were two people on either side—that was the image. So I said, 'Does the dog somehow let the people know that it's starving?' What I'm also assessing is, Is a person taking some initiative or finding some areas of personal control and not feeling so hopeless or helpless?

"The child said, 'It tries to turn around but it can't, and so the two people don't really know it's starving,' which was a wonderful representation of how this kid often felt, that he didn't know how to communicate his needs. I spent about ten minutes on that card with the kid trying to figure out how the dog could let the people know it was hungry. Some people would say, 'You're almost doing therapy.' And in part I am, but I'm also assessing, Can this kid even entertain possible solutions to problems? Because some people will say, 'No one will ever hear this dog calling for help.' That gives you an assessment of the hopelessness of the child."

What Brooks doesn't do is use projectives in the traditional manner. "When I was first in training," he says, "I would hear things like, 'A person saw a spider. This is representative of the mother figure.' And if the spider was spinning a web, it was the all-engulfing mother. I remember reading that if a person saw a lot of eyes on the Rorschach, it was representative of a paranoid stance. Research was done that showed this didn't hold true. You have to be careful about this one-to-one relationship."

This is what Brooks, in the chapter he wrote on projective testing, referred to as the "sign approach," which "occurs when one particular kind of test response is inferred to symbolize major personality characteristics." Brooks has called this sort of interpretation "irresponsible." He is equally cautious about any attempt to extrapolate a direct relationship between a child's fantasy content as shown on projective tests and his present or future behavior in real life. All the tests do is "portray the child's inner world at the time of testing." Another concern cited in the chapter is interpretation that doesn't consider "what the testing means to the child, the degree of rapport between clinician and child, the cooperation of the child, the particular coping strategies recruited by the child, the attention strength of the child, and the testing style of the clinician."

Children aren't the same in all situations, and in this respect projective test results, like IQ tests and SATs, are fallible.

What, then, did the Stony Brook diagnostic team make of Hector?

Hector had improved markedly in the hospital, and the team needed to figure out why. "If we compare him to when he came in and when he got the Ritalin, he became much more organized," Gartner says. "It wasn't like we gave him a pill and all of a sudden the fantasies went away. They went away on a course that looked like it was the effect of the behavioral program and the nursing staff—time in the program. But he became instantly more organized and more focused. The question it still begs, to me, is, If we take him back home, what now? How much of his improvement is the result of a new environment?"

"There's one way to find out," Carlson puts in. "When you all decided to put him on the Ritalin, did you feel you were taking a chance as far as 'My gosh, what if he is psychotic?' Or were you ninety percent sure you were dealing with an ADD kid who was overstimulated?"

"We looked very carefully at his reality testing to make sure he wasn't actively psychotic," Gartner says. "Even though he said he heard voices, like in the first day or so, it really was more like telling a story. After that we saw periods when his relatedness was quite good, his empathy was quite good, and he was quite redirectable in his behavior. He would tell you he was just playing. However, given the genetic history, giving a stimulant to a kid who was about to become psychotic, you would worry. So I think there was some risk involved, but I don't think the team was walking on eggshells."

"And I don't know that you're necessarily out of the woods for that yet," Carlson says.

Debbie Lane, the teacher, says, "I don't think you would have been able to engage him even with Danielle if he had been off the Ritalin, because when he was acting like that, he wasn't able to come back after just a warning. I think it did make a big difference. He was able to sort through his head the consequences better."

Carlson is interested in where the dinosaurs fit in, and she asks the others why they think he developed the dinosaur mechanism to begin with and what purpose they think it serves. "It is a kind of violence he can control," Fennig speculates. "He can control this reality, and the other reality he cannot control. He continues to be very violent, but he's not anxious about this kind of violence." Gartner feels from the boy's history that he seems to be "a bit temperamentally on the side of fantasy and being able to develop a theme in his own play."

They talk about the shooting: Hector, telling Schwabish the story, said, "Wow, right in the head!"

"He did one thing that was a little off," Carlson says. "He thought the pen was going to explode." Fennig remarks how absorbed in his fantasy play Hector was, and Carlson says, "You try to get them so focused on you that they kind of shut everybody out. One of the reasons I wanted him to give the pen back to Debbie was so he'd come back and sort of acquaint himself with the fact that he was in the conference room, and that was his teacher, and then he could leave. I was trying to keep him engaged and entertained, but one thing I was not successful in doing: getting him to interact. Sometimes kids will answer questions with a puppet in a way that they won't with you, but I didn't get very far with that. I think we saw some of that perseverative quality. He just couldn't get out of that drawing on my mouth. It was part of the flavor that made him seem like a much younger child."

Hector is simply skilled at evasion, Gartner observes. "Getting him to talk about any negative, painful affects about home—he just sidesteps the whole issue. He redirects the conversation to something else."

"I have a suspicion," Carlson says, "that his dinosaur comes out when he feels sad or out of control, but we couldn't get him to demonstrate that in any way." Carlson is concerned about the mother's new girlfriend's behavior, which is, of course, "inappropriate. I think the last thing he needs is to be overstimulated sexually or any other way." What to do with or about Mom is a major problem for the team. "We're going to send him home?" she asks incredulously.

"We don't know," Fennig answers. "We need to think of alternatives." Both Carlson and Fennig worry that the boy and his mother are very attached to each other. Fennig reports Mom worries that she herself is depressed and abusive, and Weintraub believes she might go along with a foster placement. (The team was, of course, brainstorming here; the decision about where Hector would go would result from casework with the mother.) Gartner says, "I think he's very attached, but the way he looks now is the best he's ever looked. I think there's a big enough environmental component, notwithstanding the Ritalin. To put him back in that environment, he's going to come back to visit us or visit somebody, and he's going to end up having big problems." Once Hector adjusted to the foster home, his mother could call on him regularly.

The first step is to see what happens to the boy without Ritalin: Will it affect his attention span? Will it make him hyperactive? Will the dinosaurs come back? Will everything be a little worse or a lot worse? "What will the diagnostic implications be if you take him off the Ritalin and he's fine?" Carlson asks.

"I would be very suspicious," Gartner says. "First of all, AD/HD is not the primary problem, and the environment—because he got better with environmental stimulus and because the history suggests that would have made most kids worse—that was a big part of it. If he gets worse across the board—AD/HD kids who are really wound up get very weird, act like a donkey on the floor, do all kinds of bizarre stuff—if he does stuff like that, I'd put him back on the Ritalin. And if the fantasy goes away again, it means you've got that tendency of temperament. I wouldn't use it diagnostically, though."

Carlson says, "If when you take him off the Ritalin he goes back to his dinosaurs and the hyperactivity, my hypothesis is going to be that the dinosaurs are a kind of way he has of addressing whatever it is he feels inside that ends up like looking hyperactive, impulsive, and aggressive. At some level he is aware that he is extremely distractible and isn't making sense out of things and that the dinosaur is kind of his metaphor of acting that out. It doesn't take away the fact that he still has this ADD diagnosis. What it says is that the dinosaurs are sort of a response to his internal state rather than to the external state.

"The things that are still not right about this child, even with the Ritalin, are that he is—besides his family problems—socially immature, and maybe that's just because he's been so deprived. I don't think anybody's been paying attention to the child's development, so he's largely an uncivilized child. And I don't know whether if you were to keep him in a supportive, nurturing environment, he would catch up with that the way Debbie said he caught up in school. That's why in child psychiatry—it's true in adult psychiatry too—the diagnosis ends up being a longitudinal process, not just a cross-sectional one, and depending on what happens, you get answers. The question is, Is he essentially ADD-looking psychotic or psychotic-looking ADD? The Ritalin half-answered that. Essentially he's an ADD kid who looks psychotic, and when he has something focusing his thoughts and organizing him, he doesn't look as psychotic."

The team members pack up their papers. They have spent two weeks carefully observing Hector, and after doing the best they could in this designated period of time, which some might consider luxuriously long, they have focused intently for two hours on his case. An assortment of skills has been brought to bear by thoughtful, highly intelligent people who take their task most seriously. And while some decisions about Hector have been made, the puzzle is still not completely solved.

By the time I saw Hector, I had learned enough to know that clinicians of each therapeutic orientation would follow a different formulation in treating him. I could figure out what those formulations would be, and that there would be considerable truth in all of them—and that each one, pursued alone, would be thoroughly inadequate.

PART II

FORBIDDEN GAMES

Psychodynamic Therapy

CHAPTER 3

THE PLAYING CURE

For a psychoanalysis is not an impartial scientific investigation, but a therapeutic measure. Its essence is not to prove anything, but merely to alter something. In a psychoanalysis the physician always gives his patient (sometimes to a greater and sometimes to a less extent) the conscious anticipatory images by the help of which he is put in a position to recognize and to grasp the unconscious material.

—Sigmund Freud,
"Analysis of a Phobia in a Five-Year-Old Boy" (1909)

W HEN LAYMEN THINK OF A PSYCHIATRIST, they probably imagine someone like Charles A. Sarnoff, M.D., who lacks only an accent and a goatee to serve as the prototype. (Actually, while beards are the uniform among younger men, male practitioners of the pre-baby-boom generations tend to be clean-shaven these days; Sarnoff was born in 1928.) He is a scholarly, gray-haired man with an almost whispery voice, apt to pursue the answer to any question with terrierlike tenacity; his explanations, besides citing cases, roam the cultural landscape from Aristotle to William Congreve to Michel Foucault to James M. Barrie.

Sarnoff practices in Great Neck, New York, is a lecturer at the Psychoanalytic Clinic for Training and Research at Columbia University's College of Physicians and Surgeons and until recently was also a lecturer and supervisor in child and adolescent psychiatry at Long Island Jewish Medical Center. In addition to the requisite study in adult and child psychiatry mentioned in Chapter 1, he completed two separate long training programs in psychoanalysis (of adults and of children).

71

In thirty years of practice, Sarnoff has seen enough patients to make a fair-sized longitudinal study. He is the author of two widely used textbooks on latency and one on adolescence; the term *latency* itself is a Freudian term for the years from six to twelve and a tip-off to his orientation. (Most non-Freudians use the term *middle childhood*.) While he would appear to be the epitome of orthodoxy, Sarnoff considers himself something of a rebel within his own tribe. In his later years Freud—and thus his followers— characterized latency as a period in which sexual and aggressive drives diminish so as to permit the child to be educable; Sarnoff, on the other hand, follows an earlier Freudian theory that the drives *don't* diminish but are dammed up by a retreat to fantasies that calm the child, with the same net effect. Sarnoff's books, filled with case histories from his practice, depict latency as a bubbling cauldron of psychologically significant activity and the source of adolescents' well- or ill-being.

The American Psychoanalytic Association defines *psychodynamics* as "the aspect of psychoanalytic theory that explains mental phenomena, such as thoughts, feelings, and behavior, as the results of interacting and opposing goal-directed or motivational forces." In other words the actions we show the world reflect the conflicts within us, conflicts of which we ourselves may not be aware. A child who has undergone psychodynamic therapy, Sarnoff has written, "may have learned to look for causes in unexpected places." This is a fairly sophisticated skill, available to the latency-age children with whom Sarnoff works most often (and on whom he has become, through his books, an authority). He has, however, successfully treated patients from the age of twenty-six months on, when they first acquire the ability to remember and transform their feelings into symbols. Children from fifteen to twenty-six months old, he says, are treatable with other kinds of family and play therapy.

While all Freudian therapists are psychodynamic, all psychodynamic therapists aren't necessarily Freudian (and some treat children even younger than fifteen months). Conflicts within the psychodynamic world may appear to be even more heated than those with outside orientations; that's perhaps because psychodynamic therapists fight with each other about theory but don't talk theory at all with cognitive-behaviorists, family systems therapists, or psychopharmacologists. (This refusal to interact is mutual.) I will discuss some different dynamic theories of psychological development in Chapters 4 and 5 and the way they are played out clinically in Chapter 6.

Sarnoff defines himself as a Freudian, first because of the people who trained him: "My analyst, Otto Sperling, was supervised by Freud," he says. "He was the first resident who was ever analyzed. The supervisor of my first paper was Max Schur, who was Freud's physician and administered that last dose of morphine. So you might say I was generated in the womb of psychoanalysis." He is particularly proud of the month he spent training at Anna Freud's Hampstead Child-Therapy Clinic. Second, in accord with all this training, he says it's the drives that motivate fantasies, which then contribute to the formation of symptoms. (Other orientations, even psychodynamic ones, don't assign this weight to unconscious drives.) Finally his therapy may draw on the Freudian concept of transference, in which the patient loads onto the therapist repressed feelings for others in his life. (The use of transference, however, is not exclusive to Freudians.)

It is noteworthy that Sarnoff uses words like *contribute* and *may.* "Within mental illness or human emotional reactions today, we can find a multitude of contributions," he says, "including head injuries, genetic factors, social factors, and psychological factors—and we also have to include early childhood experience." Freudians aren't monomaniacs: the master himself, for example, writing about melancholia back in 1917, said that "the definition of melancholia is uncertain; it takes on various clinical forms (some of them suggesting somatic rather than psychogenic affections) that do not seem definitely to warrant reduction to a unity."

When feelings and events are too stressful or humiliating to deal with directly, a healthy latency-age child, as Sarnoff has written, "can fall back into a web of symbols, which, woven into a kind of mythic map, can be used as guide to a land where his power and self-esteem are reinstated." Sarnoff explains the way this works by recalling the old movie *Forbidden Games,* in which "the parents die and the children see them buried and seem to be calm and able to integrate and handle things, and then something strange begins to happen in town: crosses are disappearing from catafalques and no one knows where they're going. The children have been burying birds and little mice and having play ceremonies. They're involved in the use of three-dimensional icons, which Piaget calls ludic symbols." One of the prints on Sarnoff's office wall is a Victorian scene called *The Burial of the Pet Bird,* showing a similar phenomenon. A symptom is an *unhealthy* symbol: by approaching the children through play, Sarnoff hopes first to decipher their symbols, then to help them work through their conflicts by playing them out, and finally to give the child insight into his or her feelings and behavior.

"I call latency-age children biologically celibate soldier-dwarfs," Sarnoff says, "to show the restrictions with which they live. The child is so little that if someone picked him up and he tried to hit that person, he'd be swinging in the air. And if he has any kind of sexual fantasies, he certainly doesn't have the organ capacity for carrying out his designs. Later there's a stage called ludic demise, when the play symbols are no longer used, because the children now have, say, orgastic potential available to them.

"You actually see them go through a transition. A youngster is making Play-Doh figures of robbers. One day he moves into your office and wants to sit at the desk—he's the judge, you're a robber, and you're coming to trial. I have devised one office after another in such a way that the child has two doors he can walk through, or he comes into the room and the way I stand makes it possible for him to choose whether he's going into the playroom or the consulting room." Sarnoff is as much Piagetian as he is Freudian: he may need to look up a patient's chronological age, but he never forgets how far the child has developed in symbol formation.

There is a grandeur to this view of children, and Sarnoff is a man much seized by the romance of symbols: he's the first to suggest he hasn't quite achieved ludic demise himself. In the den of his apartment near Lincoln Center in Manhattan, unseen by patients, are stained-glass dioramas he has made, filled with colorful little lead knights and centaurs doing battle; he used to build ship models with his son until Sarnoff *fils* put away childish things and so, regretfully, did Sarnoff *père*. Sarnoff is now writing a book on the structure and function of symbols in different cultures. What adult patients do see in his consulting room—if they're of a mind to pay attention—is a set of engravings of Thomas Cole's symbolic series *The Voyage of Life,* about which Sarnoff has performed some acknowledged scholarship.

When I first met Sarnoff, he lived and practiced in a large house in Great Neck, and the office also displayed several Audubon engravings of extremely vicious birds, fish, and snakes, portraying "the cruelty of animal life, how much hostility and aggression there is." Now, however, he sees child patients in an office building in Great Neck, and the Audubon series (but not the worldview it represents) is packed away. We talked mostly at the Lincoln Center apartment—he and his late wife were, not surprisingly, passionate opera fans—which features a view of the Hudson River outside and Hudson River School paintings inside.

The technique used to assess a new patient is characteristic of both the therapeutic orientation and the individual therapist. Sarnoff will order what educational evaluations are necessary, and he pointedly calls attention to the stethoscope, ophthalmoscope, and reflex hammer in his office—the competitive arsenal against nonmedical practitioners—but his main assessment tools are nonstructured interviews with the parent and the child.

He starts with the parent, both to take the usual case history and to establish a working relationship, which varies according to the child's age. "If it's latency," he says, "I'm in touch with the parents. They know how to reach me, they can call me two times a week, they can come and see me, we work together as a team. If it's an adolescent, then you do your best to keep the parent at a distance and the child is your patient."

How a therapist deals with parents is, of course, of major importance to the parents. A minority of psychodynamic therapists and analysts will have nothing whatsoever to do with parents; family therapists, at the other end of the spectrum, treat parents and children together. Sarnoff, like most psychodynamic therapists, follows the traditional "child guidance" model: he has written, "I prefer not to see parents and children together. There is danger that the alliance between adults . . . will be interpreted by the child as a sign of disloyalty, betrayal, or simply being left out."

At the same time Sarnoff, whose position on most doctrinal issues is, "I hew as close to the ideal as I can, but go as far away as I have to," says there are times when it's simply necessary to deal with an adolescent's parents. "If you have a relatively healthy neurotic child, keeping your distance can work out, but it is a perilous course when you have severely disturbed people, manipulative people. Then you have to break the rule and make yourself available to the parents. You tell the patients everything, treat them like adults, but unfortunately some of them are not adult enough to be treated that way. But it's hard to maintain a relationship with the patient if they think you're talking to the parent, so you really are in conflict."

With younger patients, while the parent is there to identify the "zone of pathology," the interview with the child is clearly the key. Sarnoff points out that the thought patterns of children differ from those of adults, and the child may even be proud of his symptoms. Sometimes play, drawings, and ludic symbols are the only medium of communication.

At present, since Sarnoff practices privately in a comfortable suburban community and doesn't work on an inpatient unit, his patients tend to be less deeply disturbed than most of the children Carlson sees, and to come from less complex environments. (His curriculum vitae does, however, include stints at inner-city hospitals and an orphanage, and he was chief of child psychiatry at the Brookdale Hospital Medical Center in Brooklyn's Ocean Hill–Brownsville for five years.)

Therapeutic assessments start, logically enough, with a concept of normalcy, both cultural and biological. (Sarnoff once worked at a clinic where an unusual number of child patients reported hearing holy voices; he discovered that in the parochial schools they attended, this phenomenon was not a symptom but a mark of status.) Predictably for a clinician who avows a strong debt to Piaget and Anna Freud, the developmental focus is central to his therapy. He needs to know whether the child has entered latency, whether he can produce calming symbols, and how far, in Piagetian terms, the child's abilities to remember and understand have progressed. "I'll ask a child to tell me about his favorite TV cartoon," he says. "If they can tell me a whole story, then you know they are reducing their sensory experience to a verbal memory system and maybe even moving into a fine level of abstraction. But so many times you'll hear them say 'I like when Bluto hits Popeye, then Popeye hits Bluto back and they fight,' and that's all. Or they take two little figurines and they have them battling each other, constantly hitting or punching, and you know this youngster is not making up a story, he's just involved in this aggressive interaction. This is perfectly all right for a three- or four-year-old, but when you get to a five- or six-year-old, you've got a problem there."

Sarnoff, as he has written, divides therapeutic problems into two categories: one set that reflects "an interaction, past or present, between parent and child . . . occurs in only one place, either the home or the school . . . requires parent counseling, and is seen as the province of the family therapist"; and another set of problems that "go with the child wherever he may roam. It seems to be written in his heart. . . . The latter requires a psychoanalytically-oriented dynamic approach, and is the province of the child therapist or analyst." The first category of problems is rooted in reality; the second reflects a distortion of reality that lives and thrives in the patient's conscious and unconscious memory and governs behavior. "People with emotional problems suffer from abnormal persistence of memory, which results from impaired mastery and processing of elements of recall," he writes. That is, the lens through which they see the world has had a filter of fantasy placed over it. The therapist's interpretations aim to dissolve that filter—the source of the pathology—by undoing the distortions stored in the patient's mind.

Sarnoff has also dealt with the emotional consequences of learning disabilities:

> ... learning is only one of the areas affected by disorders of the central processing system. Disordered cognition can affect the way a child responds to being touched, and the way he can remember, obey, and develop prudence, which is importantly informed by the capacity to hear admonitions and remember them before incorporating them into the conscience. A child who cannot recall sufficiently to bring money for lunch when visiting a museum, though having been told and being well-intended, will suffer not only from an inability to learn but also from hunger, humiliating comments, an engendered low self-picture, and a sense of inadequacy.

Patients who haven't achieved ludic demise will find a playroom that looks rather like nursery school except for the basketball hoop: it's stocked with dolls and puppets, Play-Doh, Legos, currently popular toy figures (Ninja turtles one year, wrestlers the next), a bulletin board for tacking up patients' pictures and a Mark-a-Board for writing and drawing, a child-sized couch and chair so Sarnoff can sit at the patient's level, and a pump sink for water play. ("I removed the faucet after a child sprayed me and the whole room," he says. "I had to crawl under the sink to turn it off.") What they *won't* find in Sarnoff's office—and would find in the office of a cognitive-behaviorist—is games with rules, such as chess or checkers, which Sarnoff feels (tellingly) can be used as tactics to divert his attention from the child's real problems. Some therapists will make a point of putting out toys that pertain to the issues in a given patient's life; Sarnoff's brand of play therapy is completely nondirective, and he goes wherever the patient takes him.

"I have developed this skill of being able to make almost anything out of Play-Doh and have it look like a lion, a tiger, or whatever," he says. "I'll say 'Can you guess what I'm making?' Whatever they think I'm making, that's what I'm making."

A skilled therapist can make surprisingly sophisticated concepts understandable to children. It would appear a hopeless task to convey to an elementary school child that it may not be an actual cat that he fears but his own angry feelings that he has projected onto the cat. Sarnoff does it with an object called a ghost gun, which is a sort of slide projector that throws a picture of a ghost on the wall. Inside the gun is a needle that punctures the film, so the child can "shoot" the ghost; Sarnoff can then demonstrate to the child that the shooting appears on the screen but is actually going on inside the gun and being projected onto the screen, just as the feelings inside the child's head are being projected onto the cat.

While preadolescent children don't play with dolls and puppets, they are willing to draw and model clay. Even when older children talk, they may be talking symbolically. Sarnoff describes "a twelve-year-old boy who's depressed. Back when he was five, he was in an accident with his friend. They were playing, and he threw something with a sharp point that hit the friend and paralyzed his hand. Now the boy is perfectly willing to come into therapy, and he's even a good talker. He reads a lot. He likes to read Stephen King novels, and he begins to talk about *Pet Sematary*, in which a man's child dies, he brings the child back to life, and the child dies again. It becomes very clear— every story the child tells you is about doing and undoing. He's not telling you directly about this. If I were to say, 'You're depressed because of what you did with someone as a child,' he might get up and run out of the room. He's dealing with it in a displaced manner, passively using the symbols of Stephen King.

"Little by little you keep on getting him to talk about these stories. You gather stories like this. You wait for him as he goes through all of them. Eventually he's going to get to this. You know when to ask him to tell more—what do you think the character should have done? You begin to discuss the material in a displaced form. By inadvertence, almost, you bring the material to the surface and get a kid to work on it and talk about it and deal with it as if he's talking about someone else. That's as close as the ego can get to the trauma—he may never say it, but still he achieves a certain amount of catharsis and does better."

Late latency (from age nine to about thirteen) is a time when children begin to experience conflicts between the values of their parents and those of their peers. Transient obsessions, short acute paranoid episodes, and psychosomatic symptoms, Sarnoff observes, suggest problems in "ethical individuation." Some years ago he was treating the son of a medical colleague, an internist. "This boy used to get hives before he went to school," Sarnoff says. "One evening his father took him, with his friend, to a basketball game. They bought seats that were inexpensive, and they were sitting way up in Madison Square Garden. The boy looks down and sees there are empty seats in the expensive section. He says, 'Let's go there,' and the father says, 'If you guys want to go, you can, I'll wait here.'

"The two boys begin to move out toward the aisle, but while they're doing that, my patient's face blows up in hives. His father says, 'I've got some Benadryl in my pocket,' and the boy says, 'Give me a few minutes. I want to try to analyze this.' He thinks it through, and the hives disappear. The next day his father calls me up and says, 'The boy won't tell me a thing about what's happening, but as a physician I think I have a right to know. I've been treating many hives—what's going on?' I said, 'Look, he'll have to *tell* me.' He came in and told me this: he saw a guard and developed anxiety and guilt. When he realized what the conflict was, the hives went down, and when the father asked what happened, he said, 'No, I want to save this for Dr. Sarnoff first.' That boy is now in medical school."

Parents may worry about what they perceive as the indefiniteness of psychodynamic therapy: it seems to go on and on, with no clear-cut termination point. Sarnoff—in sharp conflict with the views of therapists of other orientations—believes that just clearing up the presenting symptom is not enough, because unless the underlying problem is rooted out and worked through, another symptom will come along to take its place— "old wine in new bottles," as he puts it. "There are many external symptoms that can change with maturation, so a sado-masochistic fantasy that had been expressing itself in the form of fear of persecution—by robbers, by dogs—may appear to remit when the child goes into adolescence. But the boy has a very sado-masochistic persecutory relationship with a girl." Cognitive-behaviorists and psychopharmacologists say there are no data to substantiate the notion of symptom substitution, and family therapists might view the phenomenon in a different context, since a symptom doesn't belong to one family member alone. Sarnoff says there is repeated evidence of symptom substitution in his practice.

What Sarnoff does expect to see in addition to a solution of the presenting problem is greater success in academic and social activities, a healthier choice of friends, and developmental progress at a rate equal to that of the child's peers: that is to say, as he has written, "further therapeutic work will only produce progress that age-appropriate natural development could provide as well." This is what indicates the therapy has reached its termination point—and it is the same termination point cited by Winnicott, the British psychiatrist.

Ask Sarnoff—who started out as a neurologist and electroencephalographer—how he got into child psychiatry, and he will describe a fairly routine career progression. But when at length he is prompted to reveal his own history, it appears to the questioner engaged in a bit of role reversal that a child psychiatrist, a Freudian no less, had long been waiting to be born—had been, perhaps, repressed for some time. "You have to keep in mind that my father went blind when I was five or six," he says. "My parents went bankrupt. They lost their house, and my brother and I were put in a kind of orphanage. The man who ran it believed in breaking the child's will. I remember sitting for hours before these half-cooked scrambled eggs. My brother and I found a little kitten and brought it inside and hid it—we were so alone. So I have a great empathy for neglected children.

"As a child, I was always fascinated with tiny things and fantasies. When I was seven or eight I saw Thomas Cole's painting, *The Titan's Goblet,* and I knew it had to mean something more than what was there. It shows a goblet that stands on a hillside. At the base of the goblet, there's a little town, and water at the goblet's base flows down in a stream, past the town and into the sea. There are trees and gardens hanging over the bowl of the goblet, which is filled with little whitecaps and tiny boats plying their way across the waters of the bowl. The base of the goblet, I read much later, is a symbol of the great ash tree that commands heaven and earth in Norse mythology. But from the beginning I never forgot it: What did it mean? Even now I go to see that painting at the Met. It's my pilgrimage.

"Cole was preoccupied with large and small, the way *Gulliver's Travels* deals with large and small. He didn't just paint landscapes, he worked with what Kant called the negative sublime. What makes certain symbols sublime is that they're horrifying and overwhelming, but because they're in a painting we can see the danger and be apart from it. We can both experience danger and feel safe. This is the role of the psychoanalytic symbol.

"My mother had gotten a dental degree before she was married, but had never practiced until then, when she had to support the family. She was the person most important in determining my life. Later my parents and a cousin who was a child psychologist bought a summer camp for Mongolian idiots—as they were then called—from well-to-do families. It was impressed on me that the cousin was very bright because he'd written a book on child psychology. His accomplishments loomed large in my mind.

"My own analyst influenced me strongly. My father was a relatively inadequate person, destroyed by his infirmity, and there was very little you could identify with. Part of the analysis was a search for a father. Otto helped me to analyze out a very severe character neurosis with psychosomatic symptoms that no longer exist. I was like the Irandas of Northern Australia who come into manhood. I was born again. That's a very strong way of describing psychoanalysis, but that was my experience."

One afternoon Sarnoff and I drove out to Schneider Children's Hospital, a division of Long Island Jewish Medical Center in New Hyde Park, New York, to watch Dr. Emanuel Falcone, a thirty-two-year-old resident completing his fellowship in child psychiatry, in session with Kevin, an eleven-year-old boy. In hopes of helping other children, Kevin and his parents had agreed to let me observe behind a one-way mirror.

"You're going to see a guy today who has far more talent than I have as a child therapist," Sarnoff said. "He doesn't have my experience, but he just picks this stuff up. He can see things quickly that I see because I learned from experience." (Some weeks later, when I asked Sarnoff whether he thought psychotherapy was a science or an art, he replied, "Did I tell you Manny was a fine scientist? I did not.")

Before the session Falcone, a dark-haired man with wire-rimmed glasses and a close-cropped beard, briefed me on Kevin. "He was ten when he came to us. He had many fears of separation. He was concerned that he might be kidnapped, that his parents might be killed or injured somehow. He was afraid of going on subways either alone or with his mother because of the subway rapist [a crime story getting extensive coverage at the time of my visit]. He also suffered from obsessional thinking and some compulsions.

"He was obsessed about being poisoned or food being contaminated. Once when the food was heavily peppered, he was convinced the specks were dirt, not pepper, and the lasagna dinner had to be thrown away. It was also impinging on his functioning: he wouldn't go on Boy Scout trips using the subway. He had trouble sleeping alone, and he would often go into his parents' bedroom.

"When he came to us, he had some rituals, like repetitive handwashing twenty times a day. There's a whole obsessive-compulsive disorder involving that, which is untreatable except by medication and a strict behavior-modification approach—many people feel psychotherapy won't do any good at all. However, there were some things we saw off the path that had us hold off those interventions. He was able to relate—the key thing in psychotherapy. And the hand-washing stopped pretty quickly when a doctor and his parents explained that if he kept it up, his hands would become infected. One fear replaced another, but that's telling because someone was able to break through his distorted view of reality.

"There is worrying within Kevin's family. His father and paternal grandmother are worriers. The father checks the gas jet and rattles the front door, checking it several times before he leaves, waking up the family. Kevin used to be quite anxious about this, feeling someone was breaking into the house. What he does now is go to the window, and if he sees his father leaving or his car isn't there, he doesn't worry.

"When I started doing a little work with the family, I got a lot of mileage out of it," Falcone said. "I asked how they had been treating his worries. They didn't mean it, but there was overconcern. For example, he didn't want to go out in a rainstorm or stand on the porch when it was drizzling. They'd say, 'It's only drizzling. The odds are that lightning won't strike. You can certainly take an umbrella because even though the umbrella is metal, it would only hit the trees first.' Well, there's more worrying in that reassurance than there's reassurance in the reassurance.

"It was very hard for them, but I had them say, 'Don't be silly, just go out, hurry up back.' I said if you must allay your anxieties, do it from a window, not the door, and don't let him see you. That was a very small piece of work—I used to see them five minutes before Kevin's session and five minutes after.

"With one session a week, his response has been very good," Falcone continued. "He went with the Scouts alone on the subway, no problem. He's started to stay out till it gets darker and they have to tell him to come in, where he used to run home the minute it got dark. He's playing rougher kinds of sports. So we were going to evaluate whether to continue treatment, and at that point he started to do worse.

"We had one failure. On an overnight Halloween outing it was his job to frighten the younger Cub Scouts. When they got to the campsite, they found it had been broken into and vandalized, possibly days ago, possibly hours ago. No major damage, just graffiti. That was at the back of Kevin's mind. He dressed up in his spooky outfit and went to scare the younger kids, but he just couldn't do it. He didn't have the size or the conviction, and they laughed at him, and the little kids ganged up to beat him up. It was a humiliating experience. He's a very sensitive, empathic child. The one point in the night when he managed to scare someone, the child admitted he was scared and Kevin just couldn't bear it anymore and said, 'Now look, it's me.'

"So what happened to the anger Kevin felt toward the kids who were laughing at him, abusing him, and beating him up? How he dealt with the anger was later that night, when things were quieting down, at bedtime, he became terrified that the vandals were going to come back and beat people up, possibly kill them with knives and guns. He became uncontrollable, his mother and the scoutmaster couldn't manage him, and they had to send him home."

Falcone and Sarnoff agreed there was a kernel of truth in some of Kevin's fears, but the paranoid reactions were always triggered by situations (like the Cub Scouts ganging up on him) that gave him cause for anger; in this case, he was not alone in the wilderness but protected by scouts, scoutmasters, and parents.

In recent sessions Falcone and Kevin—who was now waiting outside—had been talking about the school bullies. One goal, logically enough, was to teach Kevin to stand up to the bully without becoming a bully himself—but the larger purpose, Sarnoff pointed out, was to "have him reach the point where he can recognize and accept his own rage, so he doesn't have to defend against it by producing fantasies that distort reality. Once you do that you can achieve a state of calm in the individual when he goes on to deal with reality itself."

Kevin proved to be an appealing boy with shaggy brown hair, jeans, a heavy sweater, and sneakers. Sarnoff and I installed ourselves behind the mirror as Falcone began to ask how the week had gone. The conversation sounded like ordinary small talk. Kevin had joined the video club to rent Nintendo games. He was fidgeting a bit, pulling his sweater sleeves over his hands and looking around the room; perhaps he was thinking about being observed. Falcone continued to chat about video games, searching for a handle. Kevin was playing with his ear.

"That," Sarnoff whispered, "is an autoerotic gesture. Something about the games made him regress." I asked if it was stage fright; Sarnoff said Kevin, now sitting on his hands, was afraid of his dawning sexual feelings. Falcone was asking Kevin what had happened in school, and they were up to Tuesday. Kevin began to tell a long story in a casual tone. He was smiling a bit, but the story was about a beating-up. Kevin's friend Bruce had been accused of writing graffiti about one of the bullies; when he denied it, the bully said he would fight Bruce after school. So Kevin and Bruce tried to duck out together, but this bully got some big kids and they cornered the two boys. Kevin's sister was there and the two of them escaped, but the bullies got Bruce.

Falcone questioned him about the incident in fair detail, almost like a cop or a reporter, and said, "Hey, that's scary. Your friend's helpless, you have to watch, there's nothing you can do." He was trying to get Kevin to admit the emotion in the situation. Finally Falcone asked Kevin what he did next, and Kevin said he and Bruce rented a *Friday the 13th* video game. (Later Falcone told me that Jason, Freddy Krueger, and Michael Myers, the villains in horror movies, are very important figures to kids in latency and early adolescence. "We use them like a Rorschach, where the child projects his own feelings onto the characters. Psychiatrists have to keep a finger on the pulse of youth," he said. "Most of us who go into our business keep the aspects of childhood close to the heart, so it's really not difficult.")

Falcone pointed out that Jason was a big bully you got to beat up in that game. "And you just got beaten up."

"I didn't want to be the big guy because the big guy got beaten up," Kevin said. "In the video game I kicked him across the street."

"When you play the video games," Falcone asked, "how do you feel?"

"I enjoy it. I get into it."

"Do you think they help kids?"

"Yeah."

"How?"

"Hand-eye coordination." Kevin was looking around. Something was getting him.

Falcone continued, "Maybe the video game stirs up the anger."

"I don't think so. It lets it out."

"So maybe that's good."

Falcone and Kevin talked more, but clearly the major work of the session was getting Kevin to understand that the video game is one way of letting off steam. (It wasn't enough, Sarnoff pointed out later; Kevin also had to learn to deal with angry feelings directly. Video game parlors, he said, are filled with men in business suits at high noon, all zapping their bosses.) One source of mild disagreement between Sarnoff and Falcone, whose background is Sullivanian (a school of psychodynamic therapy that focuses on interpersonal relationships), is Falcone's emphasis on talk over play: Sarnoff thinks Kevin is on the cusp of ludic demise and that some information will be lost if Falcone doesn't allow more play time. When Kevin gets fidgety, Sarnoff says he needs to play.

The amount of apparent filler in a psychodynamic session is notable to a lay observer, though professionals say some of this stuff will prove significant later on. "You're panning for gold," I said. Falcone liked this image; Sarnoff didn't, feeling it implied passivity and randomness. "We have to go after these golden moments," he answered.

It was long after the session with Falcone and Kevin that I sat in on the case conference at Stony Brook at which Gabrielle Carlson and her team evaluated Hector, the seven-year-old boy who played for hours and hours at being a dinosaur. It seemed to me that the dinosaur was a perfect example of the ludic symbols Sarnoff had told me about, and that while Carlson didn't use this terminology, she and her colleagues seemed to share the perception that dinosaur fantasies served to calm Hector when he felt out of control.

When I returned from Stony Brook, I couldn't resist calling Sarnoff to tell him about Hector and ask what he made of the problem; while good therapists don't diagnose by hearsay, most are willing to schmooze a bit, after the predictable caveats of self-protection. Sarnoff thought the dinosaur play showed a high-level potential for abstraction, which would give a therapist something to work with; thus it was a hopeful sign. But based on similar formulations I'd heard from him before (most notably about

Kevin), I expected him to say that unless Hector faced and dealt with his rage and sadness about his parents, he would never lead a healthy life. This time, however, Sarnoff said, "The age from eleven to fifteen is a period of increased intensity of reality testing, during which some children develop the ability to put the past behind them. He could work it through himself.

"Therapy is just a guided transit through this passage. He *could* resolve all of it on his own. There's nothing magical about therapy. I often say to parents, you could get through the Grand Canyon yourself on a boat, but it's better to travel with an experienced guide."

CHAPTER 4

ROOTS (PART ONE)

The paediatrician feels the symptom as a challenge to his therapeutic armoury. It is hoped that this will always be true. If a child has a pain, then the sooner it is diagnosed and the cause removed the better. By contrast, the child psychiatrist sees in the symptom an organization of extreme complexity, one that is produced and maintained because of its value. The child needs the symptom because of some hitch in emotional development.

> —D. W. Winnicott,
> "Symptom Tolerance in
> Paediatrics: A Case History"
> (1953)

True insight survives its first formulation.

> —Erik H. Erikson,
> *Childhood and Society* (1950)

A NONPROFESSIONAL WHO HOPES TO MAKE SENSE of the theoretical disputes among mental health practitioners must sooner or later seek a historical context for their views. When I asked Charles Sarnoff to recommend books and articles that would supply such a context, he gave me the reading list assigned to first-year fellows in child psychiatry under his supervision. It's fair to assume that a first-year fellow would already have digested the basic volumes; still, many of the names on the list were familiar, and to me its most notable feature was that none of the articles were dated after 1969. When I remarked on this, Sarnoff answered that very little psychoanalytic writing has appeared lately; that his own book on latency, first published in 1976, had not been superseded and was still selling well, and that "today one gets rewards in child psychiatry by talking about or writing about chemicals."

As I went out in the world, I found reason to differ with this assessment: psychodynamic clinicians suggested more than enough recent work to occupy my evenings. The comments of Martin Leichtman, the chief psychologist at the Children's Division of the Menninger Foundation, in a 1990 article in the *Journal of the American Psychoanalytic Association,* seemed most intriguing: Psychoanalysis, Leichtman wrote, "is in the early stage of a revolution that promises to alter profoundly the theories that have served as cornerstones of its conceptions of personality and development and change the manner in which those theories are formulated and evaluated."

Was Sarnoff simply rigid and old-fashioned? Was Leichtman melodramatic? I read much of what I was told to read, talked with other clinicians, and finally returned to chat with Sarnoff in his eyrie above the Hudson. He seemed a study in passionate ambivalence, sensibly recognizing the limits of classical Freudian psychology and yet taking offense when others outside the family (or younger nieces and nephews) reminded him of them. Sometimes he appeared to accept that psychoanalysis was a science and should appropriately evolve; other times he sounded as if it were either a religion beset by heretics (an attitude for which Freudians have frequently been criticized over the years) or an enduring literature now blitzed by trendiness. I continued to wonder just how placid or turbulent was that theoretical river that flowed outside his window, and what might be the implications for patients if either Sarnoff or Leichtman was right.

In the beginning, obviously, there was Freud. In his introduction to what is now the standard biography, Peter Gay writes

Despite decades of research and scores of studies, he remains puzzling and intensely controversial. Freud has been called genius, founder, master, a giant among the makers of the modern mind, and, no less emphatically, autocrat, plagiarist, fabulist, the most consummate of charlatans. Every worshiper who has hailed him as a Columbus has been matched by a detractor who has derided him as a Cagliostro. . . . Psychoanalysts for their part . . . have only too often treated Freud as though he were indeed the pontiff of his faith and his words unchallengeable papal pronouncements. No reconciliation of such extremes seems possible.

Readers can pursue their own answers to the challenge of evaluating Freud, outside these pages, as deeply as they care to. I will talk here only about some of his writings that seem particularly pertinent to a survey of child therapy in the 1990s, recommending skepticism to lay people when professionals either worship Freud or dismiss him.

Two particular live children stand out in Freud's writings: Little Hans, the phobic five-year-old he described in 1909 and treated vicariously through Hans's father; and Ernst, the boy with the spinning reel, who was not a patient. Hans was actually Herbert Graf, the son of Max Graf, a musicologist who had been coming to Freud's Wednesday-night seminars; Frau Graf had been a patient of Freud's. The Grafs, who were what passed in turn-of-the-century Vienna for enlightened, cultivated, free-thinking parents, "had agreed that in bringing up their first child they would use no more coercion than might be absolutely necessary for maintaining good behavior." Nonetheless, while Hans's parents clearly loved him, their childrearing practices seem horrific to the contemporary reader.

From the age of three Hans, a smart and spirited little boy, shows "a quite peculiarly lively interest in that portion of his body which he used to describe as his 'widdler.' " (The German for this word is *wiwimacher.*) At three and a half, he is found touching his penis, and his mother says, "If you do that, I shall send for Dr. A. to cut off your widdler. And then what'll you widdle with?" Hans is perpetually curious about widdlers, those he sees on animals at the zoo and those he imagines on Mummy and Daddy. Showing an early knack for empirical research, he observes, "A dog and a horse have widdlers; a table and a chair haven't." As Freud remarks, "He had thus got hold of an essential characteristic for differentiating between animate and inanimate objects."

Meanwhile, Freud continues, "the great event of Hans' life was the birth of his little sister Hanna when he was exactly three and a half." It is an event that would terrify any child. In the middle of the night, his mother goes into labor and starts groaning, and Hans is moved out of the room they shared. He has been told to expect the stork, the popular explanation for birth in those days. There's a lot of activity in the house, and then Hans is brought in to see his mother. He can't look at her, but he sees basins full of blood all around the room. He says, "But blood doesn't come out of *my* widdler."

Life proceeds, well, normally for the Graf family—Hans jealous of Hanna at first, then apparently loving; Hans fascinated, not surprisingly, by her little widdler; Hans interested in the widdler of the giraffe at the zoo and getting into scrapes with girl playmates at the family's summer house: intellectual curiosity around a widdling theme.

Then at the age of four and a half, Hans exhibits fear that a horse will bite him in the street, and Daddy seems to think it's connected with the boy having been frightened by a large penis. In addition, he begins to have bad dreams and expresses fear of losing Mummy and Daddy. When he gets into an "elegiac" mood like this, Mummy takes him into bed; his feelings for his mother have an erotic tinge. Things get worse: Hans becomes afraid to go to the park because a horse might bite him, and Mummy once again, as she had a year earlier, warns him about masturbation.

Throughout Hans's life Max Graf has been sending Freud bulletins about the child's development. The professor is interested in infantile sexuality and hopes to learn how neuroses are formed, so he has asked his friends and pupils to take notes on their children. Now the notes on Hans have become a case history, and Freud, who after all is still exploring uncharted territory, believes that since only Hans's father could get the boy to talk frankly, he will treat Hans vicariously.

Freud—whose attitude throughout the case is Holmesian, not smug— speculates that Hans's anxiety comes from the erotic longing that he has begun to repress. The obsession with horses seems not to be an ordinary fear: it exists even when there is no horse in sight and appears to have a life of its own, waxing and waning according to stresses in Hans's life. Dreams about Mummy and obsession with widdlers continue, and Freud recommends that Daddy provide some basic anatomical information— that women have no widdlers. This gets Hans back into the park, but it doesn't get rid of the fear. Finally Daddy and Hans connect the phobia with masturbation, which the boy insists he doesn't do anymore. Mr. Graf says "But you still want to," and Hans, who could hold his own with modern peers from Riverside Drive to Cambridge, Massachusetts, says, "Yes, I do. But wanting's not doing, and doing's not wanting." Freud's comment on this is a joyful exclamation point.

Most interesting and useful is Freud's footnote about diagnosis, when "we decide whether such feelings of mingled apprehension and longing are normal or not: we begin to call them 'pathological anxiety' from the moment at which they can no longer be relieved by the attainment of the object longed for." Hans's fear resembles this: it doesn't require an actual whinny to flare up.

I asked Sarnoff about the difference between fear and phobia, and he said, "There are several different levels. Fear is a conditioned response. Fear of large animals can actually be a response to being exposed to them and becoming frightened, with a reasonable degree of fear of getting back into that situation. Then there is what we call a phobic avoidance reaction: a person is afraid of flying in an airplane after seeing a plane crash. Next there is paranoia, which involves projection: I have an angry feeling, I deny it, I project it onto someone else, and then I blame it on them and may even avoid them. With Hans you had an interesting variation. You take your hostile wish toward your father and project it onto him, but you love your father and you're not going to be able to go anywhere if you hate him, so you displace the hostility onto a horse or a dog, and then you fantasize that the horse will hurt your father, the horse has the hostile wishes."

"When the child with the fear is brought to you," I asked, "how do you distinguish which kind of fear he has?"

"Sometimes you can pick it up immediately," Sarnoff said. "There's more affect associated with this than should normally be present. There's something distorted about this—they're just *too* anxious. But sometimes you'll get a patient, and you think there's a big dog this kid's afraid of, what's wrong with that, until you find out that he's only afraid of the big dog when he's with his mother and his mother's lover. He's suddenly afraid to go ice-skating with them because of the big dog, but it turns out he's afraid people will know about his mother, and he's angry at her for this whole situation." Another example of fears coming from projection is those expressed by Kevin, the boy treated by Sarnoff's supervisee in Chapter 3, on the night of the Halloween campfire.

Hans's discomfort about his various sexual urges is exacerbated by Mummy's old threat to have the doctor cut off his widdler, which has been marinating in his psyche for the past year and a half: if living things exist that do not possess widdlers, it might be possible after all to take his widdler away and make him into a woman. Thus Freud suggests that this little boy has a castration complex—hardly a bizarre idea under the circumstances.

Now we encounter the symbolizing so important to Sarnoff, who says,

"Symbols are supposed to defend against affect. If you get enough symbolization, the person is perfectly comfortable and there's no phobia. A phobia is a failed symbolic resolution to a problem: the patient will avoid a situation without giving any other reason than 'it makes me feel anxious.' " The important feature of symbolic phobia is that even if the feared object has some legitimately scary qualities, the child finds some traits in it that are personally significant, latches onto these, and becomes obsessed. Another child, who has not found this personal significance, might more easily be diverted from his fears.

Hans's phobia extends to other large animals, particularly giraffes: one night he dreams of two giraffes, a big one with a long neck and a crumpled giraffe. "The big one called out because I took the crumpled one away from it. Then it stopped calling out, and then I sat down on the top of the crumpled one." The similarity of the two animals to Mummy and Daddy—Mr. and Mrs. Graf, as Sarnoff points out—is obvious to Daddy. The giraffe, indeed, is a symbol too close to his father to offer Hans protection against his feelings ("affect-porous," Sarnoff calls it) and so he prefers horses. And these are discussed in Hans's only meeting with Freud.

At last, Mr. Graf takes Hans to meet the professor. Father, son, and therapist have a highly successful "conjoint" session, the sort that contemporary psychoanalytic psychotherapists would consider utterly taboo and family systems therapists (see Part IV) might well be proud of. They do not—as would a family systems therapist—deal with problems in the family as a whole (the Grafs, we learn later, were divorced some years after Hans completed therapy), but the therapist is able to elicit information about Hans's horse phobia and to make the connection between his fears and his feelings about his parents: "It must be, I told him, that he thought his father was angry with him on that account, but this was not so, his father was fond of him in spite of it, and he might admit everything to him without any fear." A charming, affectionate dialogue goes on between Hans and his father, and on the way home Hans asks if the professor talks to God. After the session, Hans shows substantial improvement, but since this is not an old Hitchcock movie, the condition doesn't clear up completely after one interpretation.

The case proceeds with clues unfolding and quite credible interpretations of them. In sum, at the root of this condition is Hans's effort to piece together an understanding of how babies are born, which became intense after the birth of Hanna; his jealousy of Hanna; and his oedipal feelings. In the background is the actual behavior of the Grafs: Daddy mentions that Mummy beats Hanna and threatens to beat Hans with the carpet-beater, and both his tone and Freud's are so casual about this that one must assume it was a routine practice among enlightened Viennese in the first decade of the twentieth century; and Daddy responds to Hans's tireless quest for sexual enlightenment with what seems today to be nearly sadistic evasion, precipitating an outbreak of fantastic stories from Hans, whose side Freud is unequivocally on. Ultimately, Freud prevails with Mr. Graf, Hans begins to have healthy fantasies, and the condition clears up. (Sarnoff wonders whether Freud really did cure Hans or whether Hans just moved into latency.)

The standard criticisms of this case are that the vicarious treatment of Hans through his father was unscientific; and that Freud and Max Graf altered the details to fit Freud's theories. These observations are worth keeping in mind but shouldn't nullify the value of the case and the importance of its message: there are, after all, contemporary schools of therapy that treat children's problems by working with parents, and as Freud notes, "a psychoanalysis is not an impartial scientific investigation, but a therapeutic measure. Its essence is not to prove anything, but merely to alter something." If the case is not an impeccably accurate report, it's an insightful novella built around a thoroughly credible little boy.

An obvious limitation of the case is, however, also the source of its enduring value. There is clear cultural specificity in this story: the way the most enlightened parents in turn-of-the-century Vienna reared their children is the way only the least enlightened contemporary American parents behave. In "The Sexual Enlightenment of Children," a paper written two years earlier, before he completed and reported on Hans's treatment, Freud called the riddle of the origin of children "the oldest and most burning question that assails immature humanity" and observed:

> The answers given in the nursery wound the child's frank and genuine spirit of investigation, and generally deal the first blow at his confidence in his parents; from this time onwards he commonly begins to mistrust grown-up people and keeps to himself what interests him most.

These days children Hans's age are not widely told that the stork brings babies (although most parents are still uncomfortable discussing sex with their children, and that discomfort is bound to register), but families and cultures still have taboo subjects. What stories do modern parents cook up to explain death? Adoption? Cancer? AIDS? Mental illness? Poverty? Their own previous marriages? The misbehavior of relatives? How much psychological literature and clinical practice involves undoing the conse-quences of parents' reluctance to level with their children? While the role of symbols in psychological development is a debatable issue for thera-pists, it's fair to say that most would acknowledge that family mystery and secrecy play a role in the etiology of some children's problems. It's also worth noting, however, that while the Grafs' style of childrearing was not unusual in their society—and was probably better than most families'— all children in turn-of-the-century Vienna did not develop phobias. As Freud himself mentions, Hans's "mental constitution" and events in his life contributed to the etiology of his neurosis. Sarnoff also pays tribute to individual temperamental differences in addition to cultural and family influences.

The second important Freudian child was described in the 1920 essay "Beyond the Pleasure Principle" and could be called the model for later play therapy techniques. He was Ernst Wolfgang Halberstadt, Freud's eighteen-month-old grandson, a well-behaved child who, though much attached to his mother, never cried when she went out.

> Occasionally, however, this well-behaved child evinced the troublesome habit of flinging into the corner of the room or under the bed all the little things he could lay his hands on, so that to gather up his toys was often no light task. He accompanied this by an expression of interest and gratifica-tion, emitting a loud long-drawn-out 'o-o-o-oh' which in the judgment of his mother (one that coincided with my own) . . . meant 'go away' . . . I saw at last that this was a game, and that the child used all his toys only to play "being gone" with them.

One day, Freud saw Ernst playing with a "wooden reel with a piece of string wound round it"—too large to be a yo-yo, apparently, because it might have been used to play horse and cart. But

> he kept throwing it with considerable skill, held by the string, over the side of his little draped cot, so that the reel disappeared into it, then said his significant 'o-o-ooh' and drew the reel by the string out of the cot again, greeting its reappearance with a joyful *'Da'* (there). This was therefore the

complete game, disappearance and return, the first act being the only one generally observed by the onlookers, and the one untiringly repeated by the child as a game for its own sake, although the greater pleasure unquestionably attached to the second act.

Ernst played variations of this game while his mother was out, confirming Freud's interpretation: "It was connected with the child's remarkable cultural achievement—the forgoing of the satisfaction of an instinct—as the result of which he could let his mother go away without making any fuss. He made it right with himself, so to speak, by dramatizing the same disappearance and return with the objects he had at hand." Freud credited this to "the impulse to obtain the mastery of a situation" and suggested that throwing the toys away might be "the gratification of an impulse of revenge suppressed in real life but directed against the mother for going away."

A final comment on this child belongs to one of Freud's successors, D. W. Winnicott, writing in 1941 with an added interpretive spin:

> In the play-analyses of young children we can see that the destructive tendencies, which endanger the people that the child loves in external reality and in his inner world, lead to fear, guilt, and sorrow. Something is missing until the child feels that by his activities in play he has made reparation and revived the people whose loss he fears.

Before continuing, we need to nail down some basics of Freud's theories of mental functioning that later generations of child therapists either embraced, embellished, or rebutted. This, accordingly, is what the British would call a potted guide.

Freud conceptualized mental processes in two ways: the *dynamic* viewpoint, which described the conflict between instinctual drives and restraints; and the *economic* viewpoint, which pertained to psychic energy (called *libido*) seeking discharge. At first, he believed, mental operations are governed by the pleasure principle: that is, "any given process originates in an unpleasant state of tension" and works to relax the tension by either avoiding pain or producing pleasure. As the child develops, the dominant source of sexual pleasure shifts from the oral to the anal and finally to the genital zone. The oral phase, when pleasure comes chiefly from sucking, lasts from the ages of two to three months.

The anal phase, when the child derives the greatest autoerotic pleasure and feelings of mastery from withholding and expelling urine and feces and touching, smelling, and looking at his products, begins during the second year; and the genital phase, exemplified in Little Hans's sexual curiosity and interest in masturbation, starts in the third year.

The uncontrolled operation of the pleasure principle, however, can prove dangerous or difficult in the external world, and so, "Under the influence of the instinct of the ego for self-preservation, it is replaced by the 'reality-principle,' which without giving up the intention of ultimately attaining pleasure yet demands and enforces the postponement of satisfaction . . . and the temporary endurance of 'pain' on the long and circuitous road to pleasure."

Freud had two successive theories for mapping the mind. In the *topographic* theory, expressed in writings between 1900 and 1923, he postulated three metaphorically stratified mental systems, the conscious, the preconscious ("that which is latent but capable of becoming conscious"), and the unconscious ("that which is repressed and not capable of becoming conscious in the ordinary way"). Sarnoff espouses this theory because it was taught him by his own analyst: he offers no scientific or clinical justification for preferring early over late Freud but seems to explain his preference as one might say "I'm a Methodist, not an Episcopalian, because I was raised to be a Methodist." As he puts it in his own psychiatric jargon, "When I deal with patients, I'm identifying through incorporation and introjection of my analyst, who in turn worked with Freud before 1923." Sarnoff's comments about drives and fantasies in Chapter 3 are characteristic of the topographic orientation.

In 1923, Freud switched to the *tripartite* or *structural* theory, the one more familiar to nonprofessionals, in which specific jobs are allotted to the *id,* the *ego,* and the *superego:* "[T]he ego has the task of bringing the influence of the external world to bear upon the id and its tendencies, and endeavors to substitute the reality-principle for the pleasure-principle which reigns supreme in the id. . . . The ego represents what we call reason and sanity, in contrast to the id which contains the passions."

The superego (or ego ideal) represents conscience, and much later controversy over Freud came from his theory of how it is formed, which is based on male development: the boy ultimately resolves his Oedipus complex (the desire for sexual union with his mother and accordingly, the death or disappearance of his father) by identifying with his father, carrying, as it were, the father's Ten Commandments chiseled on an internal stone tablet. (As he proceeds in life, the commandments of other figures in authority, like Sarnoff's analyst, are added to the tablet, and the carvings of parental commands become more obscure, like the epitaphs on the older tombstones in a churchyard.)

Freud believed that women's superegos were inferior to men's because girls didn't identify with their fathers. In this formulation, he endorsed and perpetuated the prejudices of his day, and insofar as this part of the theory was accepted by his followers and the public, he did considerable harm. Few contemporary Freudians do accept it without serious modifications—which also vary. A fair example of current revision appears in *Psychoanalytic Theories of Development: An Integration* by Phyllis Tyson, Ph.D., and Robert L. Tyson, M.D., a heroic, interesting, and useful effort to synthesize evolving and sometimes clashing views:

> . . . the need to resolve conflicting feelings of love and hate held toward the idealized same-sex love object is central to superego formation. For the girl, this conflict must be resolved before oedipal progression can take place. For the boy, this conflict is central to oedipal resolution.

The Tysons do discuss differences in superego formation, which essentially come about because a girl identifies with her earliest caregiver—in most cultures, the mother—while a boy must differentiate from that caregiver. Gender-based differences in psychological development have been the source of theorizing and debate for most of the century; in order not to stop this report dead in its tracks, I will leave the subject with the Tysons' summary and move on to what Freud said about parents, which has frequently been misunderstood:

> The super-ego seems to have made a one-sided choice and to have picked out only the parents' strictness and severity, their prohibiting and punitive function, whereas their loving care seems not to have been taken over and maintained . . . experience shows that the super-ego can acquire the same characteristic of relentless severity even if the upbringing had been mild and kindly and had so far as possible avoided threats and punishments.

It is interesting that the modern reader would be more likely to blame the Grafs for Hans's phobia than Freud was. To the extent that parents are tortured by *mal de mère,* Freud is not really responsible; that onus falls on some of his successors.

The Tysons point out that one of Freud's major contributions to psychology (and one that may be less known to lay people than some of his other ideas) is the distinction between primary and secondary process thinking. Primary process, what Freud called "thinking in pictures," begins, he believed, at birth. It is the language of the unconscious (or the id), which governs fantasies, dreams, symbols, and ultimately artistic activity. Secondary process thinking—thinking in words—is ruled by the reality principle (thus the ego) and, the Tysons observe, "is characterized by rationality, order, and logic."

The distinction between these two types of thought is particularly useful because, as the Tysons observe, "With a few notable exceptions . . . psychoanalytic investigation has been mostly concerned with the primary process, whereas academic psychologists have focused chiefly on the development of secondary process thinking." Later research led to numerous modern revisions of this Freudian theory of cognitive development. But a pervasive difference in therapeutic orientations—both within the psychodynamic world and between that world and others— still derives from the emphasis each assigns to objective or subjective reality. And perhaps it is here—in its solitary battle with the illusory demons that haunt us all—that psychodynamic therapy makes its most unassailable contribution. Like the Shakespearean poet's pen in a line from *A Midsummer-Night's Dream* that Sarnoff is particularly fond of, it "gives to airy nothing a local habitation and a name."

Freudian theory has also been criticized for its explanation of mental processes as the result of psychic energy seeking discharge. Numerous writers have pointed out that, as the Tysons put it, "Freud used the terms of energy—its conservation, displacement, and discharge—as metaphors for psychological functioning" because scientists in the nineteenth century believed these physical principles governed all scientific phenomena. While many of Freud's successors were turned off by the antiquated scientific metaphor, there is still clinical value, the Tysons remark, in "the idea of an instinctual drive as an idea, an affect, an impulse, a wish that has motivational impact."

Sarnoff is quite comfortable accepting a limited domain for psychoanalysis: he says, "The only thing we can do in psychoanalysis is find out the sources of behavior in the fantasy and early life and in drives. That doesn't mean there aren't other sources." But psychoanalysts in the thirties found the emphasis on the id, the drives, and the libido confining, and without discarding these earlier concepts, they began to shift their theoretical attention to the ego. "I think they began to develop a divine discontent about psychoanalysis because they were trying to make it into a universal psychology," says Sarnoff. "They came upon things that couldn't be explained on the basis of early childhood experience, so they tried to develop concepts and to understand how the awareness of external reality developed." Freud's daughter Anna studied developmental lines (see Chapter 2) and found the roots of pathology either in the failure to progress from some particular developmental level or in regression to an earlier level. Heinz Hartmann pointed out that "though the ego certainly does grow on conflicts, these are not the only roots of ego development."

Accordingly, successors to Freud both in Great Britain and in the United States began to study the first three years of life, the preoedipal period. To understand their work, we must master a few terms before we move on. An *object* is the Freudian term for "the thing through which an instinctual drive is able to achieve its aim." (Thus a hungry baby is fed or not fed by its mother, the object. Little Hans's mother was the object of his erotic longing.) While Freud applied the term both to real people and to subjective mental images of those people, later theorists tended to use the term *object relations* solely to refer to processes involving the mental image of a person. When you talk with your mother on the phone, therefore, you are having *interpersonal relations;* when you argue with your mother in your head, you are having *object relations,* as you might later discover when the same issue comes up in real life and your mother reacts in a way you didn't expect.

Except for his one meeting with Little Hans, Freud did not work directly with children, and however prophetic his observations of Ernst and the spinning reel, he never pursued them to the logical conclusion of developing a technique for child therapy. Beyond these two episodes, his formulations about children were wholly derived by reconstruction from the analysis of adults. (Critics of Freud point this fact out immediately, and even a supporter like Sarnoff uses it as the basis for his differences with the master.) The mother of play therapy was Melanie Klein, who did not cite the spinning-reel episode as her inspiration.

Klein trained as a psychoanalyst in Budapest in the second decade of the twentieth century, moved to Berlin in 1921, and finally settled in London in 1925; her mentors were Sandor Ferenczi and Karl Abraham. She continued to practice until her death in 1960, and in 1955 she wrote an account of her discovery.

Ten years after Freud published the case of Little Hans, Klein began to analyze a five-year-old to whom she assigned the pseudonym "Fritz"; the boy, it turned out later, was actually her own son Erich. At that time, Klein later remembered, psychoanalysts thought it dangerous to probe too deeply into the unconscious of pre-latency-age children. Thus in a gingerly fashion, she began discussing with "Fritz" the "many unspoken questions which were obviously at the back of his mind and were impeding his intellectual development." This was somewhat helpful, but didn't clear up the child's neurotic problems, so she began to use analytic methods and interpretations, with greater success: that is, "I was strengthened in the belief that I was working on the right lines by observing the alleviation of anxiety again and again produced by my interpretations. I was at times perturbed by the intensity of the fresh anxieties which were being brought into the open." (How one achieves a transference with one's own son—as Klein claimed to have done with "Fritz"—is, of course, an interesting question.)

So Klein consulted Karl Abraham, who told her not to quarrel with success. "This analysis," Klein writes, "was the beginning of the psychoanalytic play technique, because from the start the child expressed his phantasies and anxieties mainly in play, and I consistently interpreted its meaning to him, with the result that additional material came up in his play." Klein believed then and ever afterward that children speak in play as adults speak in words.

She continued to work with children until she encountered her next landmark cases, Rita and Trude, in 1923. Rita was not yet three but "had night-terrors and animal phobias, was very ambivalent to her mother, at the same time clinging to her to such an extent that she could hardly be left alone. She had a marked obsessional neurosis and was at times very depressed. Her play was inhibited and her inability to tolerate frustrations made her upbringing very difficult." Klein wasn't sure she could analyze a child so young, but in the first session she managed to win Rita over through some interpretations, despite the unnerving skepticism of the child's mother and aunt, who watched the session. So she continued to see Rita, who at first did nothing but obsessionally dress and undress her doll.

The intensive analysis took eighty-three sessions in "only a few months" to clear up Rita's problem—and it moved Klein to the next refinement of the technique. As long as the sessions went on at Rita's house, the girl's mother lurked malevolently in the background, and Klein decided, anyway, that "the transference situation—the backbone of the psycho-analytic procedure—can only be established and maintained if the patient is able to feel that the consulting-room or the play-room, indeed the whole analysis, is something separate from his ordinary home life."

So Trude, a seven-year-old with moderate truancy problems and a deteriorating relationship with her mother, came to Klein's house. When the child was unresponsive to invitations to draw, Klein excused herself, dashed off to her own children's nursery, and retrieved toys, cars, small dolls, bricks, and a train. Immediately a drama commenced in which two of the dolls, watched by the others, began bumping into each other and into cars and falling down. Trude repeated this game with mounting anxiety, until Klein interpreted that she and her friend had been playing some sort of sexual game, the girl was afraid the teacher and her mother might punish her, "and now she might feel the same way about me." Trude instantly relaxed and became much more friendly to Klein. After a treatment that lasted eighty-two sessions with both negative and positive transferences recurring, Trude finally got along better with her mother and began to improve in her schoolwork.

Klein's description of the playroom is retrospective, but the equipment for play therapy hasn't really changed in forty or even sixty years: playrooms look a lot like nursery schoolrooms, except that toys have a minimum of personality so that children can use their imaginations. Sinks are essential, as are materials for drawing, writing, and painting. Klein liked to keep each child's playthings locked in a special drawer, so "he therefore knows that his toys and his play with them, which is the equivalent of the adult's associations, are only known to the analyst and to himself."

When a child breaks a toy, the child is also destroying the person it represents, and Klein found her patients' behavior most revealing: the children would put the toy away for a time and then, some sessions later, would search for it, seeking to make reparation. "It was always part of my technique not to use educative or moral influence," Klein wrote, "but to keep to the psycho-analytic procedure only, which, to put it in a nutshell, consists in understanding the patient's mind and in conveying to him what goes on in it." The therapist, as in Freudian analysis, was a blank screen; Klein noticed that patients in therapy sometimes made little of the major events in their lives but emphasized "apparently minor happenings" that had stirred their emotions and phantasies. (According to Juliet Mitchell, who edited Klein's papers, "The 'ph' spelling is used to indicate that the process is unconscious"; when one is deliberately woolgathering about romance and glory, presumably, one has a more prosaically spelled fantasy.)

So far so good. But Klein, moved by the aggressiveness of her child patients, soon came to believe that "the super-ego arises at a much earlier stage than Freud assumed," and she embarked on the wildly speculative theorizing for which she is, at least in the United States, notorious. Rita, who often played "the role of a severe and punishing mother who treated the child (represented by the doll or by myself) very cruelly," was not unusual among Klein's patients. She and Trude, among others, exhibited what Klein considered the "leading female anxiety situation": the little girl made "phantasied attacks on the mother's body, which aim at robbing her of its contents, i.e., of faeces, of the father's penis and of children," and was naturally terrified that the mother—the "primal persecutor"—would retaliate. Nor did little boys escape this terrifying plight: therefore they feared castration. Klein concluded that

> the oral-sadistic relation to the mother and the internalization of a devoured, and therefore devouring, breast create the prototype of all internal persecutors; and furthermore that the internalization of an injured and therefore dreaded breast on the one hand, and of a satisfying and helpful breast on the other, is the core of the superego.

The same feelings existed in bottle-fed children and had little if anything to do with actual interpersonal relations. Klein found that

> object relations start almost at birth and arise with the first feeding experience ... that all aspects of mental life are bound up with object relations ... that the child's experience of the external world, which very soon includes his ambivalent relation to his father and to other members of his

family, is constantly influenced by—and in turn influences—the internal world he is building up . . . external and internal situations are always interdependent, since introjection and projection operate side by side from the beginning of life.

Both Freud and his daughter Anna took an evolutionary view of psychological development: the child passes from the oral to the anal to the genital stage and, in Anna Freud's theories, proceeds along several developmental lines to a healthy autonomy. Klein's notion of time was more complicated. Instead of phases, she had "positions," which were pathologically named. At first, in what was called the "paranoid-schizoid position," the child saw its mother as split into two part-objects, the good breast and the bad breast. At about six months it recognized that Mother was one individual, thus entering the "depressive position," an emotional crisis as central to Kleinian theory as the Oedipus complex is to Freudians: whether the child could identify with the good mother and repair the damage done by its destructive feelings was the augur of its future mental health. The Oedipus complex—which Klein certainly didn't discard—begins almost at birth, and its resolution is something of an anticlimax. Not surprisingly, Melanie Klein and Anna Freud are two of the most famous enemies in the history of psychoanalysis.

Klein did not treat infants and thus observe them directly; her theories come from the analyses of children aged three to six. While she is not extrapolating from adults, then, she *is* extrapolating. Her rationale appears here in one of her more baroque passages:

> It does not seem clear why a child of, say, four years old should set up in his mind an unreal, phantastic image of parents who devour, cut and bite. But it *is* clear why in a child of about one year old the anxiety caused by the beginning of the Oedipus conflict takes the form of a dread of being devoured and destroyed. The child himself desires to destroy the libidinal object by biting, devouring and cutting it, which leads to anxiety, since awakening of the Oedipus tendencies is followed by introjection of the object . . . the child then dreads a punishment corresponding to the offence: the super-ego becomes something which bites, devours and cuts.

Is there anything at all for us here? What Kleinian influences will patients encounter?

Klein has few outright followers in the United States; her devotees are more numerous in England, Canada, and South America. Most therapists in the United States believe she attributed to the infant capacities that it didn't have. "Most of the things she says people will agree with, but not with the timing of the point of origin," says Sarnoff. "Children are not capable of developing the kinds of symbols she's talking about until they're twenty-six months of age. She is retrospectively reconstructing on the basis of the behavior she has seen at a later age rather than on the basis of the child's level of cognitive skill. Children bite when they suck their thumbs. She's talking about the earliest point at which rage can be expressed through the biting of an object. But what is the earliest point at which that can occur and leave an imprint in memory that can influence future life? When you reconstruct with a patient in analysis, though, you say, 'I think this happened to you at such an age,' and they take it back to wherever you suggest because they don't remember. But they realize now that some of their behavior was informed by this type of early experience."

"So it's a sort of convenient story that works for the patient and the analyst together?" I asked him one afternoon.

"Yes," Sarnoff said, "because the analyst is not going to be rewarded for having gotten the right month. He's going to be rewarded—and the patient will be rewarded—by the patient getting better, and having the sense of 'Is this what I'm doing?' There's something called an 'aha' experience."

Klein's descriptions of individual cases are lifelike and interesting; it is her theoretical speculations and the overwrought language in which they are couched that are difficult to swallow. But her ideas about the aggression, ambivalence, guilt, and reparation that complicate object relations are valuable still, and she was the first to direct clinical attention, appropriately, to events in the first three years of life. Her shadow is longer than one might expect.

A disciple of Klein who is more palatable to modern readers and who has won particularly wide acceptance in the United States is D. W. Winnicott, who began his career as a pediatrician and was sometimes described as "the British Dr. Spock." Winnicott, born in 1896, ran a pediatric clinic for many years and treated psychoanalytic patients of all ages and social classes from the thirties until his death in 1971. His own theories both elaborate on and depart from Klein's: object and interpersonal relations are equally important to Winnicott, and he is as interested in the actual conditions in the patient's life as in the patient's fantasies. In 1940, Winnicott made his most quoted remark to the British Psycho-Analytic Society: "There is no such thing as an infant." What he meant, as he then explained, was that the infant and its maternal care were inseparable, and it was through this lens that Winnicott viewed all psychological development.

Described in the introduction to his collected writings as "a joyous and troubled soul," Winnicott emits a charm, humanity, and depth of feeling not often encountered in psychiatric writing. The title of the collection, *Through Paediatrics to Psycho-Analysis,* evokes what is inside: like the family pediatrician, Winnicott speaks lay language, but that language (and indeed, the sensibility) is strongly English and has a period flavor. (He is the only psychoanalytic writer whose patients have the "fidgets" and the "collywobbles"; Sarnoff once invited Winnicott to join him in a session with an American juvenile delinquent, who was confused indeed when Winnicott asked, "Did you ever pinch anything?") At any rate, while reading his papers one tends to conjure up a mother and infant both swaddled in heavy Shetland wool, rocking in a dark room in a drafty country manor or a dreary council flat.

While Winnicott did believe you could reconstruct an infant's mental processes from the analyses of toddlers, older children, or adults—an issue of continuing vulnerability for psychodynamic theorists—unlike Freud and Klein he spent considerable time as a pediatrician actually working with infants and had real observations on which to base his beliefs. A typical diagnostic and therapeutic tool was the "spatula game," which he wrote about in 1941 after having used it for twenty years on babies between the ages of five and thirteen months: he had watched and noted in minute detail the reactions of innumerable infants in the clinic.

The test worked this way. Mother and baby sat in the waiting room outside Winnicott's large office until they were called in. The room was sufficiently spacious to enable mother and doctor to look each other over before the mother installed herself on the chair opposite Winnicott, baby on her knee. At the edge of Winnicott's desk, within reach of the child, he had placed a shiny right-angled spatula routinely used as a tongue-depressor. He and the mother were to remain, if possible, impassive: "You can imagine that mothers show by their ability or relative inability to follow this suggestion something of what they are like at home; if they are anxious about infection, or have strong moral feelings against putting things to the mouth, if they are hasty or move impulsively, these characteristics will be shown up." Ordinarily, the mum acted just fine.

The baby was inevitably attracted to the shiny spatula. Winnicott describes a normal sequence of events, from which any deviation was significant:

Stage 1. The baby puts his hand to the spatula, but at this moment discovers unexpectedly that the situation must be given thought. He is in a fix. Either with his hand resting on the spatula and his body quite still he looks at me and his mother with big eyes, and watches and waits, or, in certain cases, he withdraws interest completely and buries his face in the front of his mother's blouse. It is usually possible to manage the situation so that active reassurance is not given, and it is very interesting to watch the gradual and spontaneous return of the child's interest in the spatula.

Stage 2 . . . in the "period of hesitation" . . . the baby holds his body still (but not rigid). Gradually he becomes brave enough to let his feelings develop, and then the picture changes quite quickly . . . the child's acceptance of the reality of desire for the spatula is heralded by a change in the outside of the mouth, which becomes flabby, while the tongue looks thick and soft, and saliva flows copiously. Before long he puts the spatula into his mouth and is chewing with his gums, or seems to be copying father smoking a pipe. [Father is played by Leslie Howard.]

The baby's behavior changes from stillness to self-confidence rapidly. Winnicott observes that nothing short of brute force could have gotten the spatula into the baby's mouth during the period of hesitation. Winnicott's efforts to move the spatula toward an acutely inhibited baby would produce "screaming, mental distress, or actual colic."

Now the baby felt he owned the spatula and would bang with it as noisily as possible, or would hold it "to my mouth and to his mother's mouth, very pleased if we *pretend* to be fed by it. He definitely wishes us to *play* at being fed, and is upset if we would be so stupid as to take the thing into our mouths and spoil the game as a game."

In stage three the baby would drop the spatula on the floor, be happy to have someone pick it up for him, play with it, and throw it down again—a game that any parent will now recognize: "[H]e drops it on purpose, and thoroughly enjoys aggressively getting rid of it, and is especially pleased when it makes a ringing sound on contact with the floor." This phase ends with the baby either wanting to get down with the spatula on the floor or losing interest.

Winnicott describes various cases of abnormally anxious babies who had been brought to him with feeding disturbances or asthma; as a pediatrician, he was acutely sensitive to psychosomatic symptoms and often wrote about them. In some cases he would take the child on his knee for twenty minutes every day, play something like the spatula game with her, and have the problem remit in a few weeks, a working-through of something rather like what Freud saw his grandson do with the spinning reel. (Winnicott was enamored of this story.) Children were so malleable at this age that you could do a lot of good in a fairly short time, but your good work might be quickly undone by the circumstances of life.

This essay contains a fair amount of thick Kleinian speculation—the hesitation, Winnicott says, is due to the superego, and he believes a child as young as seven months has fantasies, anxieties, and defenses. But he says, reasonably enough, "A child feels that things inside are good or bad, just as outside things are good or bad." He observes accurately that a four- or five-month-old infant can distinguish between different people and sense their moods. And he notes:

> The infant, if he has the capacity to do so, finds himself dealing with two persons at once, mother and myself. This requires a degree of emotional development higher than the recognition of one whole person . . . many neurotics never succeed in managing a relation to two people at once. It has been pointed out that the neurotic adult is often capable of a good relation with one parent at a time, but gets into difficulties in his relationship with both together. This step in the infant's development, by which he becomes able to manage his relationship to two people who are important to him . . . at one and the same time, is a very important one, and until it is negotiated he cannot proceed to take his place satisfactorily in the family or in a social group. According to my observations this important step is first taken within the first year of life.

The self-confidence with which the child manipulates the spatula and the adults around him is "the cumulative effect of happy experiences and of a stable and friendly atmosphere." Klein doesn't talk about this at all;

to Winnicott, the pediatrician, it is everything. Since this atmosphere, as described, is always provided by one "good-enough mother," the contemporary reader, especially the female reader, may regard Winnicott with a touch of ambivalence: he is sometimes profound and other times just arbitrary.

Here is the crux of his reasoning, which appears throughout the collected papers.

"Primitive Emotional Development"—the title of a 1945 paper—requires three processes, which were absent in the psychotic patients Winnicott treated: integration, personalization, and the appreciation of time and space and other properties of reality. Winnicott postulates that newborn infants have unintegrated personalities. "The tendency to integrate is helped by two sets of experience," he says. "The technique of infant care whereby an infant is kept warm, handled and bathed and rocked and named, and also the acute instinctual experiences which tend to gather the personality together from within . . . bits of nursing technique and faces seen and sounds heard and smells smelt are only gradually pieced together into one being to be called mother. Equally important with integration is the development of the feeling that one's person is in one's body. Again it is instinctual experience and the repeated quiet experiences of body-care that gradually build up what may be called satisfactory personalization."

Winnicott says, "It seems as if an infant is really designed to be cared for from birth by his own mother, or failing that by an adopted mother, and not by several nurses." He says that "it is a mother's job to protect her infant from complications that cannot yet be understood by the infant, and to go on steadily providing the simplified bit of the world which the infant, through her, comes to know." There is certainly a good case for this, if it is not taken with slavish literalism. But Winnicott's next remark, which seems out of the blue, is: "Only on such a foundation can objectivity or a scientific attitude be built. All failure in objectivity at whatever date relates to failure in this stage of primitive emotional development." The modern reader balks at such cosmic generalization.

Winnicott's comments about mothers are complex; his picture of motherhood is daunting. The good-enough mother "starts off with an almost complete adaptation to her infant's needs, and as time proceeds she adapts less and less completely, gradually, according to the infant's growing ability to deal with her failure." She acquires the knack for this through something called "Primary Maternal Preoccupation," a state almost like an illness that develops during pregnancy and lasts for a few weeks after the child is born: the mother is "able to become preoccupied with [her] own infant to the exclusion of other interests, in the way that is normal and temporary."

Winnicott suggests that some mothers who are good in other respects cannot achieve this preoccupation, and he implies that they are thus doomed, as we contemporary Americans would say, to play catch-up ball; as described, it all sounds rather like a Calvinist state of grace. At the same time in another paper, he supplies a long list of reasons why the mother "hates her infant from the word go," among the most amusing of which are, "He is suspicious, refuses her good food, and makes her doubt herself, but eats well with his aunt"; "After an awful morning with him she goes out, and he smiles at a stranger, who says: 'Isn't he sweet?' " and "If she fails him at the start she knows he will pay her out for ever." Ultimately, Winnicott says, "The most remarkable thing about a mother is her ability to be hurt so much by her baby and to hate so much without paying the child out, and her ability to wait for rewards that may or may not come at a later date." And he insists that pediatricians when they see a good-enough mother should get out of her way and let her grow.

Winnicott (and his contemporaries) took psychoanalysis beyond its beginnings and voiced a theme that has recurred in psychodynamic writing ever since: it suggests that Freud had the luxury of treating relatively healthy neurotics. "It would be pleasant if we were able to take for analysis only those patients whose mother at the very start and also in the first months had been able to provide good-enough conditions. But this era of psychoanalysis is steadily drawing to a close." New techniques were required to deal with ever sicker patients. Accordingly, Winnicott was known for a kind of regressive therapy in which he supplied the "holding environment" (sometimes literally) that had for some reason not been provided in the child's infancy. The patient regressed to infancy in Winnicott's care until his emotional development reached a stage at which traditional psychoanalytic methods would be helpful.

An example of the method was Winnicott's treatment of a nine-year-old boy called Philip, thrown out of a leading prep school for starting an epidemic of stealing. Philip had had a difficult birth and developed asthma at age two, around the time when World War II disrupted the tenor of family life and his father went off for a long stint in the army. Over the years he developed enuresis and a collection of other symptoms that suggested a "degeneration of the personality which was progressive." Philip's siblings developed normally, and his mother "had the ability to be closely in touch with a normal child but not the ability to keep in touch with a child who was ill, and it was important to me to recognize this as I needed her co-operation."

The stealing episode occurred after the father's return, when the family was beginning to put its life back together again. Psychoanalysis was logistically impossible, and so Winnicott, after three diagnostic sessions with the boy, decided "it would be this mended home that would carry the major burden of the therapy." He told the mother that Philip "had missed something at the age of two years and he would have to go back and look for it." She quickly understood that the boy needed to become an infant and agreed to manage this with Winnicott's help: "eventually she was able to take the credit for having brought the child through a mental illness; the home provided the mental hospital that this boy needed, an asylum in the true sense of the word."

So for three months Philip stayed home, became withdrawn and dependent, was dressed by his mother, remained in bed or behaved as if sleepwalking, ate in an uncivilized but mechanical manner, grew uncoordinated, and made funny noises. Whatever he did, no one remarked about it. It was, however, a proper English-country-gentry-style regression: "On occasions he would come out of this state for an hour or two, as when the parents gave a cocktail party, and then he quickly returned to it."

Finally Philip hit bottom: he was always tired, he drank huge amounts of water and wet his bed every night. Then one morning he wanted to get up. "This marked the beginning of his gradual recovery, and there was no looking back. The symptoms peeled off and by the summer (1948) he was ready for a return to school." None of the symptoms ever returned, and by age fourteen, he was working ahead of grade level at a demanding public school, manly, well built, and, of course, good at games. As we will see in Part VI, many residential milieus aim in one way or another to reproduce to some degree the Winnicottian holding environment.

Much of Winnicott's writing represents an effort to educate pediatricians about psychoanalytic theory, and he talks of the physician's tendency to move in immediately to cure symptoms: "Today, and we all agree about this, even a boil must not be allowed to take care of itself." He voices the psychodynamic position that "the child needs the symptom because of some hitch in emotional development" and that "in most cases cure of the symptom does no harm, and when a cure *could* do harm the child usually manages, through unconscious processes, either to resist cure or to adopt an alternative SOS sign."

Sarnoff—who is not a Winnicott fan, for reasons that remain opaque— is a firm believer in symptom substitution. He takes a similar but modified position on this issue, holding that it's not just harmless but actually beneficial to start by curing a symptom. "My attitude is that the child gets so traumatized by the symptom that they then develop a neurosis because of the symptom," he says, "so I like to get them doing well, and hopefully the parents will stay with you. I explain to the parents what's going to happen, we get the kid comfortable as soon as possible and then we go deeper. Right now I'm working with a youngster who would wet himself during the day and then he would wet at night, and it would happen particularly when his father went away. I was able to clear up the daytime wetting in about a day and a half. He'd be playing a game and he was afraid he'd lose the game so he wouldn't go to the bathroom. The night wetting is something else again. That had to do with his short stature and the rage and anger in this kid. He was a sweet little child, but the rage he had was coming out in the sessions. When the rage comes out, the internal anger should stop, so I can't figure out what the connection is.

"Before I take a case I have the youngster physically worked up—by an endocrinologist, with this child—so I'm ready to do what has to be done. I don't want to say 'Don't do anything about it, because we want to keep this scientifically pure.' That's not a doctor's role, that's a researcher's."

Winnicott is particularly well known for the conception of "Transitional Objects and Transitional Phenomena," the soothing haven between inner and outer reality, represented by the beloved blanket or stuffed elephant that is not self and is not other. It fills a human need for a "world of illusion," which Winnicott says is in later life satisfied by art and religion. It is there in "an infant's babbling or the way an older child goes over a repertoire of songs and tunes while preparing for sleep . . . along with the use made of objects that are not part of the infant's body yet are not fully recognized as belonging to external reality." This is the only Winnicott paper that Sarnoff assigns, although he grouchily suggests that

Piaget had the idea first. It is a lovely paper, but since it doesn't tell parents about behavior that is likely to disturb them, there is no reason to spend more time on it here.

Don't wash the elephant, though. The child will eventually lose interest in it.

CHAPTER 5

ROOTS (PART TWO)

In considering Freud's view therefore we have constantly to try to remember what he, a scientific worker in the field, would do if he were alive now and active in the psycho-analytic world, taking into consideration advances in our new understanding of infants.

> —D. W. Winnicott,
> "Birth Memories, Birth Trauma,
> and Anxiety" (1949)

Just as infants must develop, so must our theories about what they experience and who they are.

> —Daniel N. Stern,
> *The Interpersonal World of the
> Infant* (1985)

AT THIS POINT THE CONTEMPORARY READER may complain that a piece of the mosaic was missing from the early psychoanalytic writing we've encountered so far. Where was the cultural element in the psychic equation? It was Erik H. Erikson who focused on the role of culture in psychological development, and perhaps significantly, he was not an M.D.: he is high on the roster of lay analytic heroes cited by American psychologists responding to psychiatric disdain.

Erikson had been trained by Anna Freud in Vienna in the twenties, and his landmark book, *Childhood and Society* was, he proclaimed, "a psychoanalytic book on the relation of the ego to society"; it studied "the ego's roots in social organization." Psychopathology, Erikson said, was the result of a somatic process, an individual ego process, and a societal process, and in order to understand it, the practitioner had to do "triple bookkeeping."

A good example of Erikson's view is his study of "A Neurological Crisis in a Small Boy," the case of Sam, a three-year-old Jewish child who had recently moved to a small town in northern California. Sam turns out to be highly evocative of Little Hans. Early one morning, five days after Sam's grandmother died while visiting the family, Sam had an epileptic seizure that terrified his mother, who was instantly reminded of her mother-in-law's final heart attack.

A month later Sam found a dead mole in the back yard, was "morbidly agitated" over it, and asked his mother "shrewd questions" about death. She tried to answer, but her answers failed to satisfy Sam. That night he had a more severe seizure and was rushed to the hospital, where his condition was diagnosed as "idiopathic epilepsy, possibly due to a brain lesion in the left hemisphere." But two months later, after accidentally squashing a butterfly, Sam had a third attack, and the hospital noted, "precipitating factor: psychic stimulus." Erikson explains, "In other words, because of some cerebral pathology this boy probably had a lower threshold for convulsive explosion; but it was a psychic stimulus, the idea of death, which precipitated him over his threshold." There were no other visible triggers.

What were the circumstances of Grandma's death? She had arrived several months earlier, invoking considerable performance anxiety in her daughter-in-law, who was insecure about her skills as a wife and mother; moreover, Mother was worried about Grandma's health. Sam, as feisty, mischievous, and precocious as Little Hans, was warned about his grandmother's weak heart, and the constant restraint made the boy tense. One day, Sam's mother went out for a while leaving the two together and came back to find Grandma collapsed on the floor with a heart attack, in a setting that suggested Sam had been provoking her. The grandmother was sick for some time, and at length she died.

The suggestion of a psychic stimulus reminded Mother of Sam's behavior the night before his first seizure: he "had piled up his pillows the way his grandmother had done to avoid congestion and . . . had gone to sleep in an almost sitting position—as had the grandmother." But the mother had not told Sam the truth about the old woman's death: she had said that Grandma had gone on a long trip north to Seattle. He had cried and said, "Why didn't she say good-by to me?" He was told that there had not been time. Then, when a mysterious, large box had been carried out of the house, the mother had told him that his grandmother's books were in it. But Sam had not seen the grandmother either bring or use such a lot of books, and he could not quite see the reason for all the tears shed over a box of books by the hastily congregated relatives.

Erikson believes Sam wasn't fooled for a minute, and Sam began to make the same sort of derisive remarks that Hans had made when Mr. Graf held to the story about the stork bringing Hanna: when an object got lost, Sam said, "It has gone on a lo-ong trip, all the way to See-attle." Later, in a therapy group, he became obsessed with building oblong boxes out of blocks.

Now Erikson introduces the element of culture. Sam's parents had always had great hopes for their intelligent son, and in the past they had fostered his curiosity. In the multiethnic neighborhood where the family lived before, it was useful to be street-wise, tough, and fast with your fists. Then they moved to a wealthier town where they were the only Jewish family, and suddenly Sam was told "not to hit the children, not to ask the ladies too many questions. . . . The problem now was to become quickly what the Gentiles of the middle class would call 'a nice little boy, in spite of his being Jewish.' Sam had done a remarkably intelligent job in adjusting his aggressiveness and becoming a witty little teaser."

But Sam was constitutionally a hot-tempered child. At the time of his grandmother's visit, he had hit another boy and drawn blood and was confined to quarters with Grandma. And besides the major seizures that followed her death, he had a number of minor attacks that seemed to succeed aggressive outbursts. One of these occurred while Sam was playing dominoes in a session with Erikson, who had become his therapist two years after the onset of the epilepsy. The domino incident proved a peg for Eriksonian interpretation: "If you wanted to see the dots on your blocks, you would have to be inside that little box, like a dead person in a coffin." Erikson hit pay dirt with this interpretation, enabling a discussion of the boy's fear of death, but it was not the whole story.

Erikson had also been working with Sam's mother, and he uncovered an incident in which Sam had thrown a doll at her, loosening one of her front teeth, and she had smacked him terribly hard in return. Mother and son each felt intensely guilty over this episode. Sam's parents had believed that "as a little Jew one has to be especially good in order not to be especially bad," a notion that could be traced to the family's ancestors in Russia. Erikson suggested that aggression had a particular connotation in this family, "the children of erstwhile fugitives from ghettos and pogroms," and that "our patient had been caught in this, his parents' conflict with their ancestors and with their neighbors, at the worst possible time for him. For he was going through a maturational stage characterized by a developmental intolerance of restraint." This view, then, amounted to Anna Freud's developmental focus with an overlay of cultural anthropology.

Sam got medicine for his epilepsy and psychotherapy for his emotional problems, while his parents received child guidance, the whole package a forerunner of the best modern treatment:

> An attempt was made to synchronize the pediatric with the psychoanalytic work. Dosages of sedatives were gradually decreased as psychoanalytic observation began to discern, and insight to steady, the weak spots in the child's emotional threshold. The stimuli specific for these weak areas were discussed not only with the child but also with his father and mother so that they, too, could review their roles in the disturbance and could gain some insight before their precocious child could overtake them in his understanding of himself and of them.

Sam's mother, now prepared, was able to say the therapeutic thing to Sam: when he says, "Only a bad boy would like to jump on his mommy," his mommy answers that "a good boy might think he wanted to but would know he didn't really want to." Erikson makes a strong point that

> wording is not too important. What counts is . . . spirit, and the implication that there are two different ways of wanting a thing, which can be separated by self-observation and communicated to others . . . it made it possible for the boy to warn his mother and himself whenever he felt the approach of that peculiar cosmic wrath or when he perceived the (often very slight) somatic indications of an attack. She would immediately get in touch with the pediatrician. . . . He would then prescribe some preventive measure. In this way minor seizures were reduced to rare and fleeting occurrences which the boy gradually learned to handle with a minimum of commotion. Major attacks did not occur.

Erikson—a notably sensible man—grants that the attacks might have stopped anyway, and he emphasizes that he has not claimed to cure epilepsy by psychoanalysis. What he did do was "help a whole family to accept a crisis in their midst as a crisis in the family history. For a psychosomatic crisis is an emotional crisis to the extent to which the sick individual is responding specifically to the latent crises in the significant people around him." This anticipates family systems therapy, which we will discuss in Part IV. A characteristic Eriksonian perspective is the notion that a new cultural context made Sam, the intelligent teaser and questioner—who had coped well with his previous environment and was prepared "for the adult role of a Jewish intellectual"—maladaptive in his new community.

Erikson was an admirer of Freud, crediting him with "the first consistent theory which took systematic account of the tragedies and comedies which center in the apertures of the body," and while deploring his unfortunate nineteenth-century thermodynamic metaphors, he regarded Freud's idea that libido progresses from one bodily zone to another as a good beginning. But

> It was clear to him, and it becomes clearer to us—who deal with new areas of the mind (ego), with different kinds of patients (children, psychotics), with new applications of psychoanalysis (society)—that we must search for the proper place of the libido theory in the totality of human life. While we must continue to study the life cycles of individuals by delineating the possible vicissitudes of their libido, we must become sensitive to the danger of forcing living persons into the role of marionettes of a mythical Eros—to the gain of neither therapy nor theory.

First Erikson put Freud on a matrix chart, on which the bodily zones—oral, anal, and genital (with subdivisions)—were laid out vertically, and five modes of behavior—incorporative 1 and 2, retentive, eliminative, and intrusive—were arranged horizontally. The intersection of the zones and modes defined a set of developmental stages. Within each stage there was a spectrum of permissible childrearing behavior (permissible because it satisfied the minimum requirement of not hampering the child's survival) endorsed by different cultures in pursuit of their aims:

Some people think that a baby, lest he scratch his own eyes out, must necessarily be swaddled completely for the better part of the day throughout the greater part of the first year; but also that he should be rocked or fed whenever he whimpers. Others think that he should feel the freedom of his kicking limbs as early as possible, but should "of course" be forced to wait for his meals until he, literally, gets blue in the face. . . . there seems to be an intrinsic wisdom, or at any rate an unconscious planfulness, in the seemingly arbitrary varieties of cultural conditioning: in fact, homogeneous cultures provide certain balances in later life for the very desires, fears, and rages which they provoked in childhood.

Erikson endorsed the pervasive psychodynamic belief that emotional development requires passing through a definite set of stages in proper order: a patient with certain neurotic symptoms has regressed to or fixated at a particular infantile zone or stage. The "eight stages of man" are the crucible in which the individual's character is formed from the conflict between (in order) trust and basic mistrust; autonomy and shame and doubt; initiative and guilt; industry and inferiority; identity and role diffusion; intimacy and isolation; generativity and stagnation; ego integrity and despair. These stages progress, Shakespearean fashion, throughout the life cycle.

There is one comment in *Childhood and Society* that seems to me in particular to evoke and update Little Hans and to illustrate how parental attitudes can precipitate emotional problems in children. What is important in this description is that the effect of the adults is so subtle and nuanced that it is beyond their control, intrinsic to the human condition. Erikson starts by citing the psychologist Arnold Gesell's description of a normal fifty-six-month-old boy regarding himself naked in a full-length mirror. Then;

Let us assume that sometime during this procedure his penis becomes erect. This sexual behavior, while by no means abnormal, has nothing to do with the sequence to be photographed as normative. Such behavior was not invited to the test; it has, as it were, crashed a good, clean party. . . . In a given situation it may happen; it may not: it is not "normative." However, if it does happen and this at an inopportune moment—i.e., when somebody in the vicinity (mother, attendant) thinks it should not happen—then it may, or may not, elicit from that somebody a drastic reaction which might consist merely in a rare and bewildering change of voice or a general diffused attitude. This may or may not happen in relation to a person or at a time of the life cycle that would give the event decisive importance for the child's relation to himself, to sex, to the world. If it does, it may take a psychoanalyst many months of reconstruction in which no normative charts will be of help.

Parents need to know this sort of thing can happen, although professionals today would not consider any single incident sufficient to produce a real problem: a series of interactions betraying an ill-concealed attitude and combining with developmental and temperamental factors would be required. Beyond that, it would seem, were they to worry about it, they might drive themselves crazy.

While Erikson was directly anthropological in emphasis, other American theorists also stressed the importance of the real world to an individual's development. Harry Stack Sullivan focused on adults, not children, and so will be treated briefly here; but he influenced the entire field of contemporary psychiatry, forcing even the Freudians, as Sarnoff points out, to look beyond drives and fantasies.

In 1940, Sullivan wrote that "the field of psychiatry is the field of interpersonal relations, under any and all circumstances in which these relations exist. It was seen that *a personality* can never be isolated from the complex of interpersonal relations in which the person lives and has his being." He classified thought and action in terms of goals, which in turn were grouped into those that brought satisfaction and those that brought security. The satisfaction-bringing operations were the ones that had preoccupied other psychoanalytic schools, those that gratified such bodily needs as food, hunger, fatigue, lust, and loneliness. But "the pursuit of security pertains rather more closely to man's cultural equipment than his bodily organization." Security pursuits included goals like prestige, ability, and power.

Sullivan believed we are born "with something of this power motive in us." He thought

The full development of personality along the lines of security is chiefly founded on the infant's discovery of his powerlessness to achieve certain desired end states with the tools, the instrumentalities, which are at his disposal. From the disappointments in the very early stages of life outside the womb—in which all things were given—comes the beginning of this vast development of actions, thoughts, foresights, and so on, which are calculated to protect one from a feeling of insecurity and helplessness. . . . This accultural evolution begins thus, and when it succeeds . . . one respects oneself, and as one respects oneself so one can respect others.

In Freudian terms Sullivan was dealing exclusively with ego, the imposition of the reality principle on the pleasure principle, and he saw development as a wholly interactive process that begins with the infant's "mightiest tool, the cry." Thus he is an ancestor of Chess and Thomas (see Chapter 1) and akin to the family systems therapists (see Part IV). The process called "the foundation of the self system" is "the organization of experience reflected . . . from the significant people around one." And anticipating the interests of contemporary epidemiologists, he added, "We see here the explanation of one of the greatest mysteries of human life, how some unfortunate people carry on in the face of apparently overwhelming difficulties, whereas other people are crushed by comparatively insignificant events, contemplate suicide, perhaps actually attempt it."

How would Sullivan's approach be played out in a clinical session? Logically enough, a therapist who sees development as a wholly interactive process will behave somewhat differently from one who focuses on unconscious motivation. Sarnoff, for example, told me he doesn't believe *everything* that happens is unconsciously motivated, but "when we work in the psychotherapy situation, we act as if it were, to see what we can get out of it. We don't want to lose any possibilities."

Hand-in-hand with unconscious motivation goes "psychic determinism," the belief that each statement a patient makes in therapy governs the next statement the patient will make. "If you talk, what the person says is influenced by what *you* said, not what *they've* been saying," he continued. "That is the origin of silence in psychotherapy. Freud himself was not particularly silent till the last years of his life, when operations for cancer and prostheses in his mouth interfered with his speech and he chose not to talk unless he had to. But he knew you can influence the unconscious motivation and therefore you have to differentiate between what you have introduced and what the patient has introduced. If I say to a child, 'Do you have a make-believe about that?' I'm not introducing anything, just asking them to change the structure they're using. But if in the middle of the session I say, 'It's raining, shall I lend you an umbrella?' do you think the rest of the session will be determined only by the patient's unconscious motivation? What if his unconscious fantasy was that all people are cruel and withholding, and he's moving closer to the affects and finally the anger associated with this? It doesn't go away. He feels corrected, or it's temporarily suppressed."

Contrast this with the attitude of a therapist who believes his role is to introduce material and watch how the patient reacts to it. The relationship between therapist and patient, as Sullivan laid it out in a series of lectures to psychiatrists, is that of a "two-group" which consists of an expert and his client. The expert's stance is that of "participant-observer." Instead of just sitting there silently, he asks questions in a style that to this reporter seems most familiar: it resembles that of an experienced journalist interviewing a benign source. (Journalists sometimes find it equally useful *not* to perform these Sullivanian rescues.) As Sullivan told his audience,

If you will pause to consider the people whom you look upon as "understanding"—that is, able to handle you expertly—you will notice that they demonstrate a very considerable respect for you. . . . This respect for you, which is so impressive when experienced, not only takes the general form of endorsing your worth as a companion in the same room, but is also shown by a certain warning of any severe jolts that you might receive in the discussion, and by a certain tendency to come to your rescue at those junctures at which you would feel better if you had some information that you don't happen to have.

By the middle of this century, psychoanalysis had produced an increasingly rich literature in which scholars explored different aspects of the human drama. They told the same stories that had recurred in myth and poetry and religion and fiction since stories began, speaking of timeless struggles in a new language. Was this science? If so, it was subject to obsolescence, with each scholar's theory fair game to be entirely superseded by a better theory. Or did each theorist lay out a truth beyond science, a human truth that could last forever as long as it lived peaceably side by side with other human truths, waiting to be chosen by some and rejected by others in each succeeding generation?

These questions became—and remain—increasingly important. They lie at the heart of the debate I set up here between Martin Leichtman of Menninger, who has written of a contemporary scientific revolution in psychoanalysis, and Charles Sarnoff, who more or less believes there is nothing new under the sun. (Sarnoff and Leichtman are not aware of each other; the debate is my artifact.) And there is no better place to start looking at them than in the work of Margaret Mahler.

In 1955, Mahler, a clinical professor of psychiatry at Albert Einstein College of Medicine in New York City, and a colleague, B. J. Gosliner, hypothesized "the universality of the symbiotic origin of the human condition, as well as . . . an obligatory separation-individuation process in normal development." In brief, infants begin life with a "normal autistic phase" in which they are unresponsive to outside stimuli, and then, during their second month, move to the "normal symbiotic phase," during which they experience a "state of undifferentiation" from their mothers. Separation-individuation follows that. Childhood psychoses represent failures of the process.

Mahler and another colleague tested these hypotheses on psychotic children at the Masters Children's Center in New York. The result was a famous book called *On Human Symbiosis and the Vicissitudes of Individuation: Volume I, Infantile Psychosis.* Mahler's views on infantile psychosis have been mostly superseded by biological research, and that book is now out of print. A more lasting contribution is the product of her subsequent and corresponding study of normal children and their mothers, *The Psychological Birth of the Human Infant,* written in collaboration with Fred Pine and Anni Bergman and published in 1975.

"The biological birth of the human infant and the psychological birth of the individual are not coincident in time," the book begins. "The former is a dramatic, observable, and well-circumscribed event; the latter a slowly unfolding intrapsychic process." This process is called "separation-individuation," which means "the establishment of a sense of separateness from, and relation to, a world of reality, particularly with regard to the experiences of *one's own body* and to the principal representative of the world as the infant experiences it"—that is, the mother. This process continues throughout the life cycle, but the crux of it is completed between the fourth or fifth month of age and the thirtieth to thirty-sixth month. It actually embraces two developments: separation, defined as "emergence from a symbiotic fusion with the mother," and individuation, "the child's assumption of his own individual characteristics." Conflicts unresolved during this period can remain or be reactivated later in life.

The purpose of this study was to illuminate what the authors call the "hatching process" in normal children. Development, Mahler and her colleagues point out, does not proceed at the same time on all fronts, and so a child may walk early, enabling him to separate physically before he is emotionally equipped to cope with the independence his new skill affords. Such a child, the authors hypothesize, may panic but will not know how to articulate his feelings; his psychological development may then be arrested. Other children may be traumatized by seemingly minor events. Observation of children hatching may give clues to the origin of mild and transient disturbances as well as more lasting problems. And finally, what is the role of the mother in all this?

In both concept and method, Mahler was a pivotal figure. The preverbal period presented an obvious problem to psychoanalysts, which each school solved differently. "At one extreme, . . . Melanie Klein and her followers impute to earliest extrauterine human mental life . . . an inborn symbolic process," Mahler and her colleagues wrote. "At the other end of the spectrum stand those Freudian analysts who look with favor on stringent verbal and reconstructive evidence . . . yet who seem to accord preverbal material little right to serve as the basis for even the most cautious and tentative extension of our main body of hypotheses." The style of all psychoanalytic research was to match the child's behavior with what older patients talked about in analysis. Mahler, standing in between Freudians and Kleinians, believed that since movements, cries, gestures, and facial expressions are the sole method of communication for children who don't know how to speak, this material has particularly rich meaning at that age; thus you can make reasonable inferences about the child's feelings, provided they come from "multiple, repeated, and consensually validated observations."

At the same time Mahler's research methods were set up to "strike a balance between free-floating psychoanalytic observation and pre-fixed experimental design." The research was a longitudinal observation of 38 children and their 22 mothers in a pilot study that ran from 1959 to 1962, followed by a formal research project that lasted from 1962 to 1968. The clinic environment was uniquely natural—as the authors describe it, "like an outdoor playground setting where the children play where they please while the mothers sit on benches and talk—with their children in full-view and with the opportunity to attend to whatever mothering is required of them." Mahler and her staff watched the children "with a 'psychoanalytic eye'—informed by all of our past encounters with intrapsychic life."

Because Mahler's work originated from psychoanalytic hypotheses and was highly interpretive, it didn't rock the tribal boat; but a developmental psychologist, wedded to the highly structured and time-limited conditions of the laboratory, would shrink in horror from this method, which is basically journalistic. (A reporter who has followed a subject around for a long period of time will recognize that despite some inhibition and some showing off, there are real limits to how long and how well anyone can maintain a pose; through a succession of off-moments, the real person shows through.) For urban mothers of that period—who actually raised their children in a similar setting—the study is engrossingly lifelike.

The mothers were the well-educated, child-centered, nonworking middle-class mothers who lived in the neighborhood and were drawn in by the promises of discount nursery-schooling at Masters Children's Center; by an attractive place to gather with other mothers and children; and by plenty of helpful child-care experts around, not to mention a desire to aid research. Since the subjects were basically healthy and didn't need therapy, the mothers were given freedom to choose two to four mornings a week to visit.

While the pilot project observed babies nine months and older, it was clear that some separation experiences began earlier, so the formal study started the infants at four months and younger. What sorts of behavior did the researchers note? In the children,

We observed infants alternately melting into, versus stiffening and stemming against, the mother's body . . . the infant stiffens and distances in the mother's arms. He cannot crawl yet, but still he alternately distances and fuses with, that is, seems to melt into the mother's body—then the outside world beckons and competes with the hitherto exclusive attention to the mother. . . . As soon as the infant's apparatuses mature sufficiently, he may slide down from the mother's lap, thence he crawls, paddles, and still later walks away from the mother.

As for the mothers,

How does a mother carry her child when she arrives: Like a part of herself? Like another human being? Like an inanimate object? How does the young infant react to the mother's taking off his wraps? Once in the room, does the mother separate herself from the child physically and/or emotionally, or is there an "invisible bond" between baby and mother even across some physical distance? Does the mother know what is happening to her infant even though he is at some distance from her? How quickly, how readily, and how appropriately does she respond to his needs? Does she make a gradual transition by taking him slowly to the playpen, for example, and staying with him until he is comfortable, perhaps offering him a toy? Or can't she wait to be rid of him, dumping him into the playpen immediately upon arrival and turning her attention to other things, perhaps her newspaper or conversation, turning to the child to overstimulate him only as her own needs demand it?

Like Freud, Klein, Winnicott, Erikson, and other psychoanalytic observers, Mahler divided the first three years into successive subphases, which, in the style of Klein and Winnicott, have pathological names, a nomenclature that the Tysons (see Chapter 4) find as self-defeating and innately obsolescent as Freud's thermodynamic metaphors. To cull what is of value in Mahler from what has actually become obsolete, it is necessary to transcend the language.

Newborn infants, Mahler believed, live in a state of "normal autism." They sleep most of the time and are aware only of what makes them feel good. (Freud called this state "primary narcissism.") "The effect of his mother's ministrations in reducing the pangs of need-hunger cannot be isolated, nor can the young infant differentiate them from tension-reducing attempts of his own, such as urinating, defecating, coughing, sneezing, spitting, regurgitating, vomiting—all the ways by which the infant tries to rid himself of unpleasurable tension." At the age of two months, the infant moves into "normal symbiosis," in which he behaves "as though he and his mother were an omnipotent system—a dual unity within one common boundary."

Symbiosis begins with the two-month social smile, which other researchers had signaled before Mahler. It is enhanced by the mother's affectionate behavior, particularly that which involves eye contact—holding, feeding, talking, and singing—and is the origin of normal adults' pleasure in being hugged. The psychological notion of symbiosis is not like the biological definition, because "the infant's need for the mother is absolute; the mother's need for the infant is relative." It may surprise the contemporary nonprofessional that neither Mahler nor Winnicott before her believed breast-feeding was essential to a child's well-being, and no therapist I met—of any orientation—cited the lack of it as etiologically significant in children's psychological problems. At least one, however, cited the lack of it as etiologically significant in excessive parental guilt. Here is what Mahler had to say:

> [B]reast feeding, though important, did not necessarily result in optimal closeness of the mother and her infant. One mother, for instance, proudly breast-fed her babies, but only because it was convenient . . . it made her feel successful and efficient. While breast feeding her child, she supported her on her lap with the breast reaching into the baby's mouth. She did not support or cradle the baby with her arms because she wanted her arms free to do as she pleased. . . . The baby was unsmiling for a long time. . . . On the other hand, there was a mother who thoroughly enjoyed her children when they were infants but did not breast-feed them. During feeding she held them close, supporting them well. She smiled and talked to them, and even when her baby was lying on the diapering table, she had her arms underneath him to support and cradle him. . . . Her baby son was not only very happy and content but developed first an unspecific and then a specific smiling response very early.

If symbiosis goes well, the baby, at age four or five months, moves into the first subphase of the separation-individuation process, which Mahler calls "differentiation" or "hatching." The sign of it is the preferential smiling response to the mother. Observers saw in the infants "a certain new look of alertness, persistence and goal-directedness" and said babies with this look had hatched. At six months—around the age Winnicott's new patients were tested with the spatula game—the infants began to study their mothers, and "these are the weeks during which the infant discovers with fascination a brooch, a pair of eyeglasses, or a pendant worn by the mother."

Mahler and her team cited Winnicott here, noting that the mother's style of soothing or stimulating the child was taken over and replicated by the child, thus becoming a transitional pattern; the child also began to handle transitional objects. A disturbance in the way the infant practiced (or didn't practice) this behavior might be a harbinger of later psychosis or borderline pathology. Mahler says this "delusion of a common boundary"—a difficulty distinguishing between self and other—is "the mechanism to which the ego regresses in cases of the most severe disturbance of individuation and psychotic disorganization," known in her terminology as "symbiotic child psychosis."

As we saw in Chapter 2, diagnosis and the description of disorders is an evolving process, which draws on biological and epidemiological research and parallels the evolution of psychological theory described here. DSM-IV parcels out various aspects of what Mahler called "symbiotic child psychosis" and related conditions under the nomenclature of Pervasive Developmental Disorders, Psychotic Disorders of various types, Affective Disorders, and Personality Disorders. (The latter classification, which we have encountered in previous chapters and will meet again, is defined as "an enduring pattern of inner experience and behavior that deviates markedly from the expectations of the individual's culture, is pervasive and inflexible, has an onset in adolescence or early adulthood, is stable over time, and leads to distress or impairment.") In asking how current practitioners describe Mahler's symbiotic children, we should also keep in mind the diagnostic-camel aspect of the DSM and take it with a grain of salt: psychodynamic therapists and biological psychiatrists have been fighting about children with personality disorders for years (particularly the ones called "borderline") and won't settle their arguments soon. We will, however, see some severely troubled school-age children in Chapter 15 who are unable to soothe themselves and need help in recovering from cataclysmic tantrums. Their DSM diagnoses vary widely, but they are the children Mahler was talking about.

The most important cognitive and emotional pattern among children of seven or eight months, according to the Mahler team, is "checking back to mother," a phenomenon that evokes Winnicott's babies with the spatula. It begins with the baby studying mother feature by feature and exploring what objects—the brooch, the eyeglasses, and so on—are not part of mother's body.

The authors note what earlier writers have called "stranger anxiety" at this age and report tremendous individual differences, even among siblings, in how it appears. In the happier, more confident children, an air of "curiosity and wonderment" predominates when they study strangers; but "among children whose basic trust has been less than optimal, an abrupt

change to acute stranger anxiety may occur; or there maybe a prolonged
period of mild stranger reaction, which transiently interferes with plea-
surable inspective behavior." (For Erikson, "trust versus basic mistrust"
is at issue in the first developmental stage. Chess and Thomas, whose
longitudinal study of New York children we discussed in Chapter 1, found
"approach or withdrawal" in reaction to strangers and all other new
stimuli a temperamental factor that interacts with the environment to
shape the child's behavior.)

The next Mahlerian subphase, called "Practicing," comes in two parts:
the early phase, when the child can move away from mother by crawling,
climbing, or standing but still holds on; and the practicing period proper,
marked by actual walking. It is a period of distancing and exploring that
proved particularly salutary for the pairs who "had an intense but uncomfortable symbiotic relationship. . . . Those mothers who had been most
anxious because they could not relieve their infant's distress during the
symbiotic and differentiation phases were now greatly relieved when their
children became less fragile and vulnerable and somewhat more independent . . . children became more relaxed and better able to use their
mother to find comfort and safety." A theme that pervades the book is that
the mothers, depending on their own personalities and talents, had
phases they were good at and phases they were less good at. Events in the
children's lives—parental vacations, hospital stays—sometimes caused
temporary setbacks depending on the timing.

The salient characteristic of this phase is that as the child "begins to
venture farther away from the mother's feet, he is often so absorbed in his
own activities that for long periods of time he appears to be oblivious to
the mother's presence. However, he returns periodically to the mother,
seeming to need her physical proximity from time to time." A colleague of
Mahler's had used the term "emotional refueling": here, the authors
report, "We saw 7- to 10-month-olds crawling or rapidly paddling to the
mother, righting themselves on her leg, touching her in other ways, or just
leaning against her. . . . It is easy to observe how the wilting and fatigued
infant 'perks up' in the shortest time following such contact; then he
quickly goes on."

Sarnoff finds this idea timeless and compelling. "It's not just with a
patient—you can see it in mythology, you can see it in stories. Every time
Hercules defeated Antaeus and threw him down, Antaeus came back
stronger because his mother was the Earth, and in going back to his

mother, he got back his strength so he could go out again." As a young man, Sarnoff knew Mahler, Winnicott, and Erikson, and it is sometimes difficult to tell when he is simply taking part in the political allegiances and rivalries of the distant psychoanalytic past; but while he is somewhat disparaging of Winnicott and Erikson, he says, "I think everything Margaret Mahler says has validity and can be used in understanding behavior."

Somewhere around the age of a year, the child learns to walk, ushering in the practicing subphase proper, the happiest age of all, a six-to-eight-month period when "the child seems intoxicated with his own faculties and with the greatness of his own world. Narcissism is at its peak!" The authors were impressed by the strong symbolic meaning of walking to mothers and toddlers and its importance to children's psychological birth. They describe the child's delight in mastery and exploration and also the "elated escape from fusion with, from engulfment by, mother . . . the toddler's constant running off until he is swooped up by his mother turn[s] from passive to active the fear of being reengulfed by mother . . . [and] also reassures him that mother will *want* to catch him." Most of the children were exhilarated most of the time and became "low-keyed" only when their mothers left the room.

Pride goeth before a fall, and the psychic fall for Mahlerian babies is called "rapprochement." Around the time of or shortly after walking, children become capable of representational intelligence, symbolic play, and speech; they are in the last stage of hatching. At about a year and a half, there is "a noticeable waning of his previous imperviousness to frustration, as well as a diminution of what has been a relative obliviousness to his mother's presence." As the authors describe it, "it had already begun to dawn on the junior toddler that the world is *not* his oyster, that he must cope with it more or less 'on his own,' very often as a relatively helpless, small, and separate individual . . . no matter how insistently the toddler tries to coerce the mother, she and he can no longer function effectively as a dual unit—that is to say, the child can no longer maintain his delusion of parental omnipotence . . . his love objects (his parents) are separate individuals with their own personal interests."

All of this is what nonprofessionals call the terrible twos, marked by "shadowing and darting-away patterns," misunderstandings between mother and child, mood swings, tantrums, clinginess, and ambivalence toward mother, father, and others. This is the age at which Ernst Halberstadt devised his game with the spinning reel. The playing out of this drama, which to Mahler is the most important one in childhood, subsumes theories of Freud, Klein, Winnicott, and Erikson, among others; it occurs at a time of broadening emotional range, greater awareness of father, the beginnings of gender identity, and toilet training, events these earlier theorists found important and that, for Mahler, feed into the rapprochement crisis.

The availability of the parents at this time is crucial, Mahler believes. And she and her colleagues note, "One could see with special clarity during this period the roots of many uniquely human problems and dilemmas—problems that sometimes are never completely resolved during the entire life cycle." The authors provide, as usual, copious illustrations of how the conflicts were expressed by various mothers and children.

The final subphase is called "Consolidation of Individuality and the Beginnings of Emotional Object Constancy." What this means in lay English is that as children approach the age of three, they should have developed a personal style of doing things and a sense of themselves as individuals, and a confidence that mother, whatever her current mood, is always the same person who will be there to love them, soothe them, take care of their needs, and provide some sort of moral compass; and that the knowledge of this allows them to do some of these things for themselves when mother is at the office, the movies, or the supermarket. They have similar though less intense feelings for other important older people in their lives.

The marks of this stage of development are verbal communication, the beginning of make-believe games and role-playing, an increasing interest in playmates and adults who are not mother, a sense of time (the words *later* and *tomorrow*) and spatial relations that allow the child to start postponing gratification and tolerate short-lived separation. (In Mahler's time children started nursery school at three, for these developmental reasons; now social factors have mostly advanced this age, with still-debated results.)

Their future healthy development depends partly on how well they have managed these tasks and partly on "accidental, but sometimes fateful, happenings such as sicknesses, surgical interventions, accidents, separations from mother or father ... events of this sort in a sense constitute each child's fate and are the substance from which are formed the endlessly varied, but also endlessly recurring, themes and tasks of his particular life."

In sum, Mahler, while not dismissing the struggles of the oedipal phase, believed that children's basic personalities are formed by the age of three, and that their relationships with their mothers are the crucial factor in their development. Mothers have a difficult job: to subordinate their own inner conflicts and fantasies about the child to the task of responding to the child's particular evolving needs. Mahler, then, was part of the contemporary psychodynamic Zeitgeist in stressing the importance of real experiences in the first three years of life. One assumes she would have put the Grafs under a microscope, as Freud did not. And perhaps the dark side of Mahler, Winnicott, and their contemporaries is a vulnerability to overzealous interpretations that produced the "*mal de mère* ideology" that Stella Chess so deplored.

All the theorists we've met so far at least claimed to be extending and modifying Freud: before begging to differ, they delivered a deferential nod. In 1971, however, there appeared a theorist who pointedly reinterpreted Freud's clinical methods. He asserted that what patients were telling him did not resonate with the Freudian-style theories then in use, that analysis as it was being practiced did not suit many deeply disturbed contemporary patients, and that it was time to come up with new ways to do therapy. Heinz Kohut did not treat children, believing that the psychoanalytic method derived its data completely from what patients themselves could describe and verify (as opposed to, say, developmental psychology, which might use Mahlerian-style observation of infants, children, and mothers; this might be very helpful but wasn't psychoanalysis). Thus his theories of development are reconstructed from the memories of adult patients; but his influence has been substantial and certainly reaches into the treatment of adolescents (as we will see in Chapter 6).

Kohut, born in Vienna in 1913, had been part of the mass Jewish emigration to the United States after the rise of Hitler. He was trained in this country first as a neurologist, then as a psychiatrist and psychoanalyst after settling in Chicago, where he ultimately taught and rose to eminence and no little controversy in American psychoanalytic circles.

In an appraisal of Kohut, Richard D. Chessick, a professor of psychiatry at Northwestern University, points out that Freudian analysis and the

North American ego psychology school "take as their basis an empirical scientific orientation founded on a positivist philosophy that was considered the hope of the world at the turn of the 20th century." Mental processes were seen as natural phenomena, "amenable to empirical dissection in the consulting room by the properly trained psychoanalyst-observer who takes a neutral and equidistant position with respect to the id, ego, and superego of the patient." Whatever their differences, Freud, Klein, Anna Freud, and Mahler were part of this tradition and believed that the neutral therapist cures patients by enabling them to "work through" their unresolved conflicts.

Winnicott, on the other hand, blamed deficiencies in mothering for the development of a "false self" in certain patients; for these patients the therapist needed first to fill in the gaps, so to speak, helping them to regress and find a "true self" that would be amenable to traditional analysis. Back in the thirties, Chessick reports, other psychoanalytic writers suggested that "the classical neurotic patient seen by Freud has gradually disappeared, to be replaced by types of severe character pathology, especially the narcissistic character, with a consequent diminution of analytic effectiveness and a lengthening of the analyses."

While there was a difference of opinion in the field about this, Chessick says that DSM character or personality disorders—in the most current terminology, those "enduring patterns" of deviant inner experience mentioned earlier in updating Mahler—now outnumber the classical neuroses, which presume a strong ego and its repressive defenses (as exhibited, for example, by Little Hans and Erikson's Sam). In particular, what DSM-IV calls "Narcissistic Personality Disorder . . . a pervasive pattern of grandiosity, need for admiration, and lack of empathy that begins by early adulthood and is present in a variety of contexts" and "Borderline Personality Disorder . . . a pervasive pattern of instability of interpersonal relationships, self-image, and affects, and marked impulsivity that begins by early adulthood and is present in a variety of contexts" are conducive to Kohut's approach. His psychology of the self aims to deal more effectively with patients who lack, in his terminology, "a cohesive sense of self." (These patients, indeed, might remind us of the Mahlerian babies who haven't achieved object constancy. That is fair enough for our purposes, although professionals split hairs more minutely than this.)

Kohut's model of treatment and cure works this way. Instead of maintaining a neutral, blank-screen demeanor on which the patient projects his feelings toward others (the Freudian-style transference) or developing an interpersonal relationship which duplicates and thus illuminates the patient's other relationships (as a follower of Harry Stack Sullivan would do), the Kohutian therapist gathers data by "empathy" or "vicarious introspection." Kohutian therapists concentrate on understanding what the patients are feeling. In treating an unusually tall man, Kohut says, we "begin to feel his unusual size as if it were our own and thus revive inner experiences in which we had been unusual or conspicuous . . . only then do we begin to appreciate the meaning that the unusual size may have for this person, and only then have we observed a psychological fact." The therapist aims not only to feel what the patient is feeling but also to step back and think about the patient's feelings, the better to understand them. The emphasis is not on tallness in general but on what the *experience* of tallness means to this particular person.

The aim of this is "exhaustive empathic comprehension," which is "testable and correctable" and which Chessick says "definitely does not offer the patient a love cure." The essence of the therapy is quite similar to what Winnicott did: "In a good holding environment, minor failures in the mother's or the therapist's empathy are unavoidable, and lead the baby or the patient to absorb gradually and silently that which the mother or therapist used to do for the baby or patient." Thus the patient, like a healthy baby, gradually learns to soothe herself when her mother isn't immediately available. The therapist, as Kohut described it, "*is* the old object with which the analysand tries to maintain contact, from which he tries to separate his own identity, or from which he attempts to derive a modicum of internal structure."

Kohut's formulation of the developmental process, along with his therapeutic style, is called *self psychology*. Very briefly, he postulated that infants begin life in narcissistic bliss, which is "disturbed by the inevitable shortcomings of maternal care." (A naïve lay reader might say, "This is like when the reality principle imposes on the pleasure principle," and I would join that lay reader.) The child tries to preserve this state by creating a "grandiose and exhibitionistic image" called the *grandiose self*, and "an imagined, completely devoted, all-powerful parent," known in Kohutian jargon as the *idealized parent imago*. If development goes well, the grandiose self becomes transformed and integrated into the personality, representing our ambitions and self-esteem; and the idealized parent imago becomes integrated as our "guiding values and ideals" and our respect and admiration for others. When development goes badly because of events or circumstances in people's lives, they fail to integrate their grandiose selves, and they develop narcissistic personality disorders; or they fail to integrate the parent imago, and they go through life searching for idealized parents to maintain their self-esteem. Significant others from whom people seek and receive emotional sustenance—in healthy or unhealthy ways—are known, in Kohutian terminology, as *selfobjects*.

This is a very brief summary of some elaborate, detailed concepts that Kohut modified signficantly over his lifetime; it will do as a start for nonprofessionals who encounter Kohutian therapists. For those who don't, it is important to understand that nearly twenty-five years ago, someone got the psychodynamic world shed of its compulsory fealty to Freud. Even if, indeed, a nonprofessional with innocent eyes can see similarities between what Freud and his followers described and what this revisionist model describes, it matters that Kohut said, in essence, that the true way to respect a genius like Freud was to be willing to challenge and disagree with him; only then could psychoanalysts think creatively.

Finally it is interesting to learn that in 1976 Kohut wrote a paper analyzing the role of Freud in the psychoanalytic world. Calling Freud "a transference figure par excellence," he suggested, as Chessick summarizes it, that "psychoanalysts' idealization of Freud leads to conformity and over-caution in the putting forward of new ideas" and that "the idealization of Freud protects the psychoanalyst against shame propensity, envy, jealousy, rage, and disturbances of self-esteem; therefore any attempted deidealization of Freud would create tremendous resistances against taking an objective, realistic attitude toward Freud."

While Kohut here is talking about the individual psychoanalyst's relationship to the father figure, Martin Leichtman, the Menninger psychologist who threw down the gauntlet in Chapter 4, sees a collective historical phenomenon similar to that described by the historian Thomas Kuhn in a famous 1962 book called *The Structure of Scientific Revolutions*. Kuhn says, the early developmental stages of most sciences have been characterized by continual competition between a number of distinct views of nature, each partially derived from, and all roughly compatible with, the dictates of scientific observation and method. What differentiated these various schools was not one or another failure of method—they were all "scientific"—but what we shall come to call their incommensurable ways of seeing the world and of practicing science in it.

The different schools compete until one wins out and becomes the "paradigm" or "set of received beliefs," from which what Kuhn calls "normal science" proceeds. Scientists can now pursue research that elaborates, explores, and extends the paradigm until anomalies burst forth that are incompatible with it. When these can no longer be evaded, says Kuhn, "then begin the extraordinary investigations that lead the profession at last to a new set of commitments, a new basis for the practice of science." Not surprisingly, considerable resistance occurs before "the community's rejection of one time-honored scientific theory in favor of another incompatible with it." In order to prevail, the new paradigm must win over a majority of younger scientists; then the older schools disappear, except for a few holdouts who "are simply read out of the profession" as the new paradigm becomes orthodox. If American psychoanalysis (and thus its child, psychodynamic therapy) is in the throes of a Kuhnian revolution, Leichtman believes we would now be in the early phases of it.

To set the stage for this possibility, we need to recross the Atlantic briefly and consider the work of John Bowlby, whom Leichtman cites as a rebel in the British psychoanalytic world and a forerunner of the current American upheaval. Bowlby's psychoanalytic training was the most orthodox: he was analyzed by Joan Rivière, a leading supporter of Melanie Klein, and supervised by Klein herself. In 1950, Bowlby, then director of the Tavistock Clinic in London, was asked to advise the World Health Organization on the mental health of homeless children. This assignment led to his lifelong research on the role of maternal deprivation in the etiology of psychiatric disorders. Bowlby was not a strict Kleinian either in theory or in research methodology; what he did do was antagonize the already splintered British psychoanalytic establishment by calling for new methods of doing research.

At the beginning of his major work, *Attachment and Loss*, Bowlby contrasted his own methods with the Freudian style of theorizing, which worked "from an end-product backwards." His change in perspective, he said, was radical: "It entails taking as our starting-point, not this or that symptom or syndrome that is giving trouble, but an event or experience deemed to be potentially pathogenic to the developing personality." Bowlby was starting with the trauma—"loss of mother-figure during the period between about six months and six years of age"—and observing its results. Like the physiological researcher, he focused on "the manifold sequelae of a particular pathogenic agent."

Bowlby's prospective view was similar to Mahler's, although he was far more critical of psychoanalytic methods, which he said reported and arranged phenomena selectively. He drew both upon research that observed the behavior of children separated from their mothers and upon ethological research, believing that what was known about other animal species could give clues to human behavior. He pointed out that Freud himself had described the limits of retrospective studies, and he asserted that while the historical method has its place in the consulting room, "if psychoanalysis is to attain full status as one of the behavioural sciences, it must add to its traditional method the tried methods of the natural sciences."

Bowlby said his own work was not incompatible with the important parts of Freudian theory—that which held that psychological disorders came from the effects of trauma on the individual's constitution, particularly during the vulnerable period of early childhood; and he accepted Freud's ideas about repression and transference. What he rejected in Freudian psychology was its theories about psychic energy and drives, which were imported from contemporary scientific theories and not derived directly from psychoanalytic clinical observation. For the nineteenth-century instinct theory used by Freud, Bowlby substituted a more modern science, that of information control theory, describing how systems are modified by feedback from the environment. (This idea had considerably more influence on behavioral and family systems therapy, as we will see in Parts III and IV.) Finally, Bowlby acknowledged a theoretical debt to Klein, Winnicott, and other members of the object relations school, in suggesting that the infant's need for an attachment to its mother is even more important than the need to gratify hunger.

Bowlby, Leichtman observes, was "a relatively isolated figure in psychoanalysis" for several decades, and "the major reason for [his] isolation was probably the form of his work." That is, Bowlby challenged "the primacy of the consulting room as a means of formulating and testing theories." Leichtman portrays Bowlby, whose work has attracted increasing interest in the United States in recent years, as one of the harbingers of a new paradigm.

The presence of so many competing theories of development and challenges to the traditional psychoanalytic method of gathering information, Leichtman suggests, have raised "profound doubts about the capacity of the psychoanalytic situation to provide a satisfactory scientific account of the formation of personality." In particular, he says, "such controversies have underlined that traditional psychoanalytic methods, notably reliance on case studies, do not provide a means of resolving disputes among systems with intelligent, committed proponents. In presenting their views, psychoanalysts always select the cases they discuss and exercise extraordinary selectivity in condensing hundreds of hours of treatment into a single paper."

For the past couple of decades, a torrent of research has poured into this environment from laboratories of developmental psychology, dealing with the very subject being hotly debated by psychoanalysts—as Mahler succinctly dubbed it, the psychological birth of the human infant. But while the world of psychoanalysis, Leichtman believes, was ripe for a new standard, the work done in the lab was not yet transferable to the couch or playroom because developmental psychologists were unwilling to connect their research through "inferential leaps" to the infant's inner world. The prerequisite for psychological research to bring about a revolution in psychoanalytic thinking, he says, was "a convincing demonstration that it could provide the basis for conceptions of the subjective world of the infant comparable to those derived from reconstruction."

In 1985 there appeared a book that endeavored to do this, and Leichtman calls that appearance "an event of major import for psychoanalysis." The book is *The Interpersonal World of the Infant* by Daniel N. Stern, then professor of psychiatry and chief of the Laboratory of Developmental Processes at Cornell University Medical Center.

The book aims to open a dialogue between the developmentalists, who just observe and "choose not to make inferential leaps," and the psychoanalysts, who "continually make inferences." Since we are by now acquainted with the limitations of inferential theorizing, I won't repeat them; at the same time Stern points out that this method "works clinically" and recognizes that without any inferences developmental research is clinically sterile. Accordingly, he suggests it is now possible, on the basis of recent research, to make a good educated guess about the subjective experiences of preverbal children and that it is in the interests of good clinical work to do so, rather than taking a rigid scientific attitude that lets patients twist in the wind.

Stern wants to know, "How do infants experience themselves and others? Is there a self to begin with, or an other, or some amalgam of both? How do they bring together separate sounds, movements, touches, sights, and feelings to form a whole person? Or is the whole grasped immediately? How is 'being with' someone remembered, or forgotten, or represented mentally? What might the experience of relatedness be like as development proceeds?" These are, of course, the questions asked in different ways—and inferentially answered—by Freud, Klein, Winnicott, Erikson, Sullivan, Mahler, and Kohut.

Stern is interested in "those senses of the self that if severely impaired would disrupt normal social functioning and likely lead to madness or great social deficit." And in outlining these he supplies, for the nonprofessional, a good working definition of what madness is, certainly better than the fragmented and dry formulations of DSM-IV. The crucial four are the sense of agency ("your arm moves when you want it to") and that your actions have consequences ("when you shut your eyes it gets dark"); the sense of physical cohesion ("the sense of being a nonfragmented, physical whole with boundaries and a locus of integrated action"); the sense of affectivity ("experiencing patterned inner qualities of feeling"); and the sense of self-history ("having the sense of enduring, of a continuity with one's own past so that one can even change while remaining the same").

The absence of agency, Stern says, can lead to catatonia, hysterical paralysis, and some types of paranoia; the absence of physical cohesion can lead to depersonalization, fragmentation, and psychotic experiences of fusion; the absence of affectivity can lead to anhedonia, which we encountered in the definition of depression in Chapter 2, but which Stern applies to the more severe kind that appears in schizophrenia; and the absence of self-history to various dissociative states. These four senses, he says, are significantly absent only in major psychoses. To these he adds "the sense of a subjective self that can achieve intersubjectivity with another"; "the sense of creating organization," which Stern doesn't really define clearly; and "the sense of transmitting meaning."

Clinicians and researchers, Stern notes, agree that in infant development there are epochs of great change (he cites two to three months; nine to twelve months; and fifteen to eighteen months) alternating with periods of consolidation (Mahler and her colleagues, we remember, reported that children at around four or five months seemed to *look* different and were said to have "hatched"). When the infants have a new "social feel," parents respond by treating them differently, and a sort of synergy occurs.

In describing what can be inferred about this process from laboratory research, Stern takes issue with most of what we have learned about psychoanalytic theory so far. Here are some of his more iconoclastic statements:

> There is no confusion between self and other in the beginning or at any point during infancy. [Infants] are also predesigned to be selectively responsive to external social events and never experience an autistic-like phase. . . . There is no symbiotic-like phase . . . the subjective experiences of union with another can occur only after a sense of a core self and a core other exists. Union experiences are thus viewed as the successful result of actively organizing the experience of self-being-with-other, rather than as the product of a passive failure of the ability to differentiate self from other. . . . The period of life from roughly nine to eighteen months is not primarily devoted to the developmental tasks of independence or autonomy or individuation. . . . It is equally devoted to . . . learning that one's subjective life—the contents of one's mind and the qualities of one's feelings—can be shared with another. . . . I question the entire notion of phases of development devoted to specific clinical issues such as orality, attachment, autonomy, independence, and trust. Clinical issues that have been viewed as the developmental tasks for specific epochs of infancy are seen here as issues for the lifespan . . . operating at essentially the same levels at all points in development.

Is Stern throwing psychoanalysis and its derivatives out the window? Not at all. He is simply saying that psychoanalytic theories are better at describing childhood than infancy and shouldn't be used for the pre-verbal period. Oddly enough, that is just about what Sarnoff believes: that the phenomena described by Klein and Mahler all appear, but one can only be sure of finding them at a later age, and to use these theories to describe what goes on in a baby's head is presumptuous. Accordingly, Sarnoff says, "Because I work with children, I see parallel development. I don't see oral phase, anal phase, phallic phase. I see oral phase that continues and has its own development—the oral characteristics at each stage of life—the same thing with anality, the same thing with phallic strivings and oedipality. Each one has its own way of representing itself at different times." (At the same time Sarnoff doesn't agree with Stern's inferential leaps, and not surprisingly he questions the clinical value of laboratory research in psychology. And Stern certainly doesn't use Freudian terminology.)

The first thing that is essential for nonprofessionals to learn from Stern is that "the early life narratives as created by Freud, Erikson, Klein, Mahler and Kohut would all be somewhat different even for the same case material. Each theorist selected different features of experience as the most central." And which of these theorists a practitioner admires will surely affect the way he defines the patient's problem, even though a good therapist will not metaphorically cut the patient's feet off to fit some theoretical Procrustean bed.

According to Stern's formulation, there are four different senses of self that accumulate before the age of eighteen months. As each appears, it reorganizes the child's perception of self and other (and accordingly, his way of relating) but the previous senses remain. Children can move back and forth between them without actually regressing. During the period when a new sense of self is forming, children are vulnerable, and problems that develop are more difficult to reverse. Since any summary of this sounds vague and murky, it makes sense to examine how Stern's theory operates and sample some research he cites to substantiate it.

Phase one, which Stern calls "The Sense of an Emergent Self," embraces the first two months of the infant's life, before that famous marker, the social smile. Here he reports on a fascinating "revolution in infancy research" which has taken on the problem of how we might know what infants know. The answers, psychologists suggest, come "by readily observable behaviors that are frequently performed, that are under voluntary muscular control, and that can be solicited during alert inactivity"—that is, during the period when the infant is not eating or sleeping but lying there taking everything in.

The actions examined are head-turning, sucking, and looking. Thus one researcher who sought to know whether newborns could tell the smell of their own mother's milk "placed three-day-old infants on their back and then placed breast pads taken from their nursing mother on one side of their heads. On the other side, he placed breast pads taken from other nursing women. The newborns reliably turned their heads toward their own mothers' pads, regardless of which side the pads were placed on." Other projects have hinged on whether infants will suck faster under certain circumstances, and on whether they will look at one thing rather than another. One researcher had mothers read a verse from Dr. Seuss to their fetuses during the last trimester of pregnancy; then when the new-borns heard that passage and an equally rhythmic control passage, the familiar paragraph made them suck furiously.

Far from the imagined Winnicottian gloom of the mother and baby in the rocker in the dark, chilly English room, one pictures a jolly American laboratory scene of alert babies watching eager graduate students jiggle twelve kinds of mobiles above their heads, offer an endless, varicolored, protean parade of pacifiers, and show infinite pictures of smiley or surprised faces in changing order to see what the child will do: the interpersonal world of the Sternian infant is a thrill a minute. From this volume of compelling research Stern concludes that "infants seek sensory stimulation"; that they have innate preferences among the sensations they seek; and most important, "from birth on, there appears to be a central tendency to form and test hypotheses about what is occurring in the world. . . . Infants are also constantly . . . asking, is this different from or the same as that? . . . this central tendency of mind . . . will rapidly categorize the social world into conforming and contrasting patterns, events, sets, and experiences."

Indeed, real life is closer to that laboratory world than one would think. While it may seem to parents that their new baby does nothing but eat, sleep, and spit up, "a great deal of social interaction goes on in the service of physiological regulation": while the infant is "crying, fretting, smiling and gazing," the parents are "rocking, touching, soothing, talking, sing-ing, and making noises and faces."

Classical psychoanalysis, Stern says, has mostly overlooked this fact, portraying a "fairly asocial infant" but also "a rich description of the infant's inner life as it is affected by changes in physiological state." This is the way Freud and Mahler portray the beginning of life. On the other hand, "The British object relations 'school' and H. S. Sullivan, an

American parallel, were unique among clinical theorists in believing that human social relatedness is present from birth, that it exists for its own sake, is of a definable nature, and does not lean upon physiological need states . . . the attachment theorists have further elaborated this view with objective data" (that means Bowlby and his colleague, Mary Ainsworth). Moreover, infants have an innate capacity "to take information received in one sensory modality and somehow translate it into another sensory modality." When a blindfold is removed, they can spot the pacifier they just sucked on—and thus do not experience two different types of maternal breast, as some theorists avow. What babies acquire during this period Stern calls "the sense of an emergent self."

Next comes a sense of "core self and core others," achieved by the age of seven months: that means Stern's infants have completed this process at an age when Mahler says they are only beginning it. By this time, they have consolidated the four crucial aspects of the organized sense of self mentioned above—agency, coherence, affectivity, and history. One experiment was done in Stern's own lab with Alice and Betty, a pair of four-month-old Siamese twins connected on the ventral surface, a week before they were to be surgically separated. They were sometimes in the habit of contentedly sucking each other's fingers, and at other times of sucking their own. Stern and some colleagues started gently changing the hands around, and "Alice seemed . . . to have no confusion as to whose fingers belonged to whom and which motor plan would best reestablish sucking . . . each twin 'knew' that one's own mouth sucking a finger and one's own finger being sucked do not make a coherent self."

Two- or three-month-old infants can recognize still photographs of their own mothers; can also tell that happy Mom and sad Mom are both Mom, and that close Mom and distant Mom are both Mom; and that happy Mom and happy Dad are both happy. Stern now reports the theory of a number of cognitive psychologists on how people organize memory—in terms of episodes—and applies this to infants. "An episode appears to enter into memory as an indivisable [sic] unit. The different pieces, the attributes of experience that make up an episode, such as perceptions, affects, and actions, can be isolated from the entire episode of which they are attributes. But in general the episode stands as a whole."

An infant experiences a nursing episode in all its details and matches up successive episodes until she has stored a generalized nursing episode, a sort of mental picture of the usual nursing scene. But if something new and different happens—"the infant's nose gets occluded by the breast. The infant cannot breathe, feels distress, flails, averts head from breast, and regains breath"—this experience is stored separately from the general script. Whether the infant comes to rewrite that script or buries it in long-term memory depends on whether the occlusion recurs. Stern elaborates this theory to cover, for example, that basic psychoanalytic question of how the infant perceives and remembers its mother.

Part of the sense of a core self is the sense of "self with other." Psychoanalysts' faulty generalizations about infancy are derived from the clinical recollections of disturbed adults. In discounting the theories of Winnicott, Mahler, and others about normal symbiosis or fusion, Stern observes that "all the events that regulate the feelings of attachment, physical proximity, and security are mutually created experiences." He cites cuddling, being held, and gazing, which "can never occur unless elicited or maintained by the action or presence of an other." The ordinary game of peekaboo is "a self-experience of very high excitation" which can't be achieved by an infant alone. Mother's behavior is not always the same, while Father and Uncle Gary and Grandma also play peekaboo.

Parents by their own reactions "can regulate what affect category the infant will experience," for example: "Is that cup-banging to be taken as amusing or hostile or bad?" The parents, Stern says, socialize "what part of the private world of inner experience is shareable and what part falls outside the pale of commonly recognized human experiences. At one end is psychic human membership, at the other psychic isolation." This is their most profound function. Thus Stern talks at length about "intersubjectivity" and "attunement," to which psychoanalysis, perhaps because of the dominance of separation-individuation theory, has given inadequate attention; they are, in Stern's view, two sides of the same developmental coin.

The experiments in attunement performed in Stern's laboratory, interestingly enough, strongly evoke Winnicott and Kohut. Winnicott's good-enough mother simply "holds the situation" so her baby can "go on being" without interference and his "true self" develops. What the mother—or the therapist—does, according to Kohut, is validate the child's feelings through empathy. Stern's videotaped experiments involved a child playing with a new toy and his mother behaving as instructed by the researcher, to determine the child's reaction:

While on his stomach, he grabs the toy and begins to bang and flail with it happily. His play is animated, as judged by his movements, breathing, and vocalizations. Mother then approaches him from behind, out of sight, and puts her hand on his bottom and gives it an animated jiggle side to side. The speed and intensity of her jiggle appear to match well the intensity and rate of the infant's arm movements and vocalizations, qualifying this as an attunement. The infant's response to her attunement is—nothing! He simply continues his play without missing a beat. Her jiggle has no overt effect, as though she had never acted.

By matching the child's intensity, the mother has implicitly given the baby permission to continue as he wishes. But when the researcher instructed the mother to misjudge the baby's level of animation and jiggle his behind more slowly, "the baby quickly stopped playing and looked around at her, as if to say 'What's going on?' " Stern has performed numerous experiments with attunement, the "closeness of match" whose "violation is meaningful." What, in the laboratory setting, Stern calls "closeness of match" is really no different from what Stella Chess and Alexander Thomas, in their twenty-five-year longitudinal study of New York children, called "goodness of fit." And as we observed in Erikson's example, in life the interactions between parent and child are so plentiful and minute that human beings cannot avoid transmitting their attitudes and values to their children; moreover, inevitably, some interactions misfire.

The final domain that Stern investigates is "The Sense of a Verbal Self," which appears at fifteen to eighteen months. Language "finally permits the child to begin to construct a narrative of his own life," but it is a double-edged sword, since experiences that aren't part of that narrative are, in the Freudian term, repressed; the mechanisms for such well-known psychodynamic phenomena as denial, disavowal, and double messages are now in place.

The capacities now available to the child are immensely sophisticated: Stern describes the mental functioning required for a toddler who has seen someone make a phone call to remember and imitate that telephoning several days later. Thus in play therapy, an unhappy eighteen-month-old boy whose father had just moved out sat before a dollhouse in which the boy doll was asleep in a bed with the mother doll. The boy was highly agitated. First he took a father doll and put it in bed with the mother and the boy, but still he was not satisfied. "The child then made the daddy doll put the boy doll in a separate bed and then get into bed with the mother doll. The child then said, 'All better now.' "

As Stern observes, "The child had to be juggling three versions of family reality: what he knew to be true at home, what he wished and remembered was once true at home, and what he saw as being enacted in the doll family . . . he manipulated the signifying representation . . . to realize the wished-for representation of family life and to repair symbolically the actual situation." Stern calls this a momentous psychodynamic development.

Another important feature of this period is the emergence of "mutually negotiated meanings." This means that "when daddy says 'good girl' the words are assembled with a set of experiences and thoughts that is different from the set assembled with mother's words 'good girl' . . . the difference in the two meanings can become a potent source of difficulty in solidifying an identity or self-concept." This evokes Winnicott's spatula game and his definition of mental health as the ability to negotiate relationships with both parents at once.

Stern observes that while "the acquisition of language has traditionally been seen as a major step in the achievement of separation and individuation . . . the opposite is equally true, that the acquisition of language is potent in the service of union and togetherness."

What happens to "the traditional clinical-developmental issues such as orality, dependence, autonomy, and trust" in Stern's world? They "have been disengaged from any one specific point or phase of origin in developmental time. These issues are seen here as developmental lines—that is, issues for life, not phases of life." Stern talks at great length about the clinical implications of his paradigm and gives numerous case histories to illustrate how it can be applied clinically throughout the life-span. He says "The actual point of origin for any of these traditional clinical-developmental issues could be anywhere along their continuous developmental line . . . the therapist is freer to roam with the patient across the ages and through the domains of senses of the self, to discover where the reconstructive action will be most intense, unimpeded by too limiting theoretical prescriptions." What the therapist does, Stern points out, is "search with the patient through his or her remembered history to find the potent life-experience that provides the key therapeutic metaphor for understanding and changing the patient's life."

That, of course, is what Sarnoff says the therapist does. And as he remarked earlier, "The analyst is not going to be rewarded for getting the month right."

What is interesting about Stern's book is that however much of received psychodynamic beliefs he rejects, there is a tremendous amount of earlier formulation that he evokes and restates. What he is doing is cherry-picking. Indeed, for nearly a hundred years, some highly astute observers have been watching troubled children. What most strikes this nonprofessional reader is that in all this time the children have not changed; it is the observers—whose intelligence is undeniable—who have changed, because they watch the children through their own cultural and individual adult prisms, the better, they hope, to understand the problems. That it is Stern's prism that seems most resonant with our contemporary American culture does not diminish the accomplishments of his predecessors.

For many reasons that we will discover throughout this book, psychodynamic therapy is fast moving out of favor; this is unfortunate, for the struggles it and it alone addresses will endure. Some of its problems are of its own making: the authoritarian stance of many practitioners is not acceptable to patients in our more egalitarian world. As Leichtman writes,

> Psychoanalysis today is in a state of flux. It encompasses a host of theories which differ radically in their conceptions of personality, development, psychopathology, and treatment; the means by which those theories have been established are being challenged from a variety of directions; and the discipline is subject to so many different intellectual and social crosscurrents that the directions it is likely to take in the future may be more uncertain than ever before in its history.

What this controversy does suggest is that far from being stagnant and dated, psychodynamic therapy is a vibrant and changing field. It also means that nonprofessionals need no longer regard psychodynamic therapists as figures of authority, and—to use a jargon word from other branches of therapy—it empowers the informed nonprofessional to follow Stern's example and cherry-pick. I have tried to point out some themes that recur, restated, throughout psychodynamic theorizing. Certainly most therapists would agree with the Tysons that "we move away from the building-blocks, or 'Lego' idea of development according to which each piece of developmental experience is assumed to be built solidly on top of the preceding piece. . . . Ours is a more plastic model—made of a substance like Plasticine that never dries up—in which the shape and configuration of various cascading and intertwining strands change as evolution and development proceeds."

In the next chapter, we will meet some psychodynamic therapists whose approach is somewhat different from Sarnoff's, and thus see how various theories are played out in clinical practice. As for the theorists, it is important to remember that they were often wrong. And that they were often right.

CHAPTER 6

IN THE SERVICE OF THE EGO

We must emphasize again that the development of the sense of self is the prototype of an eminently personal, internal experience that is difficult, if not impossible, to trace in observational studies, as well as in the reconstructive psychoanalytic situation. It reveals itself by its failures much more readily than by its normal variations.

—Margaret S. Mahler,
*The Psychological Birth of the
Human Infant* (1975)

True neurosis is not necessarily an illness, and first we should think of it as a tribute to the fact that life is difficult. We diagnose illness and abnormality only if the degree of disturbance is crippling to the child, or boring for the parent, or inconvenient for the family.

—D. W. Winnicott,
"Paediatrics and Childhood
Neurosis" (1956)

"I USED TO BE A TEACHER," Michael Thompson is saying. "There's part of me that still wishes I was. I taught fifth grade and seventh grade and eighth grade, and I had two problems with teaching. One was it gave me a very big headache by the end of the day, and the other was I only cared about the kids who gave me trouble. The ones who did their homework and loved the subject and handed in everything and were well-behaved were not interesting to me. I was only interested in the kids who did nothing and acted out and after a while it became apparent that I should be a child psychologist, not a teacher. But I loved the feel of schools, and I love coming back."

Thompson, a strapping, bearded man in his middle forties with curly brown hair, is doing a superior job of wooing his audience at the École Bilingue, a French-American private school in Arlington, a Boston suburb. "I gave up teaching and went back to graduate school and got a Ph.D. and learned about children's psychological difficulties," he goes on, "and some years ago I began consulting with schools. I had all this learning, and I could impressively diagnose children. I went into schools and realized that teachers are superb natural diagnosticians. I became convinced that if I had to make a diagnosis on a child—whether or not they were normal or abnormal—and I had a choice between seeing the child myself, talking with the parents, or talking with the homeroom teacher as my only source of information, which would I choose?

"There's no contest—I would talk to the teacher. First of all you see so much. Second you are much more objective than the parents. And you have acquired a great deal of information that you may not have tallied as diagnostic but which is in fact highly diagnostic. You know far more than you give yourself credit for."

The crowd mutters a bit, and Thompson says, "I already see the reaction: 'He's setting us up, this is a trick.' And you're right, I am setting you up, it's a trick. Since you don't have any confidence in yourselves, I'm going to give you a quiz, a number of clinical cases from different schools. Read them through, take ten minutes, and rate them one to four. Work from the gut. A one is completely normal, no intervention needed. A two is normal but some adjustment has to be made in the child's environment, family or school, without calling in a mental health professional. A three is not normal: some psychological intervention is essential, and a four is more information needed. Don't cop out and rate everything a four, but if you genuinely can't decide, write down the one piece of information you'd like."

Thompson distributes a three-page handout to the faculty, who immediately produce that well-known "purposeful hum" that teachers everywhere covet in their classrooms; some of the hum has a Gallic inflection. Ten minutes later he calls them to order and continues his talk.

"People think there's a mystery about mental health, but it's simply this: A symptom is a call for help, telling us there is some pain that cannot be communicated in words. We try to look systematically at symptoms and figure out what children are trying to tell us. So here is my approach," he says, and launches into the italicized, rule-stating tone the teachers themselves use so often. "*A symptom is normal behavior that is displayed too much, too intensely, or in the wrong place at the wrong time.* For example, Freud described compulsive hand-washing as a serious symptom. Everybody washes their hands every day. For vocational reasons some people—ceramics teachers and surgeons—wash their hands twenty or thirty times a day and think nothing of it. But if you ever see someone stand at the sink and wash their hands twenty-five times in a row, you don't need a lot of other information to know there's something wrong. The person is driven by something. Hand-washing is often related to guilt—think of Lady Macbeth and Pontius Pilate—though there's a disorder that may deprive it of its content, and it becomes a neurological automatic thing."

Thompson describes a boarding-school student who exploded in study hall one day: "He got into a fight with the teacher about homework, and all of a sudden he began to heat up. He said an extraordinary number of obscenities to the teacher and read the teacher out in an astonishing way. The other kids were just riveted. He was thrown out of school because what he had done was too intense, too public. What he was saying was 'something's going so wrong that I have to use this language,' which all children use when they are away from adults, and adults use when they're not around children, but he jumped over the line and used it to an adult about the adult in front of other children. That made it a symptom. He got himself out of school and into therapy in a big hurry."

They are starting to get down to cases: how did the teachers rate number seven? " 'A kindergarten boy is afraid of the dirt on his table in school. He believes there are germs on it. He won't change seats with anyone because he believes there are "dangerous germs" on other tables. He won't eat outside with other children in good weather because he says that germs may "fall on his food." One day he left his coat at home but wouldn't wear a spare coat from the lost and found due to possible germs,' " Thompson reads. "You all do this very well. I think no one gives him a one. Two teachers give him a two." One of them, who is French, says, "I think all Americans are crazy about germs." The other, American, says, "A kindergarten boy can have a very big imagination. It could be a small fixation and not very serious." A Swiss teacher wonders if maybe the parents are fussy.

"Everyone else rates it three," Thompson says. "I disagree that this is a narrow thing. If it was only the table—but when it gets connected to the germs outside, they fall in his food, they're on his coat, that's too many germs. We're talking about a boy who is living in a world that's radically different. Science teachers often vote two: it's just a misunderstanding, a science teacher would be able to set this boy right." There's great nervous Franco-American laughter. "This is so phobic it's paranoid! It's nuts!" Thompson explodes. "This is crazy on content alone, but also on the intensity of his reaction."

When behavior is less dramatic but still egregious, Thompson looks at how long it's been going on. "If a child has always been shy and inhibited, his shyness may be constitutional and not symptomatic," he says. But a sudden change in temperament that persists longer than it should— weeks of depressed behavior, for example, or mourning that goes on longer than a year—is cause for alarm.

The conversation digresses to cases that aren't on the handout, some of Thompson's and some at the school, including a child at the École who seems to be much less mature than his classmates. Along with other types of odd behavior, "he has a problem with his meals," says a teacher newly arrived from France. "Perhaps this is is because every day he has in his lunch box the sandwich peanut but-tair and jelly." A savvier French teacher says, "Some kids *always* have the peanut but-tair." Aside from this delightful display of ethnocentricity, the teachers do okay, judging a friendless Japanese seventh-grader who spends all his free time playing the violin to please his musician mother as perfectly normal. (Thompson: "I'd give him a two, but he's not ill. He could become ill if he's allowed to live too many years without friends, and if his mother doesn't get off his back.") Thompson tricks them with a terrified fourth-grade girl who says her older brother locked her in a closet; the teachers give her a three. ("She may be a one. The situation is a three. You can't judge whether it's fact or fantasy. By law, you have to report it and the state will investigate.")

As they wrap up, it seems as if Thompson has been flattering the teachers. Like parents, they can sense when something's wrong; they're not as prone as parents to feeling guilty and thus defensive; but teachers and parents are both laymen, and assessing pathology is often tricky. Still, Thompson says, "I could learn more from talking to you for two hours about the child—whom you've seen for hundreds of hours—than watching the child myself for the same two hours." In essence, the teachers are a data base for the psychologist.

Thompson, who has a B.A. and an Ed.M. from Harvard and a Ph.D. in educational psychology from the University of Chicago, took his clinical training in Chicago in the Laboratory of Adolescent Clinical Research at Michael Reese Hospital Psychiatric and Psychosomatic Institute. He serves a carriage-trade practice in Cambridge: he is affiliated with the Cambridge Center for School Consultation, a group of psychologists and psychiatrists who consult individually for leading private schools all over the country, running workshops for new school principals (called "heads" in the private school world), teachers, and parents. (One parent version of his École Bilingue workshop is called "Between Good and Evil in Adolescence." It helps parents to spot "the too-good child: constricted, perfectionistic, overly burdened by conscience," the "anti-social child: impulsive and undisciplined, still looking for limits," and the "just-right child, experiences all of the fears of the 'too-good' child and all of the impulses of the 'anti-social' child, but manages to maintain balance and walk between the extremes.") In the past he has taught, supervised, and consulted at hospitals in Boston and Chicago with a broader clientele.

He also treats children, adults, and families in private practice. Over several years I have called Thompson from time to time, finding his teaching skill as useful to a lay reporter as it is to school communities, and finally spent several hours discussing how he applies his classical psychoanalytic training to contemporary clinical problems.

"If you had talked to me when I left Chicago in 1979," Thompson told me, "you'd have met a psychologist who was going to be a lay analyst. I have a colleague who came back from Chicago with me, moved to Boston, and became a star at the Boston Psychoanalytic Institute. He's a wonderful guy, and he's having the career I thought I was going to have. I have continued to practice therapy that is fundamentally psychodynamic, but it is now informed by so many different kinds of theories— family systems theory and Jungian theory and biological knowledge, because that's where the greatest expansion and emphasis have been in this field."

At this point Thompson went into another room to take a call from a newly referred parent. Besides the usual yeses and nos, I heard one complete sentence: "Are you and your husband able to be in a room together?" Children of divorce figure prominently in Thompson's private practice, and he said, "I make it clear to the families that we are here on behalf of the child and I want them to respond at their highest level of good behavior. I'm kind of short with them, to convey 'Don't be indirect, don't pretend you're getting along better when there'll be some secret agenda. Tell me up front who's savaging whom, so I can see all of this and I don't have to discover it, because I want to focus on the child and I want you to be clear about your shit.' Otherwise things keep blowing up because I step on some goddamned divorce issue, and the child therapy can't be done.

"I need to find out whether they will let me do a child therapy or whether they really want me to get in and write up a lot of notes so they can subpoena me to testify that one is a better parent than the other. That's custody evaluation, not therapy. If somebody says they want a therapist, I want to know if they really want a therapist. I'm terrible in court. The answer to the question I asked that woman, by the way, was no."

Thompson is a great admirer of Winnicott. He continued; "Winnicott said that children are transiently symptomatic throughout life, that everything that takes adults to the courts or the asylums has its normal equivalent in childhood, so you have children who are getting psychiatrically ill for periods of time and then getting well. But in Cambridge if your child doesn't get better very quickly you look for a child therapist, or if you are about to do something like get divorced and you're psychologically savvy, you may know that the chances of their getting symptomatic are very high. I have had people who said to me, 'Will you hold our child while we savage each other?' I used to accept that task more often than I do now because I don't believe that any outsider can really hold a child safe."

We went back to our discussion of theory, and Thompson said, "We have more arrows in our quiver now than we used to, and if you hew to analytic framework alone, you've put yourself in too narrow a band of understanding. Guntrip [a British psychiatrist of the object relations school] said theory makes a good slave and a bad master. Treating chronic depression without psychopharmacology and something of a cognitive approach is not right. But in the moment it's very difficult to be a biologist and an analyst and a family systems person and a Jungian and a Rogerian. You have to have a kind of *take* on things, always illuminating and always narrow—always a blinder, but if you have no theory at all, you get up and run around the room and say, 'Oh my God, I'm a goner.' We need some way of understanding things, and the way I fundamentally understand things is analytic."

Thompson waved a hand toward one of his bookshelves, which contained more than a decade's worth of heavy volumes of *The Psychoanalytic Study of the Child,* the preeminent annual anthology of papers published by Freudian child analysts. It had been given to him by a colleague who changed careers, saying, "If I read one more article about the dream symbol of the bee representing the mother's nipple, I'm going to go crazy myself." Thompson said he was no longer looking for psychosexual conflict, and to illustrate a typical recent case, he told me this thoroughly Winnicottian story: "I had a five-year-old boy come to me once, and his presenting problem was he was no longer going to his mother—he wasn't asking her for help and nurturance. If he got a cut, he would go to his older brother, who was ten, not to an adult. His parents were getting divorced and his father was out of the house, and he stopped going to his mother. This was a symptom, not age-appropriate behavior. The kid walked into my office and leaned against the edge of my couch. He wasn't all that tall, but he had so much poise I thought of a stand-up comedian, and he said, 'My leg hurts. Do you fix hurting legs?' I said, 'I'm not that kind of doctor,' but he had told me he was hurting in the first moment. At the same time he didn't look needy, anxious, or depressed. He was superprecocious, the kind of loyal good soldier you see in kids whose parents are divorcing, and he had sworn off being a child.

"He got into therapy, and he regressed and got younger, more boyish, more needy, more age-appropriately dependent. He also had what is known in technical terms as a regression in the service of the ego. He had gotten out too far ahead of himself, and he went back and started to use his blanket again. By that time he was six, and not all six-year-olds drag their blankets around. The mother was very excited and pleased, because of what his presenting problem had been. She wanted him to be able to take the blanket, but the teacher didn't like that stuff in the first grade."

"And the other kids would have given him a hard time," I said.

"Exactly," Thompson continued. "So what do you do when you need a regression and other kids are going to give you a shellacking for it? The mother went out and bought him a small gym bag, and he took his blanket in the bag and never opened it, but he had it with him all day at school. It's your regression in your gym bag, your hidden regression that doesn't bring social scorn or disapproval. Let's be honest, how many of us have blankets in our gym bags? We all have our *stuff*. I'm unable to go to sleep without a glass of water at my bedside, but I virtually never drink from it." I asked Thompson if the boy eventually dumped the blanket, and he said, "Yeah."

I had been reading Melanie Klein when I talked to Thompson, and her speculation about children's fantasies was making me grouchy. "They trained me to be an empiricist at the University of Chicago," he said, "and I worshiped at the altar of empirical research, but as Bob Dylan says, I know more than I can prove. There are some levels of human experience that are not available to observation or empirical description, and I think it's very good that we have a group of people who are dedicated to thinking about what things mean to human beings, when meaning becomes so idiosyncratic and invisible. I don't read Melanie Klein anymore, but I use her every week. I have a patient who gets to feeling that the good in him is going to be overwhelmed by the bad and he's segmented off the bad, but he still lives in terror. For me Melanie Klein—in all her funny language—pulled that together into useful theories about the split between bad and good, and the primitive mechanisms for controlling the bad in you before you become capable of ambivalence. It explains the kinds of panics and defenses people get into in a way that family systems theory—to which I currently am quite devoted—does not explain."

"It seems," I conceded, "that only dynamic therapists have a feel for the dark primitive side of you that comes from childhood."

"They're the only ones that tune into the ferocity and enormity of childhood feelings," Thompson said. "I knew a little boy once who was two-and-a-half or three when his younger sister was born, and this kid was remorseless with his sister and with his parents. There are two things that children never forgive you for: one is the birth of siblings, and the other is moving. They also don't forgive you for dying, but you're not around to deal with that. But this kid essentially had a two-year tantrum, and they didn't take him to a therapist. They tried to control his behavior, they tried to modify it, they tried to reinforce it, they gave him separate time, and he just kept it up.

"You can manage sibling rivalry and call it sibling rivalry and teach kids to share and try to get them to love their little sister, but this father finally sat him down and said, 'Look, Patrick, do you think if you keep this up we're going to send her back?' and the little boy looked at him and said yes, and the father said, 'That's never going to happen. I understand now that you believed that if you kept this up, you could wear us down and drive us into sending her back, and that's never going to happen.' The kid's behavior changed from that day. Now *that* is a therapy session! He made the interpretation and the behavior changed, where a million behavioral paradigms had failed, because this kid had a driving idea, that he had the will and the endurance to make his parents send this sister away."

"I'm more interested in the father who was able to figure that out," I said.

"From the father's point of view it was, 'Nothing else has worked. What does he want us to do, get rid of her?' I think parents do therapy like that all the time because parents, other than child therapists, are the ones who struggle to make the meaning. It's very painful for parents."

As I left Thompson, he said, "I have been doing child therapy for twenty years, and it still scares me when a child comes through the door and I think, 'Can I understand them? Will I be able to get inside their world? Will I know anything? Will I just end up being some kind of adult?' There's such a gap between us and children, it's so hard to go back and get into it. You have to suspend something as an adult. I see it in gifted teachers, there's a way they suspend something about themselves to be with kids and at the same time are perfectly adult. It's quite a trick. I'm always reassured when I have a nice play session with a kid, that I can still get back there."

How much of a therapist's clinical style is the result of theoretical orientation and how much is just his own personality? This question dogged my research footsteps, and so I was particularly interested in meeting Stanley Spiegel, a psychologist who wrote a courteous letter of amplification in response to an article of mine on child therapy. Spiegel, who is in his sixties, is the only child analyst and therapist on the staff of the William Alanson White Institute in New York, one of the two leading centers of Sullivanian interpersonal therapy, where he holds several teaching and supervisory positions. Spiegel's letter underlined the differences between Sarnoff's Freudian view of development and the interpersonal approach, and it pointed out that while "in traditional Freudian psychodynamic approaches the therapist does attempt neutrality . . . [in interpersonal psychodynamic therapy] the presence and identity of the therapist or analyst is a vital part of the treatment." Spiegel sent me a copy of his book, *An Interpersonal Approach to Child Therapy: The Treatment of Children and Adolescents from an Interpersonal Point of View*, and after I had read it, we had lunch at an Indian restaurant near his New York office.

When I met Spiegel, he was in private practice in New York City and in Nyack, a suburb; his clientele was somewhat similar to Sarnoff's and to Thompson's—upper-middle-class children and adolescents with low-to-middle-range pathology. Now he spends part of the year in Santa Fe and sees patients only as a consultant, continuing to teach. "I don't know whether we're seeing different problems or diagnosing them differently," Spiegel told me, "but the implication nowadays is that problems are characterological. They're not a neurotic reaction to something at a particular time, they're a personality structure that's in trouble. I think for that reason you end up with longer-term treatment. The kids we get are the ones that are in trouble, and the ones that are in trouble are usually causing trouble in school."

Spiegel's particular hot buttons seemed to be the excesses of the Freudian and biological approaches. But it is most useful to describe some principles of Sullivanian theory that he has modified to apply to children and adolescents and that he outlines clearly in his book. Spiegel believes, first of all, that the essence of psychopathology is "problems in living." He writes, "Although there may be biological components to disorders of adjustment, it is one's relationship to one's world and to other people that is of central importance to the practice of psychotherapy." Depression, he told me, has much to do with difficulty handling separation and loss: "If you have a parent who's immediately replacing a goldfish or a puppy that dies, how can children deal with real loss if they're protected against it? And if you don't have experience in separations as a child, how the hell do you handle them as an adult?"

Spiegel, who holds that personalities are shaped mainly by interpersonal relationships, accepts that temperament "may be" inherited: his complaint is that biological approaches give short shrift to interpersonal factors, and that "from birth to death one is constantly learning ways of relating to other people (as a result of prior interactions with other people)." Among modern theorists, it is Daniel Stern—"I think he provides the documentation for Sullivan"—who most impresses Spiegel.

Spiegel's view of psychological disorders derives from Sullivan's "one-genus postulate": symptoms are extreme versions of dynamic operations present in healthy people too. He sees a continuum from mental health to mental illness or, in one example, "from neatness and orderliness to obsessional and finally ritualistic behavior. Thus the carefully observing clinician is able to some degree to understand empathically the terror of the anxiety and the uncanny emotions to which he too is susceptible." While adults don't have tantrums, therapists know how they feel when something is stolen from them or when a supervisor gets bossy; they draw on this in relating to children.

As a Sullivanian, Spiegel looks for security operations— "the maintenance and enhancement of self-esteem" as he puts it, and the avoidance of anxiety—as important motives for behavior: "The search for self-worth may . . . involve stealing or inflicting pain on others; stealing might be a way of enhancing self-esteem by showing superior strength . . . if one cannot permit bad thoughts about oneself because they would lower self-esteem, one may go to great lengths to prevent these thoughts, to the point of dissociating many events and experiences in life." Spiegel says that "one's self-image is essentially the result of the reflected appraisal of others," an idea that comes directly from Sullivan. Accordingly, he takes a particularly dim view of confrontation in child therapy.

An interpersonal therapist considers himself "a participant observer in the treatment process," the issue about which Spiegel wrote me his amplification letter. Many therapists I met during my research seemed highly sensitive to the threat of "boundary violations" posed by a patient's asking them personal questions: to the nonprofessional, this seems a gross overreaction, despite numerous explanations of how a blank-screen attitude is vital to successful transference. Interpersonal therapists seem commendable to me for their refusal to label bad manners good practice. Spiegel believes "withholding information that is not highly personal would at best be rude and is in itself likely to resonate with issues of secretiveness and withholding that might well be part of the family experience of the patient. With a child it is important to recognize that withholding information in response to direct questions can be particularly deleterious, for it is unlikely that the child can accurately conceive of the classically defined role of 'therapist' as some kind of catalyst."

All these principles mark an attitude midway between that of classical psychodynamic therapy and the cognitive behavioral approach. Unlike the cognitive-behaviorists, he is interested in the meaning patients make of their lives; but he diverges from other psychodynamic therapists in attempting absolutely minimal speculation about fantasies and their origin. I was most impressed by the modesty of Spiegel's approach and the restraint of his formulations; the guts of his clinical style is interpretation through metaphor, which he believes is the most effective way to work with children. "Many years ago I practiced in the South," Spiegel told me. "The South twenty years ago would be like the North thirty years ago. What you got with adults as well as children was the great relief they felt to discover that if they talked about something, it made them better. Then I moved to New York and found the trick was to get them to shut up.

"I've just got a kid whose parents are about to divorce. They give the child all these great stories of how things are going to be wonderful, he's not gonna have one home but two. So the kid talks the right language and that's what he tells me, but when you see what's going on, through his play, through psychological tests, he's very afraid, very anxious. On top of that he's now scared to talk about his anxiety because in effect they've said you're not allowed to be anxious." It is overintellectualizing that worries Spiegel about his patients: he writes about another child, "It was my intention to help her clarify, and to put her in touch with her own feelings and to find them acceptable." As I thought about the boy, however—being sold a phony bill of goods by his parents—he also seemed to me to be a highly contemporary version of Freud's Little Hans and Erikson's Sam.

Spiegel described his limited style of interpretation with the case of a six-year-old hellion named Danny, who was busy tearing up a good public school in the suburbs. "The teacher wasn't that great," he says. "She already knows this is a kid that gives her trouble, and she says, 'Danny, can you think of a word that begins with F?' So, of course, he goes to the board and writes 'FAK.' Instead of saying 'We don't use words like that' or 'At least you got the first letter right,' she sends him right down to the principal. Anyway, the first time the kid comes into my office, he practically wrecks it in twenty minutes. It was my own fault, I had too many things in there. But I could see he was interested in capguns. He quickly showed me—which I didn't discourage—that you could explode the caps outside the gun. Okay. So we're talking about fires, the kid's interested in fires, so I introduce fire engines, cars, trucks—I'm gonna set things up with fires going on, which indeed I do.

"You wonder what does fire mean to this kid? He pretends he's putting out fires. It strikes me that there is this terrible uncontrollable force he's got going inside of him. I may be right in speculating that it's anger, but all I say to the kid is, 'You seem to be pretty good with that fire extinguisher, although some fires are awfully hard to put out.' That's as far as I go. I don't get into his head."

Children who bang toy cars together appear frequently in the literature of play therapy, and the meaning of this metaphor varies according to the circumstances of the child's life. Spiegel keeps his interpretation on the car level: with one child who was most likely reenacting fearful arguments between his parents by ramming a truck into a big car and a small car, Spiegel simply said, "Small cars can get pretty smashed up in a collision," and, "Perhaps if the little car stayed over here in the corner and out of the way, it wouldn't get damaged." Too much mind-reading, he believes, can be frightening to a child, and overinterpretation is "like having an infant consider which leg goes first when he is learning to walk. If he does this, he is quite apt to fall on his bottom." At the same time he gives short shrift to the nondirective technique of just repeating what the patient says. "Early in my training merely verbalizing and reflecting feeling was considered an acceptable and even preferred approach, but I first began to question the utility of this method when a child said to me, 'How come you say everything I say?' " Children should be aware of their feelings, so as not to dissociate them, but insight into dynamics and etiology is inappropriate.

The book contains an elaborate sample of an assessment interview with a mother and father whose three-year-old son insisted on sleeping in his parents' bedroom at night. The interview smoked out all sorts of parental neuroses and family taboos before Spiegel learned that just before the problem began, the parents had removed the guardrails from the child's bed. Spiegel told them to put the rails back for a while until the child decided he was ready to take them off. The behavior stopped immediately, and while the therapist found evidence of other childrearing problems, the parents "were not seeking any other assistance. Foisting it on them would have been inappropriate."

The dark side of the Sullivanian viewpoint appears on page 49 of the book: "In my view psychopathology is primarily a result of difficulties in interpersonal relationships and most often a reflection of parenting." Tact appears to be Spiegel's middle name; he tries to deemphasize guilt, and he admits to other factors in the child's pathology, but when I asked him, "Deeply in your heart of hearts, do you think the parents did it?" he answered, "Yes, but not out of malevolence. They did it because they're misguided or they're neurotic or they're trying to do something their own parents did or didn't do." This belief, which is a natural outgrowth of deemphasizing biological and object relations factors, may not make a large difference in the techniques of therapy—Stella Chess, Gabrielle Carlson, and Charles Sarnoff also offer parental guidance—but parents dealing with Sullivanian therapists should know it's there.

Sarnoff, Thompson, and Spiegel all treat children who are not that far removed from Little Hans, and as I talked to them, I wondered how psychodynamic approaches work for the most deeply troubled young patients; the psychoanalytic world has, of course, been asking itself this question since the thirties, and other therapeutic tribes have also asked it, in a tone that is less inquisitive than disparaging. My tone *was* inquisitive when I approached Richard Marohn, a Chicago psychiatrist who specializes in adolescents and puts contemporary theories—most notably those of Kohut and Stern—to work in treating delinquent and suicidal teenagers. His formulations, permeated with these views of development and disorder, are very different from Sarnoff's, although he is capable of acknowledging Freud and Anna Freud when he finds their ideas appropriate.

Marohn, born in 1934, is now an attending psychiatrist at Northwestern Memorial Hospital and professor of clinical psychiatry and behavioral sciences at Northwestern University Medical School; he also teaches at Cook County Graduate School of Medicine and the Chicago Institute for Psychoanalysis, practices privately, has collaborated on some research studies with Daniel Offer and Eric Ostrov (see Chapter 1), and has, over the years, run hospital and prison psychiatric units and consulted for prisons.

He is a prolific writer, and before we met, he sent me a large selection of interesting papers and book chapters published over the past twenty years. Of these, a presentation called "The Adolescent in Psychotherapy: A Developmental Perspective," which Marohn delivered before the Toronto Psychoanalytic Society in 1991, seemed particularly pertinent both to my questions and to Marohn's approach. Moreover, his discussions of adolescent problems seemed to exemplify the "one-genus postulate" I'd encountered with Spiegel: that normal, slightly troubled, and seriously disturbed teenagers face the same problems on a continuum of intensity.

While Marohn accepts the Freudian idea that an important task of adolescence is displacing libido from the parents, he vigorously challenges Mahler's belief that separation and individuation are pivotal, and he deplores the dominance of her perspective. Most clinicians, he concedes, do look at growth as a gradual process, but Mahler's terminology lends itself to "a polarized, dichotomous stance about development and an inordinate emphasis on autonomy." Healthy adolescents, Marohn asserts, don't sever ties to their parents but transform them. Both research and clinical practice demonstrate that "healthier adolescents invest in both peers and mother; it is the sicker adolescent who individuates by detaching."

At this point Marohn, like a good Kohutian, laments the inability of psychoanalysts to view Freud objectively, which has hampered them from matching up theory with clinical data. Infants derive sustenance from the ministrations of their parents and the other important adults they know; thus they learn, if they are healthy, to seek nurturance from significant others in more mature ways throughout their lives. He cites Stern and other researchers who disproved the concept of a symbiosis from which infants must detach.

Recent infant research suggests that feelings—*affect,* in psychiatric terminology—shape and organize the individual's view of the world. Practitioners, Marohn suggests, should discard theories that deem affect "a sign of immaturity, something to 'grow out of,' " and recognize that one of the important tasks of adolescence is to label and take responsibility for one's own feelings and ideas. Moreover, he puts a professional stamp of approval on what any parent with twentysomething offspring has observed, "that so-called 'adolescent' maturational tasks continue well into young adulthood."

A healthy adolescent, Marohn says, looks for stimulation and action, a propensity that evolves from the "curiosity, assertion, and exploration of infancy." It is the teenage version of Stern's "emergent self," the one that tests hypotheses about the world. As Marohn observes, "He seeks to dance, to drive fast, to listen to loud music, to read, to run, to battle, to argue, to 'turn on,' to create and play exciting music, to explore his body, to stimulate his body, and to arouse, incite, and provoke others." He suggests that as parental inhibition can turn healthy toddler assertiveness into destructive rage, the same inhibition may play a role in "adolescent bravado, defensiveness and violence." But Marohn notes that "a most effective discipline is 'grounding,' that is, taking away the 'action.' "

The other three Sternian selves are conspicuous in adolescents too: the core self seeks to define itself and its feelings and to distinguish self from other, and it "engages the other in mutual self-regulation." (That's the baby who can't play peekaboo alone.) The subjective self "seeks shared intentions and affect attunement," and the verbal self "explores new ways of 'being' with another"—reflected in a range of behavior from teenage romance to, presumably, gang membership.

Marohn tells of Lauren, a depressed high school junior who found no solace in her family and instead sought comfort in drinking and sex. When she drank, "it lessened her controls and only made it much more likely that she would cut herself or injure herself in some other way." In therapy she came to talk more about her feelings and stopped blaming others for them: she grew willing to stand up to her mother and her friends about how *she* felt. The upshot was a different way of dealing with depression: "When a girlfriend slighted her, she called her mother on the telephone to talk instead of getting drunk or trying to cut herself." So Lauren learned to take comfort from affiliation, transforming instead of severing her tie with her mother. Unhealthy adolescents must learn, Marohn says, to "use affect as a source of information." The notion of affect as a signal goes back to Freud and is also a cornerstone of cognitive therapy.

Marohn describes other cases, including a relatively healthy young man who couldn't admit to vengeful and competitive feelings that "his upright parents could never have understood." He needed other adults and peers in his life—selfobjects—to balance his exclusive relationship with a concerned but overrighteous mother and father; in therapy after his girlfriend jilted him, he began to get "a more realistic appreciation of life and people, some disillusionment and deidealization of parental values, attitudes, and characteristics."

A mark of healthy adolescence, Marohn writes, is "joy in play." A high school freshman was brought to therapy because of minor delinquency. "Initially, he 'played' with me in sessions: he showed me various skateboard maneuvers in my office, or he sat in my swivel chair when I got up to answer a knock at the door. Later, we would reverse roles. Now he continues to 'play' with me. Although he usually rides his skateboard to the office after school, we now play with ideas: riddles, computer problems, sports talk, and speculation about my income. Before too long, I suspect we will be tossing around ideas about college and future vocation."

Marohn emphasizes that information about fantasies and inner dynamics cannot be discovered empirically and can be learned only through transference. He writes: "Kohut described true psychoanalytic data as derived from introspection and empathy. As a scientist and clinician, I would hope that such data can be integrated with and tested by direct observation. Yet we recognize that these are two different perspectives, not always capable of being reconciled or integrated. As a psychoanalyst and psychoanalytically oriented psychotherapist, I try to focus on my patient's experience of his or her world." Empathizing with adolescents is tricky, Marohn remarks, for the same reason that Spiegel is cautious with giving interpretations to children: too much mind-reading can frighten the patient. Thus the therapist has to balance the real relationship and the transference relationship. The therapist of adolescents is both a transference figure and a participant in the patient's development: "He answers questions, chats, feeds, jokes, plays, asks questions, clarifies, and interprets."

I asked Marohn, who is tall and gray-haired, whether he thought suicide and homicide were two sides of the same coin and about the relationship of delinquency to poverty. "I want to correct a misconception," he said. "The data suggest that across all socioeconomic groups the rates of delinquency are the same. The difference is that kids from the lower socioeconomic groups tend to be more violent. But the propensity for adolescents to be impulsive or do things that society would say are illegal is basically the same in all classes. They're going to be doing drugs, shoplifting, joyriding in cars, minor thefts. Upper-class kids tend to be handled through the mental health road; lower-class kids tend to be handled through the juvenile court road. Girls tend to be excused for their delinquency, so that by the time a girl is finally brought to the authorities, it has escalated to a very serious issue."

"I thought girls don't get noticed till they get pregnant," I said. Marohn accepted that: "Yeah, I think the primary preoccupation society has with girls is that they get pregnant and society has a problem, or they are promiscuous, so to speak—I don't know if that term is used anymore, but I still think there is a double standard. Girls are not excused for their sexual behavior and boys are excused.

"There was a standard psychoanalytic position about suicide that if you were depressed, the way to deal with your depression was to externalize the aggression that had somehow been turned against the self. Treatment would be organized around trying to help the person get angry, and then they wouldn't feel depressed. But the data that's coming out of a lot of suicide studies, and something we have seen in our work with delinquents, is that just *because* kids were violent or angry or impulsive, they tended to be at times depressed, and they could be suicidal."

"So acting out didn't relieve the depression?"

"Absolutely not," Marohn said. "The data that's coming out now in well-organized studies of suicide, like David Shaffer's at Columbia [see Chapter 1], looking at several hundred adolescents who killed themselves in the New York area over two or three years, it's very clear that certainly depression is one of the risk factors in predicting suicide, but impulsivity is also— being impulsive or antisocial. Not attention deficit disorder— it's difficult to make a diagnosis of ADD or AD/HD after death. But they do have kids they can pretty well establish are antisocial, have delinquent propensities, or are impulsive. So the old idea that you either internalize your aggression or externalize it doesn't work as well."

I asked Marohn about deaths in car crashes, which figure in his papers, and about the idea I'd recently heard from a psychologist in a residential milieu that there may be some suicidal element in gang affiliation— walking around in the wrong gang colors at the wrong time could have a suicidal purpose. "There are such things as victim-precipitated suicides," Marohn said, although this variation had not occurred to him. "We know that adolescents love to flirt with death, and as they try to master the unpredictability of the inner world, they play it out in the outer world by taking chances, facing risks in varying degrees. Games of skill and daring become important, but in the more impulsive and violent kid, there are some pretty dangerous games—playing chicken, putting themselves in dangerous situations, challenging and provoking people.

"One of the things adolescents have to come to grips with is their mortality: preadolescents really don't have an appreciation of what death is all about. But adolescents—to different degrees, depending on their level of cognitive development—think about the meaning of life and what death is all about in a way that hasn't been done before. Certain adolescents are testing their mortality and seeing how far they could go."

Marohn reviewed his formulation of the three most important tasks of adolescence—consolidation of the sense of oneself, transforming ties with one's parents, and integrating one's emotions, which include sexuality: this is the context in which he views his patients' problems. "We don't know why adolescents psychologically have to move away from their parents or why they are so uncomfortable with their ties to their parents," he said. "The most satisfactory explanation was that given by Freud, which is that the sexuality that the adolescent begins experiencing is a strong, vibrant, consciously felt sexuality, whereas earlier, oedipal sexuality didn't have this forcefulness and was readily repressed. As a result the adolescent can no longer have the attachments he had to his parents as his primary relationships. So the exploration of sexuality has to be experienced outside the family."

"Suppose," I said, "nature made human beings adaptive, and suppose you simply think an adult has got to move out and not be dependent on parents. Would you need all that oedipal stuff to explain it?"

"There are other ways of thinking of this from a more socially oriented perspective, in terms of the need for different relationships, the need for affiliations that are more at one's level, twinship kinds of experiences, but that doesn't explain the anxiety and turmoil that some adolescents experience when dealing with affectionate feelings for their parents," Marohn answered.

I pressed him a bit further. "Not the anxiety of being alone, the fear that their parents will die?" But Marohn was firm: "I don't think so." And he reiterated his concern about the overemphasis on separation. "In our good old American way, we talk about people becoming independent and autonomous, we set up this independent being as a kind of objective and ideal. We try to talk with patients as though they needed to be able to stand on their own two feet and not acknowledge how standing on our own two feet is enabled by having relationships that affirm us and sustain us.

"They're not necessarily holding us up like crutches, and kids increasingly as they move through adolescence are able to develop certain psychological and emotional skills that they previously had to rely on others to perform for them: their capacity to organize, to introspect, to verbalize, to plan, to be aware of affect states, to distinguish one emotion from another, to comfort themselves, to regulate their self-esteem—all competences that enable one to develop a sense of oneself."

I asked Marohn what happened to his teenage patients who were unable to proceed with these tasks, and he told me about two cases. "One boy was so terrified of moving along in adolescence that he needed to develop a facade of braggadocio, of being a tough macho kid, and at the same time he was desperately unable to function in school because psychologically he was so disorganized, he simply couldn't focus on the material. He would develop rationalizations for this, namely 'School is for sissies, there's no reason to learn'—this is not an uncommon attitude that many tough kids have, and there's certain subcultures that support this— gangs and so forth.

"So we bring this kid into the hospital—he had been in gang fights. We recognize that he's violent, it's difficult to get close to him, he would occasionally get into fights with the ward staff if they told him it was time to go study. But after he had calmed down, he seemed to be doing well on the unit, and he was ready to go to school. We had a school at the other end of the building, and the kids would be escorted over there. He didn't do too badly in school, but we noticed that his behavior on the unit had deteriorated.

"It took us a while to figure this out, but what we thought was happening was that this kid was so psychologically limited that in holding himself together in school, he became emotionally exhausted. He had little or no capacity left to control himself. So we decided that for this kid, the answer was to have school for him on the unit. Instead of taxing him with the need to go to the other part of the building and meet with other kids and control himself, he got private tutoring and started learning.

"If you want to relate this to the tasks of adolescence, he was unable to begin taking over those functions that the mother had performed because some very basic early mothering experiences had been denied him, and he didn't have the fundamental framework. Unless there was some intervention, this kid would stay basically an infant or a child all his life. He would have an adult body and probably have adult jobs, and he might get into seemingly adult relationships, but he would really be functioning at a very infantile level.

"I'm in a sense condensing hundreds of cases I've seen over the years: we're basically talking about a kid who was born to an adolescent mother who had little capacity herself to organize, comfort, soothe, and regulate herself. Who in some ways experienced a pregnancy and a child as a way of nourishing herself and probably didn't do too badly with the child until he started showing his own identity and self and his own orientations. The kid who's six months old needs a different kind of mother than the kid who's six years old, and mothers have to be able to make these kinds of shifts. But if the mother herself is locked into some very primitive level of organization for which the child serves very important purposes, then she may need another baby to take care of, and this kid begins to be cast by the wayside.

"More often than not you see this problem in the inner city, but you can also see it in upper-middle-class white families in the suburbs. And the constitutional givens, including the nature of prenatal care, are tremendously important. We can't predict how well someone's going to do solely on the quality of the parenting."

Marohn then offered me a case from the other end of the spectrum. "We have," he said, "a young girl from a very fortunate background who is doing beautifully in private school, but who begins making suicide attempts. They seem to be related, on the surface at least, to her parents being away. Although earlier this was not an issue for her, it began in adolescence—they'd be on vacation or she'd be in summer camp. The family seems to be a happy, intact family. Both the parents are professionals doing well.

"But from her thirteenth year she starts making suicide attempts, necessitating hospitalization. She starts talking increasingly about the barrenness of life, that life has no real meaning for her. She makes another suicide attempt after a girlfriend turns on her and jilts her in some kind of fight over a boy. On the surface at least, the suicidality seems to be related to losses. Why should this be? It seems that this girl had fairly adequate mothering. We can't be sure, but a big factor for her was not the inadequacy of the parenting, but for whatever reason this girl is terrified of adulthood. She seems, in every competent step—whether it's getting A's in school or eventually going off to a superior college, which she's destined for—she has the sense that she's going to be standing there in adulthood all by herself."

"This sounds like an anorectic in the making," I said.

"That's not happened," said Marohn. "Anorectics have the tremendous anxiety about maturing, maturing sexually, but they also have the peculiar focus on the need to control, partially to control mother, partially to control their bodies. This girl's not been so concerned about that. Primarily it's the tremendous fear and anxiety about what it's going to mean to be on her own, and her competence gives her little solace. Early in life it was important to her, and she could revel in it and enjoy the adulation and the praise of other people for her competence, her good looks, her intelligence, her balance, and so forth. What she now begins recognizing is that it's this competence that is going to move her away from childhood. She's going to have to give up Mommy, and it's terrifying to her. Why this girl from this privileged background has that kind of anxiety, I don't know. There may be more than you can know about the mother-daughter relationship."

"Where's Dad?" I asked.

"Dad is very much in the picture," he said. "But he has a tendency to minimize her problems because he looks on her as this very charming, accomplished young woman. It's hard for him to appreciate how she could be so self-hating when she seems on the surface to be so well-liked. Again, there may be constitutional differences. The weakest area in our field is to explain how people get to be the way they are. If we were good at this . . . we don't have predictive capacity in the behavioral sciences, partly because the variables are just too many. So when we get into explanations, retrospective explanations, we tend to be somewhat deficient."

"Which gives parents a big problem, because they don't know how to process what's happened to their kids," I said.

"The parents will generally tend to feel somehow they're responsible," Marohn answered. "But it's very hard to demonstrate that the parents are indeed responsible. I think what I would want in parents is some kind of *flexibility*, some capacity to respond as much as possible to what the kid needs at the moment. It's very hard to do. This girl is now in process, so it's hard to say how it's going to come out. She's now in a treatment facility. What you're looking for in similar cases is to establish a treatment relationship that one uses to help her move into adulthood. Gradually through the losses she will experience in the treatment relationship, she will derive certain psychological capacities that will help her move into adulthood. It becomes a kind of alternative parenting.

"Because when a girl thinks suicide or threatens it, the parents become discombobulated. They can't take the risk of saying 'I will let you struggle with this.' They've got to step in and do something. So it's almost like an asthma attack—you get that secondary gain. With asthma, initially you may have an allergy, but after a while you realize—unconsciously—the tremendous psychological value it has, how well it works to be able to regress and have someone locked into taking care of you.

"Therapists," Marohn continued, "have to take those kinds of risks. That's partly what we're trained to do."

It seemed a fearful responsibility: I recalled the stories we read so often about suicidal teenagers who have been in therapy. "They don't do it out of the blue," I said.

"There are some kids who simply don't tell you," Marohn answered. "I know as a therapist working with suicidal adolescents and adults that I have to take risks. I can't, every time someone talks about being suicidal, pop them in a hospital. I have to recognize that there are real problems the person and I have to struggle with, and maybe we need to talk more on the phone or have more frequent sessions, but I can't take the struggle away from them. They may need to use medication, to adjust to medication. Working with suicidal people is tricky. There's always the problem that someone who is hell-bent on suicide, no matter how much they care about the therapist, may say 'I'm not going to tell him because he'll interfere.' But it would be much less scary to a therapist than to a parent who has to do something, or who dismisses it and says 'He's just doing that for attention.' "

"Suppose I'm sixteen," I said, "and I stretch out here on your couch, and I say 'Sometimes I think there's nothing in life to look forward to, and I want to get out of it.' What are you likely to say to me?"

"It depends where we are in our relationship," Marohn said. "If this is the first two interviews where I'm trying to get a sense of where you are psychologically, I'm going to ask a lot more about it. I'm going to ask whether you have a plan. There's a difference between somebody taking aspirin and somebody getting Dad's handgun. Guns work very effectively. A gun does what it was intended to do; it's a very competent product. So you have to assess the lethality. And the level of fantasy: some kids have ideas that they'll be reunited with a parent who has died, or that they might be reincarnated. The fantasy adds to the risk: it tells you how impaired their reality testing might be. When someone says 'At last my pain will be over,' you tell them they won't be there to enjoy it. If they're religious, religion teaches that they're going to be punished for this act.

"You don't hear religious factors very often; more often you hear 'I'm not gonna do it because it would devastate my parents.' Then you've got to be concerned, because moments come up when they're in a rage and they don't care if they devastate their parents, or they would even like to do that. Another common fantasy is 'When I'm dead, everyone will realize how bad they've been to me.'

"If the same issue comes up when you've worked with someone for a while, it's the nature of the relationship you have with them that's going to carry them. Oftentimes the most important thing you can do is simply to listen and to acknowledge to them how painful it is. Many of us who go into this field because we started out in medicine, we always want to *do* something, and that may be the worst thing. They need to have somebody in their lives who can listen to their pain, without getting so nervous about it that you have to quick go do something."

We talked a bit about teenage sexuality, and Marohn, in sum, said, "There's no way teenagers are going to say no to sex. What you can get them to do is understand about being responsible sexually. I don't see sexuality as different from the other tasks of adolescence, where the adolescent needs to be able to identify emotions."

As we wrapped up our session—which Marohn, of course, did with deftness and aplomb—he said, "There was a time that I felt I needed to know all the street names for all the drugs, and that I also needed to be up to date on all the rock groups. I lost that. There was no way to keep up with it, and I no longer feel that's an issue. I find it's no problem with my patients. When I could do that stuff, it was impressive to them, but now I just say, 'Tell me about this group, I don't know it,' or 'What's that drug you were just talking about?' They're not bothered.

"It's the person that's so threatened by that lack of knowledge, who has to phony it up, that's got a problem. Kids want you to be direct and honest. They value things being said to them without their having to acknowledge that you're right. They have to have the option of saving face by not saying 'You're absolutely right. We both recognize what's going on, but don't expect us to acknowledge it openly,' which is a kind of respect for them as a person."

PART III

REVISING THE MAP

Behavior Therapy

CHAPTER 7

"SHOW THAT I CAN"

The reign of the white rat in the psychological laboratory ended at least a quarter of a century ago.

—B. F. Skinner,
About Behaviorism (1974)

Man is disturbed not by things but by the views he takes of them. . . . It is the act of an ill-instructed man to blame others for his own bad condition; it is the act of one who has begun to be instructed, to lay the blame on himself; and of one whose instruction is completed, neither to blame another, nor himself.

—Epictetus,
The Enchiridion (A.D. first century)

PERHAPS THE MOST CHARACTERISTIC PHRASE of Philip C. Kendall, Ph.D., is "My *belief* is . . ." That idiom (which would be foreign to Sarnoff) labels him as a cognitive-behaviorist, a member of a school "identified as much by its epistemological dedication to the search for rigorous standards of proof as its alignment with any set of concepts," according to a recent article in the *Journal of the American Academy of Child and Adolescent Psychiatry*. In the real world Kendall has beliefs that come from his clinical experience, but he is always careful to separate those from conclusions supported by research data.

Kendall, born in 1950, holds a cornucopia of titles at Temple University: professor of psychology, head of the Division of Clinical Psychology, director of clinical training, and director of the Child and Adolescent Anxiety Disorders Clinic. He has published innumerable journal articles

175

and is the author, co-author, or editor of twenty-one books on cognitive-behavioral therapy for children, practices privately in Ardmore, Pennsylvania, and is a past president of the Association for the Advancement of Behavior Therapy, the chief professional organization in his field.

As Sarnoff's personality seems to fit his therapeutic orientation, Kendall's manner is equally evocative. A tall, dark-haired, fair-skinned man with horn-rimmed glasses and the requisite beard, he suggests a science teacher who also coaches the tennis team. And he does say, "I'm an interpersonal, psychological coach, and I'm going to find out if the backhand's good, if the serve is good, do they volley well, do they focus, and wherever they need the help, that's where we're going to put it." Kendall's aura of common sense is one that many parents, especially those turned off or intimidated by the idea of psychotherapy, would find accessible and reassuring.

A parent made uneasy by ludic symbols, repression, selfobjects, and the whole abstruse psychodynamic conceptual canon—and not even convinced his daughter is clinically depressed—might support therapy once she's been evaluated by the arsenal of standardized tests that Kendall and other cognitive-behaviorists use, such as the Self-Perception Profile for Children, the Multidimensional Measure of Children's Perception of Control, the Children's Negative Cognitive Error Questionnaire, the Children's Attributional Style Questionnaire, the Hopelessness Scale for Children, the Matson Evaluation of Social Skills with Youngsters, the Loneliness Questionnaire, the Children's Reinforcement Schedules, the Beck Depression Inventory, and the Life Events Checklist.

Patients who sign on with Kendall needn't worry about endless therapy. "We use time-limited chunks, sixteen or seventeen sessions, and at the end we say, 'Where are we now?' If we feel we need more, we renegotiate. I say, 'Okay, you came in wanting to make friends and not get in trouble. You're getting in trouble less in school but still haven't made friends. Let's work on that for sixteen more sessions.' I even give the kids certificates when they finish. They accomplished something. They didn't go to tennis camp so they don't have a better game to show, but they went to a psychologist and completed a program."

Traditional behavior therapy aims to change a behavior by manipulating the stimulus and the response. Because pure behavioral intervention is effective only for certain problems (and because some of its benefits may not last), many professionals have moved toward *cognitive*-behavioral therapy, which attempts "to change behavior and feelings by changing thinking patterns," as the *AACAP Journal* article defines it. Nearly 70 percent of the membership of Kendall's organization now labels itself cognitive-behaviorist.

Like psychodynamic therapists, cognitive-behaviorists believe that mental disorders arise from distortion of the meaning of experiences. They differ about the reason for the distortion and the way to set it straight. In a chapter of a book Kendall edited on cognitive-behavioral procedures for child and adolescent therapy, he wrote:

> Consider the experience of stepping in something a dog left on the lawn. Your first reaction ("Oh, sh—") is probably a self-statement that reflects dismay. . . . Individuals then proceed to process this experience. . . . Some may attribute the misstep to their inability to do anything right; such a global internal and stable attribution often characterizes depression. . . . An angry individual, in contrast, might see the experience as the result of someone else's provocation ("Whose dog left this here—I bet the guy knew someone would step in it!"); attributing the mess to someone else's intentional provocation is linked to aggressive retaliatory behavior. . . . An individual who brings an anxiety-prone structure to the misstep experience . . . would see the threat of embarrassment and the risk of germs, and process the experiences accordingly. Anxious cognitive processing of the experience might include self-talk such as "What if somebody notices the bad smell, they'll think I'm dirty." "What if germs get into my shoes and then to my socks, and my feet? Should I throw these shoes away?"

Later in this chapter Kendall wrote, "Knowing that we all, figuratively, step in it at times, what is needed is a *structure for coping* with these unwanted events when they occur." Cognitive-behavioral therapy aims to provide that structure by helping children analyze whether their perceptions are justified, modeling the way to deal with stressful situations, and giving them opportunities to rehearse a competent response. While a good flexible psychodynamic therapist will offer some help in coping strategies, Sarnoff describes this as "what one does while waiting for insight to arrive."

Kendall, on the other hand, says, "I think other schools pay too much attention to cause. Once they find a cause, then miraculously things will get better. I don't believe you can find an exact understanding of cause. We want to get as good a handle as we can, because fifteen to twenty-five percent of the time, it will help us design a more accurate intervention. Then we want to move forward." At the same time Kendall, who is about as flexible as Sarnoff, would not disdain an obvious symbol. He described one client with bulimic symptoms as "saying I can't stomach it."

Kendall points out that cognitive therapy is not effective for disorders like autism and schizophrenia and prefers straightforward behavior therapy for retarded children. (All these clients lack the requisite ability to communicate about their thoughts and feelings. As we will see, pure behavior therapy can also achieve limited but useful gains for autism.) At the other end of the spectrum, he says, "a child might come in for what's labeled depression by the parents but really is adjustment to the loss of the grandparents, who both died of cancer within six months of each other. He's allowed to be depressed for up to a year. He doesn't need therapy, just support. But if he starts thinking, 'Oh, I did it. It's my fault because they told me to clean my room and I didn't,' then we can provide some help in correcting that false belief." The clearly educational flavor of cognitive therapy makes it most suitable for children of school age.

Unlike the stripped-down, beaten-up playrooms of dynamic therapists, Kendall's office—he maintains a private practice at his home—is traditionally furnished with a wing chair, mahogany tables, an oriental rug, a rocker with a needlepoint cushion, and adult books. It seems to belie his informal manner but reflects both his therapeutic bent and his original specialty in treating hyperactive children. "It sets the tone for you to behave," Kendall says. "If I have a child who can't sit still and I put him in a room with a million opportunities not to sit still, that's tough. I bring him in here, I set the expectation that we're going to do some work. The first ten minutes we talk, and I take out the workbook or whatever and say 'Don't forget we're going to start our work.' Gradually over time I just point to the clock and they go, 'Oh yes, we've gotta start our work.' Then the last ten minutes we play computer games or hangman or draw pictures. The fun activity is a reward for work."

Most therapists play with children, but the purpose of play differs with each orientation. "I often play cards with impulsive kids," Kendall says. "Here's a book, *The Official Rules of Card Games.* Impulsive kids will start a game and switch the rules in the middle, and it's frustrating for their peers. So I say, 'Let's look it up. I'm not telling you to do it my way or your way, let's see what the rules say.' So when we play, we play by the rules, we can't switch in the middle, we don't change games, even though we don't have to play the same game all the time."

When a client is referred to Kendall, he will first meet three times with the child. "With a hyperactive kid," Kendall says, "I'd say, 'Hey, we've got some things we have to do today. First we've got to get to know each other, and second I have some materials and pictures and some games or tests, I want to see how you do on those, and I want to ask you what you like and don't like. The deal we made with your mom is, we're gonna meet for three weeks, and if we can identify some things to work on, and if we both like each other and you want to try it, we'll pursue it.

"Some parents say, 'This kid is hyperactive.' I get him in here, he's six years old, he's wiggly, but a six-year-old should be wiggly, and he's no worse than an average kid. The parents' expectations are that the child should sit still in church for three hours, but that's developmentally inappropriate. If that's my conclusion, I'll get them in and say, 'I used these tests, here's a distribution of scores nationally, here's where your child fits, right where most kids fit. I wonder why you think he's hyperactive—what do you see that I don't see?' They might tell me, and I'd say, 'This is my opinion, but if he were to behave in your home as he did in my office, I don't think that's a disorder. Maybe there's more energy than you'd like, and maybe you'd like to reduce your stress, but he seems to be within the borders of normal behavior. Maybe we can ask you to try and tolerate it a little more.' That happens two out of ten times in the case of hyperactivity."

Kendall also uses parent-and-teacher questionnaires that evaluate the child's behavior against a nationwide norm; like Michael Thompson (and like most professionals), he rates teachers' opinions high because the teacher has met enough children to provide a good standard of comparison.

Precise measurement is an important part of cognitive-behavioral therapy from assessment to termination. Kendall would not use a Rorschach in assessing a patient. "The Rorschach is an assessment of fantasies and perceptions, so if a child looks at the ink blots and sees guns and bullets, someone could say, 'That's aggressive,' and if at the end of the treatment he didn't see guns and bullets, the therapist would say, 'Aha, I reduced aggression.' They've actually reduced aggressive fantasies and perceptions, which isn't my goal. If I want to reduce aggression, I take the number of fights the client gets into before therapy and see if there are fewer fights at the end." Since he is cognitive, however, he would use the Thematic Apperception Test—the one where the child is handed picture cards and asked to make up stories about each. "I learn about the child's cognitive structure or template," he says. "I learn about the way he perceives social situations by using the pictures.

"I think the cognitive-behavioral approach is an attempt to keep the empirical side of behaviorism, the let's-look-at-the-data side," Kendall explains, "but with a tremendous willingness to say, 'Yeah, there's a lot of richness in the psychodynamic theory, and people can have denial, information processing that's defensive and that causes them to see the glass as half full or half empty. That's all exciting to our group, but we want to do it empirically, we want to test it out, we don't just want to have a religious belief in it.

"What the dynamic people can I think be faulted for is their failure to take the next step in evaluating what they're going to do. They don't say, 'Let's bring in that outside judge and see if it made a difference.' The therapist and the parents are both invested in the outcome. So we might ask the teacher to rate the child's peer group. If school personnel rated this cluster of kids, the child's friends before therapy, as 'risky and dangerous' and rated the group the child hangs out with afterward as 'socially appropriate and acceptable,' that's a significant improvement."

The essence of Kendall's therapeutic techniques is laid out in the treatment manuals he and his students have written for impulsive children and for anxious children. In the anxiety manual, for example, the authors describe seventeen sessions. The therapy delineated here is notably different in ambiance from the psychodynamic approach, in which the therapist most often remains a cipher (even a Sullivanian like Stanley Spiegel, while he would courteously answer the child's queries, is unlikely to volunteer anything). Adult and child ask each other get-acquainted questions, and "it will be helpful throughout the treatment if the therapist is comfortable with the child's asking personal information about her and with providing answers to appropriate questions." The down-home flavor of the therapy should be pleasing to most kids; it would engage some parents and turn others off.

Clients begin by learning to identify anxious feelings and the somatic responses to them. After each session they take home a Show-That-I-Can (STIC) task. The first of these is to write down "a brief example of a time when he feels really great—not upset or worried. The child is asked to try to think and focus on what made him comfortable and what he felt and thought at the time. To help the child understand the assignment, the therapist should provide an example of a time when she felt really great and should describe it in terms of what she felt and thought." When they complete the STIC task, the children earn two points, which can be used to purchase rewards the child and therapist agree on—small toys, books, or games in the earlier sessions and later on, time spent playing a computer game or going out for ice cream with the therapist.

The sessions continue with role-playing and storytelling exercises that show the child how people express their emotions physically. The child picks a real or fictional hero and with the therapist makes up stories about how the hero would cope with worry and overcome challenges. Gradually, child and therapist discuss situations in which each of them feels anxious and describes their feelings. The therapist is noting which situations are most taxing for the child, and the child is keeping a journal between sessions. Children learn to recognize their own symptoms of anxiety—butterflies in the stomach, flushing, trembling—and pick up relaxation techniques and self-talk to invoke when they feel tense. The therapist keeps in touch with the parents, who may be involved in some homework assignments.

The course moves from understanding feelings to figuring out coping strategies (" 'I expect . . . to happen,' or, 'I am afraid . . . will happen.' How else can I think about it? What else could happen?"). In later sessions the children begin a graduated series of custom-tailored *in vivo* exercises, in which they're exposed to situations that might make them anxious and, with the therapist nearby, get them to practice their skills. Finally, the children make a thirty-second TV commercial in which their hero copes with a tense situation.

The Anxiety Disorders Clinic at Temple is a federally funded research project to test the effectiveness of these techniques and to learn more about anxiety disorders in children; it has been, Kendall points out, the first major clinical trial of cognitive-behavioral therapy for these disorders. "The majority of children identified for psychological help fall in the category of externalizing problems," he says. "They act out, they aggress, they wiggle, and it affects people around them. Other kids are referred because they don't do well in school. But a problem I think is understudied is the kids who are anxious or depressed. They don't bother anybody. You ask the teacher, 'How's Bobby?' and she says, 'Terrible. He acts up, he's rough, he needs help.' You ask 'How's Billy?' 'Oh, he's fine.' 'Does he have any friends?' 'No.' 'Does he ever talk in class?' 'No. But he's fine.' Billy's sitting in the back thinking, 'If I raise my hand, lightning will strike me dead.' " Kendall's grant proposal cites a study reporting anxious symptoms in 10 to 20 percent of school-age children.

Forty-seven children were treated in the first clinic study, 27 initially and 20 more in the waiting-list control group. Children were assigned at random to one of four doctoral candidates who had been trained in workshops and were supervised regularly. Most of the subjects of this and later studies were (and are) nine to thirteen years old. Sessions are taped, and the treatment is free. When I first visited the project, it was three months into the two-year clinical trial; after the trial there was a year of follow-up studies, and when I returned, Kendall and his students were writing up the results.

The children had been carefully screened to make sure they conformed to research requirements: they had to show one of three anxiety disorders listed in DSM-III-R. One of these was Separation Anxiety Disorder ("excessive anxiety, for at least two weeks, concerning separation from those to whom the child is attached"); another was Social Avoidant Disorder ("excessive shrinking from contact with unfamiliar people that is of sufficient severity to interfere with social functioning in peer relationships and that is of at least six months' duration"); and the third and most common was Overanxious Disorder ("excessive or unrealistic anxiety or worry for a period of six months or longer"). The latter two have been subsumed in DSM-IV under the heading of "Generalized Anxiety Disorder," which is perfectly exemplified by the descriptions the clinic staff gave me.

"The classic thing we see in our kids is they worry about absolutely anything and everything," said Fran Sessa, who did the screening. "They may hear about a plane crash and suddenly become very worried about a relative having to take a plane somewhere. A lot of the kids are very bright—they're on the gifted and talented track. You'd think with the type of therapy we're doing that would be easier, but they are almost like little adults. They've either forgotten how to be a kid or were never allowed to be one. They come on with this pseudomaturity, and it's very difficult to work with them because you want to treat them like twenty or thirty, not nine or ten."

I watched the tapes of two separate screening interviews: one with Bill, a bright, husky eleven-year-old who met the criteria for Overanxious Disorder, and the other with his parents. Dad seemed morosely frustrated, Mom volubly strung out as they answered detailed questions about Bill's anxieties on the Child Behavior Check List, rating some reactions on a scale of 1 to 4.

"He's very hard on himself," said Mom in a heavy Philadelphia accent. "He would get into these moods where he'd go in his room and just lie down because he was so upset with himself. Then he put the blame on us for everything. I know how it feels 'cause it used to happen to me. He would come home with a lot of homework, he would get so panicked— 'How am I gonna do it?' He gets himself so crazy about it, you can't say to him, 'Well, Bill, sit down and do this first.' "

"Has he ever gotten himself sick from worry?" Sessa asked.

"Terrible headaches," Mom said. "He makes it like his head's going to fall out. Sometimes he'll get a nosebleed."

Dad said, "He gets tired. He never had a headache at school, never at camp, only at home."

"Does he need more reassurance than the typical kid needs?" asked Sessa.

"I don't reassure him a lot because he gets a big head," explained Mom. "He'll put his brother down, he gets a little obnoxious."

"He's too smart," Dad said. "He's not straight A's anymore, but he used to be the one who'd take a book and read to the class."

"What does he worry about in social situations? Would he try to avoid situations because he's worried?"

"Yeah," Mom said. "At camp this summer he was very self-conscious about the way he looked when he had to go swimming. He went, but he felt very in conflict. He was wearing the same bathing suit every day, because that was the only one he looked all right in. He's not an easygoing kid at all, he's hard, he doesn't just roll with the punches."

While the headaches appeared only at home, apparently Bill found cause for apprehension everywhere. In the mornings, he asked his mother over and over what jacket to wear. He was afraid of thunder and lightning and bees and moths and slugs, and he ran on for half an hour before getting an injection at the doctor's office, after anticipatory hysterics the night before.

Bill sat through his own initial interview with visibly furrowed brow.

His voice was very soft, and he was not too forthcoming. "When Bill showed up for this interview," Sessa said, "he brought a backpack I couldn't lift, all stuffed with books. He was worried about spending too much time here and not being able to do his homework for the night."

Bill had by now had two therapeutic sessions, Sessa told me, and showed himself to be a typical anxious kid. "The therapist asked him to write down one good experience a week. Bill came in and had filled up the entire notebook with good experiences because he didn't know which good one to pick, and he was afraid of showing the wrong one to the therapist."

Anxiety is an equal-opportunity disorder; some children at the clinic have nothing in common but their symptoms. Tyrone was a fifteen-year-old African-American boy from a public school in North Philadelphia. He had been sent to an annex that dealt with the school's problem kids: he was at risk for dropping out and possible delinquency. "He has this negative peer group that pulls him to stay out of school," said Kevin Ronan, the student therapist who worked with Tyrone. "In addition he's very fearful of going to school, particularly at the beginning of the year. He has a real hard time just showing up. His fears tend to revolve around failure, having people find out that he's no good. He's phobic on a lot of specific things—dogs, airplanes, and subways. Those things his mother had initially targeted to work on—they're kind of easy—but after tossing it around in our supervision sessions, we decided a more appropriate focus was getting him to attend school regularly and helping him to become more adaptive in his environment—to be able to say no in a simple fashion.

"His mother is a very nice woman, very supportive of him, but she's not outstanding at setting limits. I think his mother's done a good job of giving him moral values. He abhors drugs. He's very much into sports, and that's helpful in our therapy. His favorite player is Magic Johnson. Sometimes we talk about what Magic Johnson would do in a situation, how he'd get psyched for it." (At the time I talked to Ronan, Magic Johnson had not yet announced he was HIV positive. Even then, there was certainly some risk in choosing a sports figure as a model: the nightly news showed regular reports of one or another athlete getting into trouble—and of course there is no hero in any area of public life who's safe to gamble on these days.

But when I returned to the clinic, Magic's life story had changed. What would this mean to Kendall's anxious client? "It was a risk," Kendall said. "But you have to use coping hero figures, not mastery hero figures. A mastery figure is somebody who does everything perfectly, like God or Christ. Our hero figures are people who cope with difficulties themselves. So Magic ran into a tough situation, and he screwed up. Now he's trying to save other people, spreading some wisdom that might be helpful, and he's also looking fairly optimistic about how he's going to deal with it. He's a coping model, and that's fine.")

I listened to a tape of Tyrone in his twelfth session, in which Ronan was focusing on Tyrone's school attendance and getting an afternoon job. "He's very fearful of the whole process, what to wear, how to get an application, how to get an interview." When Tyrone said he went to school, he might mean he went to one class for a whole week, so Ronan tried to pin him down. "Well, I mostly go every day of the week," Tyrone said. "What is the problem with going to school? What is keeping you out of school?" Ronan asked Tyrone. "I been tryin' to figure it out since this all began. If I could get a tutor I would get a private tutor and stay at home." Ronan thought one problem with anxious kids is "their anxiety is sort of clouding them, and they can't focus on exactly what it is that's bothering them. We're trying to help them relax a bit so they can sort it out."

Tyrone was now on a treadmill trying to catch up with what he missed and move along with new work, hoping to pull his grades up to a D. "I don't know if Tyrone's telling me the God's-honest-truth," Ronan said. "He's prone to not immediately coming out with the truth. He'll say, 'I've been attending school for three weeks straight.' Hopefully you're going to brush it over, but when you say specifically, 'Did you go to this class?' then he'll back off and say, 'No, I couldn't make it to that class.' I called yesterday morning at seven-thirty to make sure he was up and getting ready for school. That was part of our agreement last week, to call him nightly in order to see how his day at school went, so after the weekend I called Monday morning."

Ronan asked Tyrone, "When you get up in the morning, what are you thinking about when you don't go to school?" and Tyrone answered, "That's mostly on my mind if I can make it this morning." Tyrone is worried that his mother will push him out the door. It's tough just getting out of bed, and when he gets out of bed, it's tough seeing if he's actually going to go to school, and when he gets to school, it's a struggle to stay there. "Can I take a guess?" Ronan asked Tyrone. "Will you tell me if I'm right or wrong? When you start something new, you get nervous about it, you need to warm up?" "It's like a car battery that's gone dead," Tyrone said. "This is like when I first got into seventh grade, but it's totally different. I got more freedom."

With all this the boy didn't sound unsaveable, and Ronan said, "That's why I have chosen to stay with him when he was skipping therapy so much. There was a point where we could have said we've gotta make a contract here—if you don't show up for so many sessions, that's it. But I think these kids need particular follow-up, and you've got to be really persistent with it."

Going to school was Tyrone's *in vivo*, which Ronan cited as the reason he could call up even if it seemed to be pushing the research boundaries a bit. But while the therapy is cognitive-behavioral, there are clear social and family issues as well: Ronan wanted to get the boy's mother to go to the school and try to have him switched into a more structured program. "We're holding to the integrity of cognitive-behavioral treatment but not necessarily going blunk blunk blunk down the manual."

Just like Tyrone, Vicki, who was eleven and lived in the suburbs, also had trouble getting to school, but when she didn't want to go, her parents just carted her there. Vicki was a perfectionist, and she'd painted herself into a corner: she was afraid she might fail, and because she'd always done so well, everybody would laugh at her. In the audiotape I heard, Vicki and her therapist, Elizabeth Kortlander, were going over how Vicki approached a homework assignment. "She has a tendency to keep going on something even if she feels she should stop," Kortlander said. It was the eighth session, and Vicki had learned the FEAR acronym: "Feeling frightened? Expecting bad things to happen? Attitudes and actions that will help. Results and rewards."

"I had this space project, and I was working on it for a long time," Vicki said, "and like we had to go make a copy for something, and while we were in the car coming back, I had a funny feeling in my stomach, and I tried to like, brush it off . . ."

Kortlander asked her about the funny stomach feeling. "I pull my hair when I'm a little bit anxious," the therapist said. "When you feel anxious, catch yourself, take a deep breath . . . try it now."

"I said to myself like, calm down, I took some deep breaths," Vicki continued. "Like, I said to myself, you did enough of the space project."

"You're sort of jumping ahead," said Kortlander. "Do you know what you were feeling before you did that nice job of calming yourself down? Do you know what you were thinking of? The social studies? You were expecting not to get it done if you didn't put all this work into it? I want to catch the thoughts that were leading you to put all that work into it."

Vicki—who was Kortlander's first patient—was making some progress; she decided to move from the space project to writing a story, which was what she enjoyed. Her tone was not depressed but cute and perky. "That's something you have to watch for," Kortlander said. "She's so good at being a perky cute girl and doing everything perfectly. Every week we have these STIC assignments, and she always does them just right. So I said, 'In the next few weeks, when I tell you to do something, you have to make the choice not to do it.' That's very hard for her. She'll have to come to the session with her notebook without the assignment. We'll look through what's hard for her in that situation."

A fairly typical *in vivo* at the clinic might involve a girl who can't order food in a restaurant or ask for help in a bookstore. "The first thing you do is here on this floor, with an adult who is prepared for her visit," said Martha Kane, another therapist. "You work out a situation where the child speaks to that person—asks directions or borrows a pen. Once the child commands that, you go to the next step, which might be approaching someone who's not prepared for her coming, and you have to deal with that element of surprise. Then you gradually have the child and therapist going into a bookstore, just being there. Then the child goes in without the therapist, beginning to navigate around the bookstore; if the panic hits, you're close by. Eventually you get to a point where the child goes into the bookstore and interacts with the adults while you're out of sight."

Anyone who spends time at the clinic and talks to Kendall and his students is likely to suspect that the compelling part of their therapy lies in the extra commitment and skill of the therapist—that is, the part that's not in the manual. To some extent Kendall has come to terms with this.

"Way back, manuals were *verboten*," he says. "You couldn't put therapy on paper. Then the behaviorists said you can't study it without a manual, and the graduate students became mechanical. Now we've backed off from rigid adherence to manuals. They're a guideline—you operational-ize as best you can. And when you're doing research, you tape the sessions to see that the therapy doesn't deviate too far." In particular, therapists learn to apply the model to clients' individual crises that come up during the treatment, and to vary the speed somewhat according to a child's abilities.

When I returned to the clinic two and a half years later, Kendall was feeling good. He and his students had analyzed the progress of the clients (all behaviorists, cognitive and otherwise, refer to the children they treat as "clients"; sometimes the word is extended informally to encompass the children's families as well) at the clinic against that of the waiting-list control group—that is, a group of children who are equally eligible for clinic treatment but won't get it until after the original subjects have completed the course. Behavioral researchers choose this method of control because it's as close to placebo as they can get: that is, as Kendall explained, "If you think of all the variables that could account for outcome—the expectancies, the assessment testing, the passage of time, the effects of measurement tests, and the treatment—a waiting-list group has everything except the treatment." He was pleased to report that the treated group had shown remarkable gains. "There was improvement across the board on self-report measures, parent report measures, fear measures, and coping ability. At the beginning of therapy, of course, all the kids qualified as having a DSM-III-R anxiety diagnosis, and many kids had multiple diagnoses. At one-year follow-up, sixty percent no longer qualified as having any diagnosis. That means, of course, that forty percent still do, so we're not perfect."

I asked Kendall what he'd learned in the past couple of years: Was there, first of all, any particular silver bullet? What distinguished the kids who were still anxious from the kids who weren't? "We've looked at all the obvious things," he said, "and there was no difference in gender, race, age, initial severity, co-morbidity [the presence of more than one disor-der], or family involvement. One study not yet completed is listening to the tapes of therapy and counting the frequency of different events—number of therapist encouragements, number of child involvements, time on task—to see if any of them predicts. The first half of the treatment is educational and the second half is *in vivo* exposure. We're now measuring at the middle of the treatment and at the end to see which half is more effective, and for the subjects we have so far, the second half is more effective. It's those *in vivo* exposures that are like the silver bullet, but if you want to be a methodical scientist—and I do—what that says is *in vivo* exposures following an educational phase seem to be the active ingredient. We don't know if they would be without the educational phase, and we don't know if an educational phase that went on longer than eight weeks would be comparable."

"Maybe if people did talk therapy for two or three years . . . ," I suggested.

"I wouldn't put my bets on that," Kendall replied. "This is a bit anecdotal, but the student therapists will say, 'The child isn't ready yet, I don't know if he can handle it,' and we say, 'It's time! Whatever it is he feared, let's go do it!' And two weeks later the therapist says, 'Wow, he did it! I couldn't believe he did it!' The therapists want to protect, much as the parents have wanted to protect. They don't want to take risks, and yet it seems the risk-taking and the child's accomplishment in that risk-taking are very potent. The kids explain that success to themselves, and it makes them think differently."

Kendall told me of another discovery that seemed to have implications for nonprofessionals—for the parents and teachers and pediatricians trying to decide or advise whether a child's behavior suggests the need for therapy. "We also watched kids who came to the clinic thinking they had an anxiety disorder but didn't qualify, and we looked at normal kids, siblings of Temple undergraduates. We had them 'tell us about yourself for five minutes' while we videotaped them. So if you have an anxious child and you say, 'Katie, I'd like you to tell us about yourself, here's the camera and microphone, take five minutes and make eye contact with the camera. Here's a page of hints,' and then you leave the room, that's a stressful experience for an anxious kid. You'd think they'd show some behaviors that would differentiate them from the normal kids. Well, we counted as many behaviors as we thought would be relevant, and there were *no differences*."

"Stage fright is universal?" I asked.

"The anxious kids and the normal kids and the kids who didn't quite qualify all showed some anxiety. The behaviors we coded didn't really separate the groups. So fidgetiness or gratuitous body movements or failure to make eye contact didn't predict who would or would not be identified as an anxiety-disordered child. But—after they were all finished, we asked observers to rate on a one-to-five scale just how anxious they thought each kid was. Based on these global ratings, they were able to separate who were the anxious kids and who weren't, even though on specific counts they couldn't. There is something that separates these groups, because observers can do it."

"You can't define pornography, but you know it when you see it?" I asked.

"So to speak," said Kendall. "We have to define the codes better, or we have to come up with other things to observe, because the categories we had—which were almost exhaustive—didn't pick it up. I think the answer is within-group variability. Some anxious kids got jittery, some got stiff, some did what they were supposed to but looked uncomfortable. What they did didn't make the difference, but the intensity did."

"So an anxious kid with rigid posture is more rigid than a nonanxious kid?"

"Yes," Kendall said. "The ratings pick up on that more than the counts do."

"Everybody's scared of taking tests to some extent, everybody is a little tense, but the intensity of your tension would characterize you?" I asked.

Kendall said, "And the anxious kid would get tense buying an ice cream cone."

In essence, Kendall was rephrasing Michael Thompson's axiom—"A symptom is normal behavior that is displayed too much, too intensely, or in the wrong place at the wrong time"—a theme that recurred throughout my experience with therapists. In most cases the children I saw who were clients (or patients), if they were not medicated, looked or sounded different from the children I knew who were not clients or patients. At the same time, from Kendall's quantifying diagnostic point of view, "for internalizing problems like anxiety and depression, interview of the parent and the child works much better than observations. Observations are great for externalizing problems like acting out, hyperactivity, and aggression." Logically enough, behavior disorders can be identified by watching children behave, but a trustworthy, precise measure of how a child feels is achievable only through conversation. "When an anxious kid comes into the clinic," Kendall said, "he may just look like a bit of a goody-goody, but you wouldn't pick up the anxiety until you talk to him and hear all the things he's afraid of."

Another discovery Kendall made was that "anxious kids compared to normal kids engage in the kind of self-talk you would expect to help reduce anxiety, but it's not functional. They'll say, 'Okay, take-a-deep-breath,' but they won't do it, or they'll say 'I shouldn't be nervous,' but it doesn't have any meaning, they don't understand it. They come in with a variety of potential coping strategies that they don't know how to use, and it only gets them more nervous. I think maybe a parent or teacher said to them quickly, 'Oh, just relax,' and they don't know what that means. They don't know there's a difference if you sag your arms and take a deep breath and change your speech pattern."

"Where do you think the anxiety comes from?" I asked innocently, trying to sound neither too psychoanalytic nor too medical.

"I'd pick three primary contributing factors, not necessarily in order of dominance," Kendall said. "There's certainly a predisposition for some people to be more rather than less high-strung. I'd call it temperament, and I'd say it doesn't produce a disorder, it just produces individual differences that make some people more at risk than others.

"Second, I'd say the family pattern—I won't call it family causal agents, I'd call it modeling. But Mom and Dad provide explanations for behavior that are models for how the child will explain behavior for him or herself. So if the kid says, 'Omigod there's a bug!' and the parent goes, 'Omigod a bug,' all of a sudden the kid's alarmed when he sees bugs, whereas other parents might pick it up and say, 'Yes, a bug, we'll have to throw it out, squoosh it and throw it away,' or 'We'll have to put it in the yard. Bugs are okay outside, we just don't like them in the house.' Or perhaps a parent who was more intellectual would say, 'Look at that, a twelve-legged pterodactyl. Let's get a book and look it up.' There are lots of ways to respond to a bug, and the way the parent models it, the emotional tone and intensity, I think, is a potent reason why some kids have anxiety and distress.

"We had thought that the parents of an anxious kid would be more psychologically controlling, but that doesn't seem to hold up so far. It's very much their conditioned emotional responses to situations that set the tone for the child."

"Then," I suggested, "any one of us by this collision of circumstances could produce a child who has all sorts of problems, and there's nothing we can do except not be ourselves."

"There's a lot we can do once we know," Kendall observed. "You do have to be a little different from your natural tendency. If your natural tendency is to be aggressive, mean-spirited, and physically abusive, you have to walk around saying, 'I'm getting really angry, I want to hit, but I'm not going to hit.' Then your child's going to pick up that when you get angry, you talk to yourself, or you say what you're not going to do. When they see that, that's what they're more likely to copy."

A third possible etiology of anxiety disorders, Kendall said, is "the unexplained occurrence of a traumatic event: you're walking down the street, and someone shoots the kid standing next to you. We had a serious problem in our community when the plane carrying Senator Heinz crashed [in a schoolyard]. My friend's daughter was killed, and some other kids were burned. I've been contacted a disproportionate number of times about children in a certain age range who are still having nightmares about that. It's my preference not to see neighbors—it's hard to tinker with people's lives when you also have to interact with them on other levels, and I also don't want my own kids to be confused about what Dad does with other children—so I refer them out. But the kids seem to be having nightmares about the fact that anything can happen: the safety of this little suburban community can be impinged upon. This is the first time they've come to the realization that things can happen that you can't control."

We had been dancing around nature-nurture issues, an activity I enjoyed pursuing with therapists of different orientations throughout my research. In explaining the cognitive-behavioral approach, Kendall had said to me, "There are eight or ten variables in explaining psychopathology. Some we can control, and some, like genetics, we can't. So we take the things we can control and intervene, and take the others, recognize their impact, and put them aside temporarily."

In 1992, Kendall and seven of his students published a book on the project, *Anxiety Disorders in Youth.* The official report on the first phase of the project appeared in the February 1994 issue of the highly respected *Journal of Consulting and Clinical Psychology*, which had subjected the paper to its usual rigorous standards of peer review. The minuteness of measurement standards is impressive: in addition to the plethora of rating scales completed by parents, teachers, therapists, and observers, for example, there is an independent assessment of how each child perceives the therapeutic relationship, which is rated on a seven-item, five-point scale that asks, for example, to what degree the child liked, felt close to, felt comfortable talking to, and wanted to spend time with the therapist. This rating was later tied to each child's outcome. It turned out the differences between therapists at this clinic—all of whom scored high—weren't hugely significant, and those that existed didn't much affect whether the child made and maintained gains. Absent a group of notably chilly therapists whose results might offer either a dramatic contrast or none at all, Kendall is willing to guess that a good relationship is necessary but not sufficient for success. That is hardly surprising: it's the position any practitioner might be expected to take.

As I completed this book, Kendall and his students were deep into their second study, which treated "co-morbid" children, those whose diagnosis uncovered some other problem in addition to anxiety: Did this therapy make inroads into curing both disorders? At the same time, the clinic had just completed a successful pilot study for a third phase, which would involve treating parent-child pairs in tandem.

"Do you want to know whether that's better than treating kids alone?" I asked Kendall. "Whether it lasts longer and generalizes better?"

"That's correct," he said, "with an exception. You're taking what's called the 'horse-race approach.' We're asking, What types of problems and what types of children are best treated by these different approaches? A family that's overinvolved, where the parents can't get out of the kids' lives, may be better with a child-focused treatment. The result of that is that when the parents are automatically pulled out, the independence and autonomy-granting take place as part of the treatment being child-focused. In other contexts where smothering or overprotection are not features of the home environment, it may be better to have the whole family as the treatment unit." I had been guilty of the layman's big mistake in evaluating therapy: the notion that one approach is ever the best one for all clients. As my own research progressed, I made that mistake less and less often; but it is a difficult idea to give up.

The development of Kendall's interest in child psychology seems as appropriate as that of Carlson and Sarnoff. He went to a boys' parochial high school where one of the priests gave a fascinating course. "He didn't *call* it psychology, there was some name like "Religion and Society," but he showed us Ingmar Bergman films and talked about Freud and *The Feminine Mystique* and adolescent development. Boy, was that an exciting course! To sit and understand, even at a preliminary elementary level, that there were people who thought about the mind and how it worked!

"I took more exciting psychology courses at Old Dominion University and at the same time volunteered to work with children who were having problems. This one middle-class kid had a school problem. We played basketball and went for walks, and I said, 'Hey, if you want to do better at school, here's an idea, try it.' He liked that. He didn't like what had happened to him in the past, which was he went to a tutor who tried to drill the information into his head, and his parents had sent him to a psychiatrist who tried to analyze a lot of his life. What I think I did in that one fortuitous instance was just develop a relationship and give some good advice without forcing it.

"When I found there were some preliminary nascent theories in psychology that were consistent with that, I said, 'Yeah, I like that.' My initial investment in psychology was behavioral, but it wasn't the behavioral change agent outside setting up a contingency-reward system for everybody else. It was collaborating with the patient, the client, to set up some ways they could reach their own goals. It was using behavior *with* the client rather than doing behavior *to* the client."

Cognitive-behavioral therapy suits Kendall because it's directive and enactive rather than a slow process of interpretation and discovery like psychodynamic therapy; he suggests the matching of a therapist's personality with his orientation is no accident. "My personality is energetic, so we're doing things. It would be hard for me to keep myself neutral, distant, and reflective in what I would call an obsessive way on some historical parenting relationship issue. That would be frustrating for me because I'd say, 'Hey, you don't need to do that. We've got some ways to move right ahead.' "

I was curious to know how a cognitive-behaviorist might have treated Freud's Little Hans: while Kendall had read some Freudian theory in graduate school, he was not familiar with the case histories, so I gave him a quick rundown on the client's problem. While the active, energetic style of his therapy was evident in contrast to Sarnoff's more reflective approach, there were some similarities in their formulations. For example, when I asked Kendall whether he differentiated between a fear and a phobia, he said, "A fear is typically considered to have a certain realistic quality. If you're atop a tall building and the wind is blowing, being afraid is entirely reasonable if it's not excessive."

"Being superafraid is still reasonable?" I asked.

"If the threat is there. A phobia is likely to show similar physiological arousal and distress, but isn't based in reality. Children may show fear of horses, but a horse isn't even there. Let me walk you through a possible treatment approach. When you say 'cognitive-behavioral,' you do in fact involve these two systems. First, what does the child say to himself when exposed to a horse? 'My God, there it is, it's gonna kill me'? Or 'This thing eats people?' Whatever it is, we want to know that self-talk. Another thing would be, How does the child cognitively process that? Does he walk away thinking, 'I was a bad boy because I didn't touch the horse'? 'I'm a scaredy-cat because I didn't'? 'I'm not gonna be loved by my mom'? What are the processing features? What conclusions, what attributions does the child make? After displaying phobic reactions to the horse, does he attribute it to himself in some way, like 'I'm a failure, I'm no good, I'm incompetent'?

"Lastly, and I think that is important, what does the horse mean for this kid? Not necessarily in the symbolic sense, but in the sense of what else is associated with it, what situations go with it?"

"It sounds to me," I said, "as if you're going to psychoanalyze this kid. How do you get this information out of Hans?"

"The first part, getting at the self-talk," Kendall said, "would use *in vivo* experiences. You go to the park and you pet the horse, and the child is standing next to you, and he says, 'I won't do this!' and you ask, 'What are you thinking to yourself?' You don't do it in fantasy, and this is the behavioral part, you do it in the real situation. We're not going to psychoanalyze him in the sense of looking for repressed conflict or internal conflicts between id, ego, and superego, but we'll look for how the child thinks about the feared object, what does it mean to them in the sense of how they interpret it."

"When you've got all this information," I asked, "what are you going to do with it?"

"Again there are going to be three or four different pieces," Kendall continued. "There's modeling. If you want to be able to improve the child's abilities by demonstration, if you demonstrate entire success, jump on the horse and ride off, the child's going to think, 'It's easy for *you* to do, but I'm afraid of horses.' So the modeling has to be a gradual exposure—not just showing correct performance but showing strategies to overcome fear as you approach.

"The second part of the behavioral would be *in vivo* exposure. You keep repeated trials, petting, interacting with horses. The third one is attaching rewards to those behaviors."

"What about the other things going on in Hans's life? He's jealous of his baby sister, he watched the birth, saw the blood, was told about the stork. Are you going to deal with that at all?"

"It depends," Kendall said. "If, in the coming-to-understand part, we find that he isn't really afraid the horse is going to bite him or step on him, what he's really afraid of is that he has no access to his mother, that might come out. It's possible—I won't say it's going to be a simple task—that the child during the inital, educational stages of the treatment is going to say, 'I'm afraid of this too' and 'I'm afraid of that,' and they're trying to get your attention and involvement with them. Then you don't have the same situation.

"You have a situation where you want to manipulate the parental attention, and that would have a different effect on the fear of horses. If maternal attention is part of the problem, it's often a good idea to get the mother involved in the *in vivo* exposures. Even though it's not 'family therapy,' the family plays a role in overseeing the exposures and, in fact, witnessing some success."

In vivos are characteristic of Kendall's private practice: he doesn't make house calls or visit schools (although he does talk a lot with parents and teachers), but he and his clients are often out and about. "Last night, for example, I saw a client and we went for a walk," he told me. "This is an adolescent who has some difficulties with interpersonal things. He's always bossy and pushing and shoving and abrasive. So we go for a walk to the local deli, and he buys a snack. I only spend a small amount of money. He used to just say, 'I'm gonna get this and I'm gonna get this and I'm gonna get this.' But over time he's now different in the store. He says, 'Okay, what can I get?' I say, 'Why don't you try to get one thing?' 'Can I get a soda too?' 'Okay.' He now asks and interacts in a reasonable manner, picks something that isn't fifteen dollars off the shelf, doesn't say things like 'I have to have the best!'

"He says, 'I'll just get a snack today.' He can probably go into that store on his own, and he won't be thrown out by the manager. So after twelve or fifteen times of *in vivo* exposure, his behavior has changed in that context. Then last night, when we were walking back afterward, I said, 'Gee, you know you were real loud. I think some of the people at the tables noticed that. I think that might make some adults with you feel uncomfortable, and they might snap back at you.' I don't hammer at it, and the next week we might go back, and I might say, 'Hey, you know you weren't real loud that time, that was nice. I felt comfortable with you.' We're doing the *in vivos*, and we're processing it together. 'How did that make you feel?' "

"Is this going to generalize?" I asked.

"I don't think it's going to generalize to getting along with kids in an athletic activity, or to being with his family at a holiday dinner, because there are going to be a lot of other pressures, but as we work, these things will be driving it. We'll take a scheduled break for a couple of months so he can develop a little bit, percolate on what happened, and come back with a new angle."

"He can presumably say, 'If this happened in the deli, maybe it'll work on the baseball field'?" I asked. Kendall crossed two sets of fingers. "I think that's the hope," he said, "and sometimes it works. But you have to program it, be more systematic. You have to say, 'Look, you did real well here, but you're getting into fights on the baseball field. Do you mind if I tell your coach to monitor how you're doing? He can just keep a little index card and write it down and let me know.' Then I've bridged the gap. I've told him we're going to try and generalize, to use these skills in another setting, and I'll monitor it. Then I think we'll get there."

Research projects like the anxiety clinic follow a narrowly prescribed format; in private practice clients often appear with multiple problems, and Kendall is willing to address several at the same time. "A hyperactive child may have problems with friends, so I would teach problem-solving strategies to reduce the impulsiveness, but we would often engage in this around peer activity." He will treat people off and on for a couple of years and will sometimes work with the parents, either additionally or instead. "In one case," he says, "the parents were recently separated and about to divorce. The father was pressured and driven in his work and his child-rearing, while the mother was more relaxed. The child was showing some symptoms at school, and the school people wanted to put him on Ritalin. I did some assessments and diagnosis and recommended that the mom not put the child on Ritalin, that this was a really smart kid who was going to need a lot of activities in the classroom because he was a thoroughbred—he was just a *very smart kid*. The parents should spend some time repairing their relationship so there would be consistency between them, I said, and the teacher needed to put more time into educating the kid and less into medicating him into submission. We'll check up in a few months and see how all that's going."

Like all therapists who work with individual children, both Kendall and his student therapists at the clinic often run up against a client's family problems. "There are two tines in the fork when you have accurately identified interactions with the parents that are maladaptive," Kendall says. "One strategy is to teach the child to distance himself from it, to say, 'That's my parents. I don't have to believe them if they say I'm the worst person on the face of the earth—that's their problem, not mine.' The other tine in the fork is you change the environment. Do you get the child to adjust to the world they live in in a healthy way, or do you change the world they live in to make it healthy? We have these artificial boundaries. Family therapists say religiously that the whole family has to be in treatment. Child-focused therapy says religiously you just treat the kid. Then everybody sort of bends those boundaries a little bit in the middle.

"I'd like to look at the role of parental involvement in different disorders and the outcomes. For conduct disorder I think increased involvement and responsibility may be ideal; with anxiety disorders reducing parental involvement and giving the child more control may be ideal. It could be the thrust of a decade of research and writing, to see if people should modulate the degree to which they involve families based on the nature of the problem they're trying to treat."

I asked Kendall what turned him on these days, and he said, "The sophisticated individualizing of a program. I no longer think—not that I ever really believed it strongly—that one thing is going to work for everybody. I get turned on by the ability to identify the individual cognitive styles that allow us to hook in and have our procedures work. When we have our supervisory meetings and I see the therapists making suggestions that come from prior clients, that's good, they're using their experience and finding out what works. But what I really like is when they say, 'Here's where this kid is coming from, here is their template for viewing situations, therefore I'm going to come at it this way to hook them in.' I like that even better."

It seemed the boundaries were blurring. If psychodynamic therapists were becoming more empirical, cognitive-behaviorists were blending their empirical view with what they gleaned from clinical practice with each individual child. To watch intelligently where their journey might be leading, it is necessary to understand where it began.

CHAPTER 8

REBELS AND REVISIONISTS

Give me a dozen healthy infants, well-formed, and my own specified world to bring them up in and I'll guarantee to take any one at random and train him to become any type of specialist I might select—doctor, lawyer, artist, merchant-chief and, yes, even beggar-man and thief, regardless of his talents, penchants, tendencies, abilities, vocations, and race of his ancestors.

—John Broadus Watson,
Behaviorism (1924)

In a strict 'radical' sense of the term, a 'behaviorist' is a scientist who restricts his inquiries to publicly observable events and conscientiously avoids inference. . . . Using that definition, I would contend that there have been more unicorns than behaviorists.

—Michael J. Mahoney,
*Cognition and Behavior
Modification* (1974)

"ASK ME IF I BELIEVE IN THE UNCONSCIOUS," ordered Philip Kendall one balmy spring morning as we sat in his office in Weiss Hall, the psychology building at Temple University. The office, like Sarnoff's, was chock full of meaningful artifacts, but these were not the symbolically pregnant art-works of the psychoanalyst; they were stacks of spiral-bound papers and printouts and proposals fresh from the oven, awaiting digestion and disposition—grades, grants, comments—crying "Me! Me! Me!" and covering every available surface, giving literal significance to the phrase "everything's out on the table." Sarnoff's artworks, I thought, were the lodestars of his professional career, and whether he was writing or seeing patients, they fixed his gaze on what he believed to be the eternal verities. Kendall's waiting papers were a reminder too, of all the work that was yet to be done, the data that weren't in yet.

But today, with a secretary holding the calls and only an occasional knock from a graduate student in administrative crisis, Kendall was expansive, reflective, and a bit puckish. "Okay," I complied. "Do you, Mr. Interlocutor, believe in the unconscious?"

"Not that I'm aware of," he said.

If at least some psychoanalytically trained therapists are becoming more cautious in their inferences and newly open to the implications of current research, so are many behavioral therapists questioning the universal undiluted application of experiment-based theory: perhaps the clinic and the lab need each other more than they supposed. To comprehend how this came to be—how Philip Kendall, sort of, accepts the unconscious, and what it means to him and his tribal colleagues to do so—we must go back in time and think once again about scientific revolutions.

Cognitive-behavioral therapy is about twenty years old and is an outgrowth of behavior therapy, which came into its own in the fifties and sixties as a revolt against psychoanalysis—which, to be accurate and fair, was itself a revolt against the "normal science" of the turn of the century: Freud and his disciples fought hard for respectability. But in the sixties the flavor of revolution—the quest for a new standard, the idealism and zeal in promoting it—pervaded behavior therapy. For an understanding of this, I have drawn on an account by Daniel B. Fishman and Cyril M. Franks, two behavioral psychologists at Rutgers University; on some theoretical work published over the past twenty-five years; and on conversations with Kendall—a member of the more cynical generation that followed and tempered the rebellion—who described the world that unfolded to him as a young graduate student, a junior academic, and finally a shaper of that world.

I found the work of many behavioral theorists dry and difficult to read. To anyone who reveres the beauty, simplicity, and precision of English at its best, behavioral writing sticks in the craw, and the notion that ideas are more serious when presented in jargon makes the hackles rise. If behavior theory is widely misunderstood, its purveyors have themselves to blame. In reading behaviorists' books, then, I had much to overcome—

yet the books held important ideas that justified (more or less) the effort required to get at them. I shall do my best to translate; I hope readers will come along with me, but if the journey is too arduous, they are free to skim.

Echoing Kuhn's book on scientific revolutions, Fishman and Franks point out that all approaches to psychotherapy are surrounded by some paradigm that includes basic theoretical assumptions, data that support them, clinical techniques, values and ethics, and a sociological, political, and historical context. To comprehend the orientation it is necessary to know something about all these underpinnings; for example, everything Kendall said in Chapter 7 reflects the cognitive-behavioral paradigm. A psychoanalyst—or indeed, a Skinnerian behaviorist—would not make the assumptions he makes.

From the seventeenth until shortly after the first half of the twentieth century, Western science—including psychoanalysis and psychology in general—was based on the belief that there is an objective truth that can be confirmed by detached, rational observation. Originally, behavior therapy was an exaltation of this empirical standard, to which, behaviorists held, psychoanalysis didn't measure up.

The term *behaviorism* was conceived by John B. Watson, director of the Psychology Laboratory at Johns Hopkins University. In "Psychology as the Behaviorist Views It," a famous 1913 tract in the *Psychological Review*, Watson sought a redefinition of the psychologist's territory. He declared "no dividing line between man and brute": thus experiments on laboratory animals could be extrapolated to yield information predictive of human behavior. Attacking "mentalism," he denied the existence of " 'mind' and 'mental states'," held emotions to be reduceable to glandular secretions and muscle movements, and asserted that human behavior was almost exclusively determined by environmental, not hereditary or biological factors. Twelve years later, Watson did report on the emotional reactions of infants reared under experimental conditions and concluded that the only basic instincts were fear, stimulated by the loss of physical support and by loud sounds; rage, stimulated by the restraint of bodily movement; and love, stimulated by stroking. By conditioning these responses, one could transfer them to different stimuli, and a complex emotional organization would be built up.

Watson's ideas about conditioning drew on the work of Ivan Petrovich Pavlov and Edward Lee Thorndike. Pavlov was the Russian psychologist we all learned about in high school biology, a contemporary of Watson's, who discovered what is now called the conditioned response by training dogs to salivate when a bell rang. (Fishman and Franks point out that the term *conditioned* was actually a mistranslation of *conditional*, which meant temporary and highly responsive to the environment, as distinguished from innate reflexes like the sneeze.) In 1913, Thorndike, an educational psychologist at Teachers College of Columbia University, formulated the "Law of Effect" (later called "operant conditioning"), in which subjects could be induced to choose their future response to a particular stimulus by the manipulation of prior punishment and reward. Pavlovian (or "classical") conditioning and operant conditioning were the foundation of American behavioral psychology for the next fifty years. But throughout that time behaviorism was a research mode, not yet a point of departure for therapy.

The next big name among behaviorists—perhaps the name most familiar to outsiders—is Burrhus Frederick Skinner of Harvard. Like Freud, Skinner has been widely misunderstood; to grasp the basics of the behaviorists' world, it is necessary to clear up some misperceptions before we explore where later theorists diverged. Indeed, as the source from which all tributaries of behaviorism flowed, these ideas merit our immersion. Skinner's first book, *The Behavior of Organisms*, appeared in 1938; I have chosen to examine a 1974 work, *About Behaviorism*, written after the theories had had thirty-six years to evolve.

In his introduction Skinner refutes some common errors about behaviorism. Here are a few of them: that it neglects innate endowment and argues that all behavior is acquired; that it represents a person as an automaton or puppet who does nothing but respond to stimuli; that it doesn't account for cognitive or creative processes or for intentions; that it assigns no role to a sense of self; that it is superficial and cannot deal with the depths of personality; that it limits itself to the prediction and control of behavior and misses "the essential nature of being a man"; that its achievements in the laboratory cannot be duplicated in the outside world; that it manipulates people in an antidemocratic way and is thus subject to abuse by dictators but not to use by "men of good will"; and that "it is indifferent to the warmth and richness of human life, and . . . incompatible with the creation and enjoyment of art, music, and literature and with love for one's fellow men."

The source of this misunderstanding, Skinner suggests, was Watson himself. In pioneering a new approach to psychology, the founder made strategic errors by "attacking the introspective study of mental life" and by advancing exaggerated claims without data to support them. At the same time Watson deserves credit as "one of the first ethologists in the modern spirit." Pavlov had used dogs as subjects and Watson white rats because results obtained from this kind of study were easy to reproduce, but the transfer to humans was questionable and made for "hasty interpretations of complex behavior."

Having thus disarmed his most banal critics, Skinner proceeds with a jesuitical explanation of what he does and doesn't accept. Earlier "methodological" behaviorists reasoned that since we can't anticipate what someone will do by looking at his feelings, we should "abandon the search for causes and simply describe what people do": in this spirit anthropologists report customs, political scientists report voting patterns, and economists collect statistics, all of which allow them to predict behavior on the basis of what people have done in the past. Methodological behaviorists avoid "mentalism" by bypassing feelings and considering "only those facts which can be objectively observed." As Skinner points out, "most methodological behaviorists granted the existence of mental events while ruling them out of consideration."

Radical behaviorists—Skinner's brand—are, oddly enough, a more moderate lot. They are willing to consider feelings as a clue to predicting future behavior, but not as a cause of it. For example, the old proverb "A burnt child dreads the fire" recast by a radical behaviorist would read, "A burnt child avoids the fire" and might be followed by the explanation, "To ensure the child's survival, Nature has equipped her with a set of responses that society has trained her to call 'dread' and which are now activated when she approaches a fire. These responses may be taken as a clue that she might have been burned sometime before, but we should be warned that the feeling she describes as 'dread' may not be identical with the feeling her brother describes as 'dread.' "

While reflexes—breathing, suckling, excreting, and indeed, sneezing—are involuntary physiological reactions to conditions inside and outside the body, behavior in general is a response to *contingencies*—that is, consequences that may be rewarding or punishing. Seeking a mate, for example, is a response to *contingencies of survival* necessary to preserve the species. (While eating and sleeping are also governed by contingencies of survival, the survival here is that of the individual.) But seeking a mate in a singles bar, a bookstore-café, or a personals column (or not seeking a mate in one of these places) is a response to *contingencies of reinforcement*, the mechanisms that lead an individual to adapt to the current environment: one chooses or avoids behavior that has been successful or not successful in achieving a goal in the past. This choice is the result of operant conditioning. Skinner emphasizes that we are susceptible to reinforcement because of its survival value and not from any associated feelings. The feelings are "merely collateral." It is useful to remember, because it became one of the cornerstones of behavior therapy, that "When reinforcement is no longer forthcoming, behavior undergoes 'extinction' and appears rarely, if at all."

What follows from all this? Skinner observes that the way we respond to contingencies—and the particular contingencies that move us—are in our history. Since they are not conspicuous at present, they are readily overlooked. "It is then easy to believe that the will is free and that the person is free to choose." The person is not free: everything we do is a sort of sneeze, but we can't always spot the pepper. And much later in his book Skinner remarks,

> It is often said, particularly by psychoanalysts, that behaviorism cannot deal with the unconscious. The fact is that, to begin with, it deals with nothing else. The controlling relations between behavior and genetic and environmental variables are all unconscious so long as they are not observed, and it was Freud who emphasizes that they need not be observed (that is, conscious) to be effective. It requires a special verbal environment to impose consciousness on behavior by inducing a person to respond to his own body while he is behaving. If consciousness seems to have a causal effect, it is the effect of the special environment which induces self-observation.

So Skinner and Freud touch; and touching, strike sparks; and striking sparks, spring apart.

This is the foundation of Skinner's theory, through which he is able to reconceptualize thought, motivation, feeling, the self—and incidentally, love, art, religion, and all phases of human endeavor. It is essentially a new language, in its own way extremely precise, a language in which behavioral psychologists, particularly those between the ages of forty and sixty, were scrupulously trained: words that imply "mentalism" are, as labeled in the nervous humor of the field, "X-rated." For example, in the chapter headed "Thinking," Skinner says, "Thinking is behaving. The mistake is in allocating the behavior to the mind." Thus the Skinnerian term for thinking is "covert behavior," defined as "completed behavior which occurs on a scale so small that it cannot be detected by others . . . it was a mistake for methodological behaviorism and certain versions of logical positivism and structuralism to neglect it simply because it was not 'objective.' . . . It does not explain overt behavior: it is simply more behavior to be explained."

One sees the terms *covert behavior* or *covert events* ("ideas" in lay English) in the writings of behaviorists, and their use of this language is one reason their books and papers are so tedious to read. (Revisionists like Kendall display a nice dry sense of humor in their writings, but it is hard to overcome this early training, and they have never learned—or are too inhibited—to soar.) But Skinner makes a good antidote to Melanie Klein and a generally useful corrective for the wilder psychodynamic speculations. Moreover, the idea that "maladaptive" (a less-charged and therefore more useful term for what other orientations call "pathological") behavior continues because it is in some way reinforced is essential for lay people from parents to policymakers to remember; it has innumerable applications, which we will see throughout this book. Skinner himself uses the failure to enact gun control laws to illustrate the way a preoccupation with mental causes gets us off the hook in not changing the environment. And through the medium of this difficult and circuitous language, Skinner expresses a new formulation of the causes and effects of human actions, one that ought to join the other formulations we consider useful.

In his summary Skinner points out—jesuitically, again—that organisms don't just respond reflexively, which would make them robots: "But stimuli do not *elicit* operant responses; they simply modify the probability that responses will be emitted." The implications of this are the basics of child care that all parents believe they are pursuing but (viewed in a behaviorist light) do not practice as skillfully or subtly as they might. Indeed, like other psychological theorists Skinner remarks that the baby learns, early on, to control his parents. Next the child advances to controlling his peers, and finally he figures out how to use these acquired techniques in self-control. This points the way for behavior therapy: a child who can analyze his own behavior will be able to control it better.

Skinner does say that "the same basic processes occur in both animals and men," but there are "enormous differences in the complexity of their repertoires." He contends that "the objection to arguing from animals to men and women is in part an objection to extrapolating from laboratory to daily life, and the point applies as well when the organism in the laboratory is human. The setting in the laboratory is designed to control conditions. . . . Obviously we cannot predict or control human behavior in daily life with the precision obtained in the laboratory, but we can nevertheless use results from the laboratory to interpret behavior elsewhere."

Finally he reiterates that "there is nothing in a science of behavior or its philosophy which need alter feelings or introspective observations. The bodily states which are felt or observed are acknowledged, but there is an emphasis on the environmental conditions with which they are associated and an insistence that it is the conditions rather than the feelings which enable us to explain behavior."

While John Watson had promoted behaviorism mainly as a reaction to the introspective data-gathering methods of contemporary psychology labs, it's fair to say that an anti-Freudian viewpoint was almost as old as the general circulation of Freud's ideas. From the late thirties on, however— around the time that Skinner first published—there began to be additional incentives to develop some alternative approach to therapy. Psychologists at university laboratories, in accord with their training, sought a means to introduce testable hypotheses into psychoanalysis, which was then the sole form of therapy available. And once clinical psychologists went out into the world, they could practice only under the direction and at the sufferance of psychiatrists: those with behavioral science backgrounds were restricted to testing, and psychodynamically trained "lay analysts" were not quite respectable, despite Freud's efforts on their behalf. It was no wonder psychologists objected to the "disease model" of mental disorders: as Fishman and Franks observe, "The treatment of psychiatric disturbance remained fundamentally a medical problem in which the non-medical psychologist was, at best, a useful ancillary worker."

Psychologists at the University of London's celebrated Institute of Psychiatry at Maudsley Hospital, led by H. J. Eysenck, questioned the efficacy of psychoanalysis and the rigor of psychodynamic formulations. In searching out a basis for a new approach, they settled on Pavlov as a point of departure for a therapy amenable to empirical verification. The movement toward behavior therapy (a term coined by Eysenck) grew internationally throughout the sixties. It gained further impetus from the Zeitgeist, which rebelled against all sorts of authority: that of Freud theoretically, that of doctors institutionally, and that of analyst over patient clinically. "The 1950's and 1960's was [sic] a pioneering era, an era of ideology and polemics in which behavior therapists strove to present a united front against the common psychodynamic 'foe,' " write Fishman and Franks.

A representative sample of behavior therapists' thinking in the late sixties can be found in *Principles of Behavior Modification*, a textbook published in 1969 by Albert Bandura, a professor at Stanford University and a leader in the field; it was required reading for Kendall in graduate school. It is appropriately fiery. Bandura starts by saying that mental illnesses in ancient times were "believed to be manifestations of evil spirits . . . which had to be exorcised" and suggests that the "quasi-disease model . . . widely employed" credits psychopathology to "a host of inimical psychodynamic forces (for example, repressed impulses, energized traits, psychic complexes, latent tendencies, self-dynamisms, and other types of energy systems) somewhat akin to the pernicious spirits of ancient times."

But labeling behavior pathological was a social judgment affected by "the normative standards of persons making the judgments, the social context in which the behavior is exhibited, certain attributes of the behavior, and numerous characteristics of the deviator himself." For example, intense behavior that makes others uncomfortable tends to be considered pathological more often than low-keyed behavior, but there is no evidence that the "internal processes" that govern the former are less healthy than those that rule the latter. Intention is an issue: "Delinquents who strike victims on the head to extract their wallets expediently are generally labeled semiprofessional thieves exhibiting income-producing instrumental aggression. By contrast, delinquents who simply beat up strangers but show no interest in their victims' material possessions are supposedly displaying emotional aggression of a peculiarly disturbed sort . . . in many cases . . . the behavior is highly instrumental in gaining the approval and admiration of peers and in enhancing status in the social hierarchy of the reference group. . . . Certain subgroups simply value and reward skillful 'stomping' more highly than musical virtuosity."

Among the other objections Bandura mounts to the disease model are its circularity (people are deemed to have schizophrenia because they behave in a certain way, and they behave that way because they're schizophrenic); it promotes the use of drugs as a quick fix; it requires medical training to practice therapy, and medical training does not equip one to effect necessary social change; people who believe they're sick don't take responsibility for changing. There is some validity in all these comments; it's especially useful to recognize that indifference to the sociological elements in psychological disorders is still a limitation of many medical practitioners.

Among Bandura's criticisms of psychodynamic therapy are that its goals are vaguely defined and that psychoanalysts may change clients' entire belief systems without really improving the problems that brought them to therapy. Behavior therapists, on the other hand, focus on just those presenting problems, or what psychodynamic therapists call "symptoms." The idea of symptom substitution so basic to dynamic therapy—that if you just cure a child's bed-wetting, he will only replace it with some other symptom—is untestable because "it fails to specify precisely what constitutes a 'symptom,' when the substitution should occur, the social conditions under which it is most likely to arise, and the form that the substitute symptom will take." He attacks the notion that a transference relationship is necessary or even useful to effect a cure, questioning whether it generalizes to the rest of the client's life and suggesting that "those who lead emotionally impoverished lives often become more interested in securing positive reinforcement from their therapists than in solving their interpersonal problems. Personality changes are further obstructed if therapists, due to limited satisfaction in their own nonprofessional relationships, use their clients as a substitute source of gratification." The comment about the therapists, not backed up by evidence of how widespread this phenomenon might be, appears to be no more than sniping.

Bandura pulls apart Freud's analysis of Little Hans, an argument that doesn't merit inclusion here because a Freudian and a behaviorist could debate Freud's analysis all night, both be right within their separate conceptual frameworks, and settle nothing. (I have, however, in the interests of highlighting the distinctions, asked clinicians of different orientations to suggest how they would treat the case of Little Hans—and their formulations appear throughout this book.) In other arguments though, Bandura has struck some telling blows; while analytically trained practitioners might respond to them, the psychodynamic world has in general not engaged in public dialogue with behaviorists on these issues. Although the passion has died down and some positions have been modified as behaviorists discovered the limits of their own approach, these beliefs, marking the original rebellion, underlie their tribal orientation and dictate the meaning of departures from it.

In laying out the social-learning theory for which he is famous Bandura states an important theme in the behavioral world. Thus: "behavior that is harmful to the individual or departs widely from accepted social and ethical norms is viewed not as symptomatic of some kind of disease but as a way that the individual has learned to cope with environmental and self-imposed demands. Treatment then becomes mainly a problem in social learning rather than one in the medical domain."

If clients of behavior therapists exhibit something like symptom substitution, it suggests the particular behavior modification program was simply ineffective or that the client has not been taught "prosocial" behavior to replace the deviant responses. An interesting example of this is a case in which "an extremely withdrawn boy spent approximately 80 percent of his time in solitary activities in isolated areas of the nursery school." (The quantitative description of the symptom is highly characteristic of Bandura's orientation. Kendall would frame it in the same terms.) It turned out that the teachers "unwittingly reinforced" this solitary behavior by fussing over the boy, empathizing with his loneliness and trying to get him to join the group, but on the few occasions when he did comply, they took no particular notice. With behavior training, "the teachers stopped rewarding solitary play with attention and support. Instead, whenever the boy sought out other children, the teacher immediately joined the group and gave it her full attention. In a short time, the boy's isolation declined markedly and he was spending about 60 percent of his time playing with other children."

Therapists must subtly manipulate the techniques of reinforcement: for example, continuous positive reinforcement discourages clients, while intermittent reinforcement encourages them to persist. Punishment successful in the lab often fails to transfer to real life because life presents more options; during the period the punishment is working, a therapist must teach the client more acceptable behavior and reinforce that. And sometimes even if parents learn to practice effective reinforcement, others in the child's life won't play. As Skinner also pointed out, behavior (for good or ill) is extinguished by the failure to reinforce it; the simplest example of this, as parents will recognize, is that five-year-olds keep saying "doody" only as long as it achieves the desired provocative effect. Bandura adds that clients often experience problems because they don't know how to reinforce themselves: they hold excessively high standards.

Bandura was not a strict Skinnerian: by the time he wrote his book, the wall against "mentalism" had crumbled. In this vein he writes, "There exists ample evidence that one cannot account satisfactorily for human behavior while remaining entirely outside the organism, because overt behavior is often governed by self-generated stimulation that is relatively independent of environmental stimulus events." That is to say, something we can't figure out is going on in there, and until we come up with a miracle scanning device, we "will have to rely upon an individual both as the *agent* and the *object* of study."

Bandura says there will be very different conceptions of behavioral change depending on whether the therapist assumes that people respond automatically and inexorably to external events or that some inner response alters a stimulus. (That is, do people think for a minute about what has just happened to them and then respond in some characteristic way?) In what Bandura does not quite venture to call "cognitive therapy," the clients play a more active role and therapists question them at length. Research shows that people do much to construct their own rewards and punishments. Bandura believes a comprehensive theory of human behavior must encompass "stimulus control, internal symbolic control, and outcome control"—the events in people's lives, what they make of them, and what they do as a result—a point with which one could hardly quarrel.

Kendall had never been a fan of Skinner: in a note he wrote me about the books that had shaped his thinking, he called Skinner's work "very influential in my development in that it was the 'bible' that others adhered to and the 'source' that I criticized." Bandura's book, on the other hand, was " 'on target' but restrictive—it didn't go far enough into the clinical realm nor did it fully develop the role of cognitive functioning in adjustment and maladjustment."

So as we sat in Weiss Hall on that May morning, I asked Kendall if his second generation of behaviorists was pulling back from the antipsychoanalytic rebellion of the first, moving closer toward the center.

"One could say that each therapy movement is a reaction to a prior movement," Kendall agreed. "Psychoanalysis being extremely nonempirical and nonscientific and rich in theory, what's your most likely revolution? Something that's atheoretical, very empirical: behaviorism. Once you've gone to that extreme, what are you likely to react to? 'Gee, there's no theory, there should be some,' and 'Gee, it can't be just empirical, you have to take into account other factors.' So there's a bit of a movement back as you describe it.

"In graduate school at Virginia Commonwealth University, I was working in a juvenile delinquent training school," he went on. "We had set up the ideal behavioral intervention, with kids who were incarcerated by the state, didn't have a good family background, were lacking interpersonal skills, and were at risk for careers in criminal institutions. We set up a beautiful behavioral system.

"If you got up in the morning and got dressed, you got points. If you buckled your belt and tied your shoes, you got points. And if you got enough points, you got prizes: the prizes would be new sneakers, a trip to the canteen, a ride in the go-cart, and a weekend home. We had diamond level and opal level, so you could move up with more privileges and become a staff assistant to help with the program for the newcomers.

"An interesting thing happened along the way to the forum there. New sneakers became out—what was cool was to have old sneakers. I'm riding home from this school, which was a good twenty miles from the university, and I'm thinking, as soon as we set up the contingencies, they twist them around. We'd get kids who would work diligently to get to the next level, but they wouldn't want the highest level because that meant a weekend home, and they didn't want to go home. At the institution they had three meals a day, a bed to sleep in, and an activity on each day of the weekend. If they go home, they're in a room, often abused by a mom or dad, neglected, ignored, unfed. So we had to change a lot because of the way the delinquents processed this experience.

"That's when I read *Cognition and Behavior Modification* by Mike Mahoney, who had been a student of Bandura's and was working at An Achievement Place, a similar kind of behavioral program for at-risk delinquents. He'd had a parallel experience. It really wasn't that radical, among the small group of people where I was working, to say, 'Wait a minute, let's have them be in charge of their own program. They'll arrange the contingencies, and we'll pay more attention to how they process the day-to-day activities we arrange.' It didn't seem that radical, but when we went to conventions, we found other people thought it was really controversial."

I had been hearing that delinquent kids rode roughshod over token economies (residential establishments like the one Kendall described), which were, on the other hand, effective for autistic children. "Exactly," Kendall said. "I think over time the behavioral movement, which was and continues to be successful, has found its niches. For autistic kids it's ideal. It's not for the psychopath-in-training. It's not for the delinquent, because their game is to manipulate. If you try to control them and they try to control you, it becomes butting heads."

Bandura's book, I suggested, had a very sixties flavor. "One of Mahoney's books, also, was called *Power to the Person*, which I think smacks of the sixties attitude," Kendall said. "You reject the idea that psychology or science or society controls you, and you simply learn the contingencies that affect you and arrange them for your own preferred outcomes."

"In the inner city?" I asked.

"I would think the majority of people can't do that, can't control these contingencies," Kendall said. "Although it was intended to be for the people, it was really for a very select group of them."

I had encountered psychodynamic therapists who described delinquents as believing their lives were controlled entirely by others, while all *they*, the delinquents, did was react to what was done to them; in the behavioral world this is called "external locus of control." Did the two tribes agree on something? "I like the notion of our agreeing," Kendall said, "and if you look at the research and at the delinquents, they do tend to have a more external locus of control. However, if you go into their environment, their locus of control is accurate. They don't get to choose what food they eat, they don't get to choose their bedtime or where they sleep, they can't rearrange their furniture—all the things that would make them internal in locus of control. So they're quite appropriate in their perceptions of the environment. Let's change the environment, give them a chance to rearrange their rooms, choose their foods, pick a bedtime, and with that they'll develop an internal locus of control."

"Provided they're incarcerated."

"If they're not," Kendall said, "you go in and change the family. We are guided by the same theory, but we're involving the family more and more."

This is jumping the gun, but back in the seventies, clinicians were discovering the limits of pure behavior therapy and trying to modify it. As Pavlov, Watson, and Skinner were waiting to be seized by the Maudsley psychologists, so was Albert Ellis now sitting, as it were, in the wings.

Ellis had been trained as an analyst but found classical psychoanalysis and analytic therapy ineffective and unscientific. He looked at a number of other contemporary therapies and considered them equally inadequate, and he wanted to incorporate some behavioral techniques. Thus he began experimenting in 1953 and came up with rational emotive therapy—shortened acronymically to RET—in 1955. Since as Ellis later wrote, he was "allergic to the passivity of psychoanalysis!" RET was highly emotional and confrontational. (Kendall and other partial admirers thought it was suitable for use in New York City but ill adapted to the Deep South.) While it was admittedly not for children, Kendall and others thought they could modify it for use with an elementary-school-age population of average and higher intelligence.

Ellis held that emotional disturbances are caused by the interaction of biological and environmental factors; most "seriously disturbed individuals have strong innate . . . tendencies to over- or underreact to environmental influence and to exaggerate and/or minimize the significance of many events . . . of their lives." People choose to disturb themselves, Ellis said (in the ultimate expression of internal locus of control), so they have the choice to undisturb themselves. Tempering his optimism slightly, he conceded that "virtually no humans are (or are likely to be) consistently and totally rational or undisturbed."

The best way for people to change, he held, is by understanding the irrational, counterproductive beliefs by which they make themselves neurotic; with such beliefs an individual is a sort of ticking time bomb, waiting for some incendiary event to precipitate self-defeating consequences. Ellis even drew up a list of "twelve irrational ideas that cause and sustain emotional disturbance." They are

(1) *The idea that it is a dire necessity for an adult to be loved by everyone for everything he does . . . (2) the idea that certain acts are awful or wicked, and*

that people who perform such acts should be severely punished—instead of the idea that certain acts are inappropriate or antisocial, and that people who perform such acts are *behaving* stupidly, ignorantly or neurotically and would be better helped to change. (3) *The idea that it is horrible when things are not the way one would like them to be* . . . (4) *The idea that human misery is externally caused and is forced on one by outside people and events*— instead of the idea that emotional disturbance is caused by the *view* one takes of conditions. (5) *The idea that if something is or may be dangerous or fearsome one should be terribly upset about it*—instead of the idea that one would better frankly face it and render it non-dangerous and, when that is not possible, accept the inevitable. (6) *The idea that it is easier to avoid than to face life difficulties and self-responsibilities* . . . (7) *The idea that one needs something other or stronger or greater than oneself on which to rely* . . . (8) *The idea that one should be thoroughly competent, intelligent, and achieving in all possible respects* . . . (9) *The idea that because something once strongly affected one's life, it should indefinitely affect it* . . . (10) *The idea that one must have certain and perfect control over things* . . . (11) *The idea that human happiness can be achieved by inertia and inaction* . . . (12) *The idea that one has virtually no control over one's emotions and that one cannot help feeling certain things.*

While Ellis used some therapeutic techniques one might rightly question (assigning a shy woman to pick up men on buses, in elevators, and in the supermarket, for example), I couldn't wait to tack the twelve irrational beliefs up on my bulletin board, the better to keep myself in line; but it seemed that if reading Ellis was enough for me, I was probably a fairly rational person most of the time, and when I was being truly irrational, Ellis most likely wouldn't help. Kendall agreed. "The irrational person who's in need of the treatment is likely to go, 'I don't do that,' " he said. "Their lack of self-knowledge is part of the problem. If they're asked at pretreatment, 'Do you believe you must be liked by everyone?' they'll say no, but they might behave in a way that betrays the fact that they want to be liked by everyone. Part of the treatment is getting them to recognize that."

So Ellis wasn't perfect, but he made a good point of departure for a theorist seeking a middle ground between psychoanalysis and behaviorism. Such a theorist was the slightly senior colleague Kendall mentioned earlier, Michael J. Mahoney, then an assistant professor in the psychology department at Pennsylvania State University. Mahoney launched his 1974 book, *Cognition and Behavior Modification*, with the comment, "From birth to death, only a very small percentage of a person's behaviors is publicly observable. Our lives are predominantly composed of private responses to private environments—ranging from monologues in the shower to senile reveries . . . the pursuit of controlled scientific inquiry in this area is not only empirically justified but ethically prescribed."

Mahoney had been encouraged in his cognitive research by Skinner, whom he admired. But he also recalled student days when his instructor, only half joking, had ordained the banishment of the word *mind* from the classroom, so that even "remind me" became "re-cue me" and "slipped my mind" became "has left my current behavioral repertoire." Enough was enough, suggested Mahoney, deploring "the extreme semantic contortions sometimes employed to avoid covert or mental terms." While most behaviorists, even Skinner, had since modified the extreme positions of early theorists, there was still a legacy of aversion to "mentalistic terms" as "unscientific and hence bad." Cognitive concepts, being mentalistic, were also bad. But "humans do not passively observe some 'true reality.' On the contrary, each individual actively constructs his own private reality by selectively attending to a very small percentage of available stimulation and by organizing this select input according to a complex system of rules."

At the same time methodological behaviorism, described by Mahoney as the preference for empiricism over introspection and data over doctrine, "has not only endured but proliferated." "Right-wing" behaviorists, the Skinnerians, admitted neither inference nor statistically based research, tolerating only operant experiments on single subjects. "Left-wing" behaviorists—Mahoney counted himself one—were more flexible about methods and inferences "so long as an empirical utility is demonstrated": that is, so long as the researcher could justify his approach and the conclusions he drew from it. The left wing was bringing in a new lingo: they talked of a *"mediating variable,"* something that goes on inside a person's head that affects her response to a stimulus. These variables come in several flavors: for example, there are some that scientists have not yet observed but might someday—for example, the idea that schizophrenia is the result of a biochemical deficiency—and others that are simply impossible to verify by observation, like the idea that cigarette deprivation increases the tendency to smoke.

As Mahoney noted, Skinner and his followers observed stimulus and response and declared that whatever happened in between—inside the skull, that is—was unimportant to study. Obviously, this worked for animal and some human behaviors because, in scientific terminology, it was "parsimonious." Explaining the principle scientists call Occam's razor, after William of Occam, the fourteenth-century theologian, Mahoney said, "The principle of parsimony states that one should avoid unnecessary inferences and nonessential complexities in explaining behavior." The simpler, more conservative hypothesis is always preferable. But he asserted that "the principle of parsimony has no formal logical defense—Mother Nature doesn't owe us simplicity." Accordingly, Mahoney said, "An inference is justified if, and only if, it increases predictive accuracy or conceptual breadth."

What, then, characterizes cognitive-behaviorism as Mahoney and others laid it out in the seventies (a view that contemporary researchers have elaborated but not changed much)? The epigraph from Epictetus that heads Chapter 7 (and that, Mahoney reports, has been a rallying cry for cognitive-behaviorists) is a good start. Mahoney cites an extensive research report by Bandura (along with other work) that shows how people—to use an apt slang term—psych themselves up. "Subjects asked to imagine sexual stimuli display marked sexual arousal; those given pleasant or relaxing covert tasks exhibit calmer parasympathetic activity. Dramatic fear responses can be produced simply by cueing thoughts of an aversive stimulus."

He also draws on Bandura for the importance of modeling. "The average television viewer or newspaper reader can acquire a range of debilitating fears through vicarious classical conditioning," most notably fear of snakes, and clinics regularly report clients who fear flying but have never flown. Modeling has been helpful in eliminating both shyness and phobias like the one that paralyzed Little Hans. As Kendall pointed out in Chapter 7, choosing the right model is important for the effectiveness of the therapy; and in any case there are limits. As Bandura observed, "Factory workers would not long persist in their labors if their only reward were the occasional observation of a fellow worker receiving a paycheck."

Where do cognitive-behaviorists differ from psychodynamic therapists? Besides using simpler, more down-to-earth formulations, they don't work with the unconscious. They eschew notions like libidinal cathexis (the focusing of some imagined psychic energy) and repressed impulses that form the iconography of psychoanalysis but are "beyond the purview of even their owner . . . most inferred mediators in cognitive-behavioral research are observable by a 'public of one' (the person who is experiencing them). They need not be inferred by their owner." In other words, a cognitive-behaviorist will not explain your actions with motives you never knew you had. Moreover, cognitive-behaviorists believe personality traits can be changed by manipulating the environment; traits are not just inborn internal causes of behavior. Mahoney then reviews the various techniques developed for dealing with events inside that mysterious black box called the skull.

The first of these is what is called *covert conditioning*. It takes the Skinnerian view that covert behavior (which in this language always means thinking, not spying for the CIA) is the same as overt but more difficult to observe; it can be changed by similar conditioning techniques. In Mahoney's description, "The skull becomes a rather crowded Skinner box in which such conventional principles as reinforcement, punishment, and extinction are said to describe the patterning of private experience." A good argument for this is "method" acting: a researcher found that method actors were better able to control their physiological responses than were the old-fashioned John Gielgud or Spencer Tracy types. They did this by "the imaginal re-living of stressful experiences."

Among the earliest techniques for covert conditioning was *counterconditioning*, exemplified by the celebrated experiments in "systematic desensitization" by Joseph Wolpe, a South African psychiatrist, during the fifties, in which the therapist asked the client to imagine a series of fearful scenes and rank them in a hierarchy of terror; then the client got training in deep muscle relaxation; and finally he learned to pair the unpleasant imagining and the relaxation. The therapist hoped to weaken the bond between fearful stimuli and anxious responses. Systematic desensitization has been used with children afraid of the dark, as well as for pain tolerance, natural childbirth, and our old friend snake phobia. Some research suggested, however, that just imagining fearful situations was not always as effective as encountering them. Hence the *in vivos* that are so important to Kendall's therapy.

Some other techniques of counterconditioning are *thought-stopping*— that is, interrupting one link in the response chain, a procedure sometimes helpful with smokers, who might learn to say "Stop!" the minute they begin to think, "It's time for my after-breakfast cigarette"; *covert sensitization*, in which clients imagine nausea, pain, and social ridicule in connection with a problem behavior like excessive drinking; *covert reinforcement* (you imagine asking for a raise and then rewarding yourself with a dish of ice cream); *covert extinction* (you rehearse taking the test in your mind and gradually feel less anxious about it); and *covert modeling* (you watch someone handling snakes). Researchers are almost infinitely fussy about studying the best way to do covert conditioning—that is, working to modify what goes on inside the black box—but in the end Mahoney believes that the technique is wedded to the lab and yields only modest results in the clinic.

I asked Kendall why early behavior therapists seemed to see the whole world as if it were Ireland before Saint Patrick arrived. "Why were they so preoccupied with snake-phobia?"

Kendall gave out a tense laugh. "It's very sad in my mind, and a definite step backward that behaviorism made its impact based on studies of nonclients, snake-phobic college students. That to me is an embarrassment in our history. It was important in the development of strategies and in outcome research, but it doesn't carry the day anymore. One could argue—I wouldn't—that if you live in Wyoming and you're a phone worker, you need to deal with snakes, but a better argument is that these studies are analogs. Clients have similar behavior patterns: some people are afraid of snakes and others are afraid of intimacy, and if we learn how to treat snake-phobics we can generalize to intimacy-phobia. I'm not enthused by it."

"In one study," I said, "the stuff generalized from snakes to slugs but not to tests."

"I'm going to be a little harsh about the myth of generalization," Kendall said. "It was a claim that behaviorists made, a claim that cognitive-behaviorists made. It's not a claim that I will make. It's a myth to believe that if we train snake-phobics, they won't be afraid of slugs, spaghetti, or penises. A more contemporary view that maybe will hold water down the road is that if you're afraid of snakes and intimacy and something else, we complete the skill-building around one and then the next one and the next one. You need repeated treatment for multiple problems. After multiple experiences it will begin to transfer."

"So," I continued, "in a kind of Ellis-like way, you say, 'Things that used to frighten me now frighten me less. I'm not afraid of snakes, or tests, or slugs, so . . .' "

"You got it," said Kendall.

The next type of cognitive theory Mahoney describes works from an information-processing model: instead of being a Skinner box, the brain is a giant computer, and the individual is a busy and active processor of his own experience. Research in this area resembles that of artificial intelligence, focusing on issues like how data are stored in memory; some of Daniel Stern's theories, reported in Chapter 5, suggest this. (This approach is not palatable to Skinnerians, who would rather see humans as complex animals than flesh-and-blood computers.) Man's relationship to his environment resembles a cybernetic feedback loop; he is not a Skinnerian tabula rasa, and accordingly, neurosis is a massive information-processing failure.

One fly in the behavioristic ointment, according to cognitive theorists, is that contingencies are often misperceived. Mahoney repeats an anecdote that illustrates how: A mother, disenchanted with psychoanalysis, consulted a behavior therapist to stop her two young sons from constantly swearing. The therapist, stating two basic tenets of behavior modification, advised her first to use immediate and severe punishment every single time the swearing occurred, and second, in the interests of modeling, to be sure both sons were present whenever one son was punished. The next morning at breakfast, the older child said, "Pass the fucking Cheerios." The mother immediately lunged across the table, hit the offender, and knocked over the boy and two chairs with him. After the younger brother had helped his mother put the chairs back in order, she sweetly asked him, "And what will *you* have?" And the little boy, pleased to indicate that he'd gotten the message, replied, "You can bet your sweet ass it won't be Cheerios!"

Mahoney points out (in behaviorist jargon) that people hear what they want to hear, and that tends to be whatever might support their fallacious assumptions. Paranoid patients do this, Mahoney says; another example would be anorectics. Insight isn't enough: "Extensive investigations with emotionally disturbed children, delinquents, and psychiatric patients have shown that these individuals often lack the skills necessary for the generation of appropriate problem-solving options."

Mahoney suggests the therapist needs to help the client correct misperceptions. To Ellis's twelve core irrational ideas he adds some "common distortions in the thought patterns of distraught clients" reported by Aaron T. Beck and Arnold Lazarus, two other highly respected cognitive therapists. Since these distortions are as important to cognitive therapists as "problems in living" and "developmental stages" are to psychodynamic therapists, they merit a summary here. Beck called attention to *arbitrary inference* (interpreting "an unreciprocated letter as evidence of personal rejection"); *overgeneralization* ("failing in one heterosexual relationship implies total social incompetence"); *magnification* (what Ellis calls "catastrophizing"); and *cognitive deficiency* (ignoring important aspects of a situation, failing to put the information together, failing to learn from experience). To these Lazarus added *dichotomous reasoning* (seeing every issue as black or white) and *oversocialization* ("failure to recognize and challenge the arbitrariness of many cultural mores").

"Cognitive restructuring" for children includes mnemonics like Kendall's FEAR and STIC acronyms, as described in Chapter 7. (Mahoney uses similar ones with adult patients.) But as Mahoney reported in his 1974 book, research studies were promising but not sufficient, and his own clinical experience suggested some limits—the same as those Kendall raised. He believes Ellis's appeal to logic is just one technique for accomplishing the most important job: to modify maladaptive thinking.

The next step beyond appeals to logic is self-instruction. Mahoney points out that the importance of "private monologues" has been noted for centuries in various cultures; in recent years self-talk had acquired some of the taint of pop psychology through the writings of Émile Coué ("every day, in every way, I am getting better and better"), Dale Carnegie, and Norman Vincent Peale, and serious scientists had failed to do serious evaluations. But some good research on "covert speech" in children had been done by the Russian psychologists A. R. Luria and L. S. Vygotsky and by Donald Meichenbaum at the University of Waterloo in Canada. While much work in self-instruction had related to our old friends snake-phobia, test anxiety, and speech-giving anxiety, in general, Mahoney says, self-instructional training is empirically far more promising than Ellis's RET. The difference between self-instruction—which is quite similar to what Kendall's Anxiety Disorders Clinic does now without the *in vivos*—and "positive thinking" is that self-instruction is less global and much more specific, emphasizes graduated performance tasks instead of vague optimistic prattle, and is more cautious in its claims.

A branch of cognitive theory deals with "attribution," of which one aspect is the "locus of control" I discussed in Chapter 7. Mahoney observed that the way we try to solve our problems is influenced by what we think caused them: that is, "If our obesity, smoking, or depression are seen as caused by heredity, addiction, or a disease, we may be less likely to instigate an active self-improvement enterprise," a statement with, if anything, more resonance today than it had when Mahoney wrote it. The broader application for parents and children is that what clinicians think caused a problem directs their therapy, which is why we are taking the time to study different orientations. Mahoney noted research showing that individuals with an internal locus of control (called simply "internals") performed better than externals and were more likely to benefit from therapy, and that "institutionalized psychiatric patients, prisoners, and various minority groups" were often more external than normal control populations (sometimes for good reason, since they actually *had* less control over their destinies).

Mahoney's experience working in a group home duplicated Kendall's. In particular he told of a rebellious six-year-old enuretic boy named Aaron, for whom carefully tailored contingencies were ineffective. Then "one night I serendipitously said, 'Aaron, do you want to take your shower in the upstairs or the downstairs bathroom?' " and Aaron, who usually threw a tantrum, smiled broadly and said, "Downstairs." Since Aaron showered downstairs most of the time anyway, Mahoney was surprised at his compliance and performed "a series of ministudies which varied the presence or absence of choice and the type of choice involved. . . . Aaron's data were impressively consistent—when we gave him a choice, he complied enthusiastically. When we did not, he countercontrolled."

Mahoney remarks that "the human organism responds to a 'constructed' reality"—for example, that the glass is half full or half empty— and what reality people construct affects, most dramatically, why some do better than others. He asks what cognitive-behaviorists—most recently Kendall and his students at the Anxiety Disorders Clinic—have been asking ever since: "What is the difference between saying something to yourself and believing it?" There is plenty of speculation on how people change beliefs, but little clinical data: most of the efforts in this direction, Mahoney ruefully observes, have been confined to market research and political advertising. There is, he says, ample anecdotal evidence of the "cognitive click" (which is Sarnoff's "aha!" reaction), but some beliefs change gradually. A proper clinical program should focus both on beliefs and on behavior.

Mahoney's description of what therapy ought to do is noteworthy for its difference from the psychodynamic view: his therapy is exploring an entirely different mental turf. It is, he says, "an apprenticeship in problem-solving," with the therapist as "a technical consultant." The apprenticeship aims "to train *personal* scientists—individuals who are skillful in the functional analysis and systematic improvement of their own behavior." He sees therapeutic sessions as Socratic dialogues in which clients are encouraged to explore the data, form hypotheses, test them, come up with a choice of solutions, carry out assignments to try them out, and evaluate their progress. While all of this is geared to noninstitutionalized adults, Mahoney invited colleagues—thus Kendall—to modify it for children and adolescents.

At around the same time as Kendall read Mahoney's book, he acquired a preprint of the other book he considers crucial in shaping the way he works today, *Cognitive-Behavior Modification: An Integrative Approach* by Donald Meichenbaum, ultimately published by Plenum Press in 1977. Although he didn't actually meet Mahoney and Meichenbaum until sometime later, he was enthusiastic enough to get to know them over the phone.

Meichenbaum's particular interest was in "the thinking processes involved in performing a task, rather than merely the assessment of the product." In his doctoral research he had worked on an operant training program in which schizophrenics in a hospital were trained to use "healthy talk." Later, when the researchers examined the subjects on what they'd learned with an interview and some verbal tests, some of the schizophrenics, quite spontaneously, instructed themselves to "give healthy talk; be coherent and relevant." This self-instruction seemed to focus their attention on the task. Meichenbaum was sufficiently intrigued to explore the role of self-talk in problem-solving.

Soviet psychologists, as Mahoney had pointed out, had described the way children think out loud when first mastering a problem; then they internalize their instructions. Other researchers, including Meichenbaum himself, observed similar behavior: one psychologist, leaving three-to-seven-year-olds alone to do puzzles, discovered the younger children talked out their solutions loudly and distinctly, but as children got older they tended to mutter and move their lips; and the more self-talk the children did, whether externally or within, the better they were at puzzle-solving. Meichenbaum offers numerous illustrations of the fact that private speech initially makes things easier and then drops out of the repertoire once people master the task.

Meichenbaum, like Mahoney, asserts that behavior therapy techniques, as originally designed and carried out, have overemphasized the importance of external events and underemphasized how a client perceives and evaluates those events. At the same time "what a person says to himself . . . is explicitly modifiable by many of the behavior therapy techniques. . . . We can use . . . techniques, such as modeling, imagery manipulations, and conditioning to alter the client's internal dialogue" as well as his actions. Meichenbaum reports that behavior therapy works better, lasts longer, and is more likely to generalize when supplemented by self-instruction.

Several decades earlier American behaviorists had tried to adapt Freudian analytic techniques to learning theory: the client, they said, labeled his feelings, and the labels became learned responses that guided his future reactions. In essence, if you learned to stop saying you were anxious, you might relax a bit. Then Skinner contended, as Meichenbaum reviewed it, "that one controls his own behavior in precisely the same way that he would control the behavior of anyone else, through manipulation of the variables of which behavior is a function." As we've seen, Skinner considered thoughts just a more subtle kind of behavior. For operant behavior therapists, there's a vicious cycle in which people tell themselves they're afraid of snakes, tests, or intimacy and therefore avoid fearful encounters, and then the avoidance reinforces their fears.

Meichenbaum had been testing the theories of Wolpe and Arnold Lazarus called "anxiety-relief conditioning," in which the researcher administered a persistent electric shock to a client until the client said "calm," whereupon the shock was immediately turned off. One did this from ten to thirty times a session at thirty-to-sixty-second intervals, in hopes of teaching the client to relax himself by saying "calm." In his first study Meichenbaum tried this with phobics, in competition with a "self-instructional rehearsal" group that didn't receive the shocks and were simply taught to say "calm" and "relax" in fearful situations, and a waiting-list control group. The anxiety relief group—the people with the electric shocks—did significantly better than the others in altering anxious feelings and behavior.

But the clients who improved the most in the first study claimed they had "covertly employed other coping verbalizations," which in English means they embellished a bit, telling themselves, "Relax. I can handle the snake. One step at a time." So Meichenbaum embellished too with the next group of subjects, teaching them the same sort of phrases and hinging the termination of the shock on the client's repeating the longer mantra. Moreover, Meichenbaum made the shock a sort of punishment: first the therapist said, "Snake"; then the client was asked to express his fearful thoughts, and as soon as he did he got the shock; then the client made the coping statements, and the shock was turned off.

At the same time Meichenbaum set up a control group that received "inverted anxiety relief": that is, the therapist said, "Snake," and the client said, "Relax. I can handle the snake. One step at a time," whereupon the shock was turned on; as soon as the client said something like, "It's ugly; I won't look at it," the shock went off. To Meichenbaum's enormous surprise, both of these groups became less fearful, and each of them did much better than the group that got traditional one-word Wolpe-Lazarus statements. Other studies appeared in which clients got aversive conditioning without the shock—by being asked to imagine fearful scenes or unpleasant images that were unrelated to their particular phobia—or the inverted conditioning Meichenbaum had tried. The results were equally effective. The studies were showing no consistent relationship between the type of covert conditioning and the response.

So Meichenbaum asked the clients who had received inverted anxiety relief what they thought was happening. It turned out that they believed they were delivering the coping statements ("I can handle the snake") in order to prepare themselves for the shock and using the fearful statements as a signal to turn off the shock. In essence, the clients "were learning a set of coping skills that could be employed *across* situations, including confronting the phobic object." So Meichenbaum started teaching coping skills, which he called "stress inoculation training."

Meichenbaum neatly differentiates between pure cognitive therapists like Ellis and Beck, who "listen for the *presence* of maladaptive self-statements, assumptions, and beliefs," and those like himself who listen "for the *absence* of specific, adaptive cognitive skills and responses." In lay English; having a distorted view of the world is only one part of the problem; the other is simply being ignorant of how to help oneself. At this point Meichenbaum expresses the ideas we have seen practiced in Kendall's therapy: one assesses the client's internal dialogue—the way he interprets what's happening—and how that dialogue affects his feelings, his physiological responses, and his ultimate behavior. (The point of calling this a "dialogue" and not a "monologue," as Meichenbaum most crucially later states, is that not only do people talk to themselves, they also listen to what they are saying.) Some examples of this include how a student taking the SAT interprets the early departure of others in the room, or how another student explains her failing a test ("the test was unfair" or "I didn't study enough," both of which might actually be true). We are back to attribution theory and locus of control.

Meichenbaum reports a fascinating illustration of the way attitudes can affect physiology—not a new idea to the modern reader after Norman Cousins's books on self-healing, and certainly not a clear-cut link. Back in 1962 a team of psychologists interviewed patients with psychosomatic complaints (ulcers, asthma, and hives) about what had been happening in their lives just before the last attack, and they tied each patient's thought processes to the appropriate disorder. Then they hypnotized a group of healthy subjects and asked them to feel the attitudes expressed by various sick patients. The hypnotized normals experienced the same symptoms as the patients they'd been matched with.

Inner speech, Meichenbaum says, alters not only behavior but also *cognitive structures*—that is, the way one interprets the world. All of this is most similar to Daniel Stern's "sense of a verbal self" (see Chapter 5), which "permits the child to construct a narrative of his own life"; and in fact it evokes the basic psychodynamic distinction between "object relations" and "interpersonal relations," those with the mother as imagined and those with the mother in real life. It is a theme that recurs throughout the theoretical canon of every therapeutic orientation, one more illustration of the way intelligent trained observers describe the same phenomena in different languages. The goal of therapy, in Meichenbaum's view (and indeed in Mahoney's and Kendall's view), is to trigger a "virtuous cycle" in which inner speech, cognitive structures, behavior, and the consequences of behavior work together to achieve a beneficial outcome.

Meichenbaum applied his theories to work with impulsive, hyperactive children, who notably lack the ability to plan their actions. He studied the private speech of impulsive preschool children and found it differed in quality, not quantity, from that of their reflective peers. The impulsive children's private speech was "self-stimulatory" (word play, animal noises, singing), while the more mature reflective children's was "self-regulatory." Other researchers had also shown that impulsive children do not spontaneously analyze what is happening to them or make useful rules to guide themselves in learning. Meichenbaum devised a program in which an adult modeled a problem-solving task while talking it through; next the child followed the adult's instructions; then the child talked himself through the task; then the child whispered the instructions to himself; and finally he thought it through while doing it. The adult had demonstrated defining the problem, concentrating on it, directing his own responses, reinforcing himself, evaluating his own performance, and correcting his mistakes. The training proceeded through increasingly difficult assignments.

The results were promising; alumni of the program did better on IQ tests than the placebo and assessment control groups. A month later more than half the kids were still talking to themselves while solving problems. Meichenbaum continued to fine-tune his training. Other self-instructional programs had achieved similar results, but none had been studied over the long term. And Meichenbaum asked, "I wonder if we are merely rediscovering the potency of reasoning."

Kendall, Mahoney, Meichenbaum, and their colleagues continue to explore that potency. As we will see in the next chapter, the territory of the cognitive-behaviorists—the realm of the ego or Freud's "secondary process thinking"—is a fruitful land that psychodynamic therapists traverse hurriedly, like tourists whizzing through Iowa on the way to the coast. While the psychodynamic therapists alone have thought carefully about the dark irrational mental processes, they have given short shrift to the way human beings filter and organize information, an area the cognitive theorists have studied in detail. At the same time much of the groundwork of cognitive theory was done with electric shocks, snakes, and other unrealistic situations; the results that cognitive-behaviorists measure are narrowly focused and still relatively short term. The psychodynamic tribe claims a lock on profundity; the cognitive-behaviorists insist they've cornered the market in rigor. In a sense each tribe is exalting its own limitation.

CHAPTER 9

ENLARGING THE REPERTOIRE

*Human beings attend to or disregard the world in which they live.
They search for things in that world. They generalize from one thing to
another. They discriminate. They respond to single features or special
sets of features as "abstractions" or "concepts." They solve problems by
assembling, classifying, arranging, and rearranging things. They
describe things and respond to their descriptions, as well as to descriptions made by others. They analyze the contingencies of reinforcement
in their world and extract plans and rules which enable them to
respond appropriately without direct exposure to the contingencies.
They discover and use rules for deriving new rules from old. In all this,
and much more, they are simply behaving, and that is true even when
they are behaving covertly. Not only does a behavioral analysis not
reject any of those "higher mental processes"; it has taken the lead in
investigating the contingencies under which they occur. What it rejects
is the assumption that comparable activities take place in the mysterious world of the mind.*

—B. F. Skinner,
About Behaviorism (1974)

KENDALL'S COLLEAGUES, NO LESS THAN SARNOFF'S, attach significance
to a child's history. But they don't portray that history as the source of
traumas or unresolved conflicts that block development; rather they view
it in terms of what the child has or hasn't learned that governs her
behavior. On the cognitive side, children with behavior disorders may
have a "skills deficit": no one has taught them—or set an example of—
constructive ways to solve problems and cope with disturbing feelings.
On the behavioral side, their families, schools, or friends may have

presented a system of punishments and rewards that—however subtly or inadvertently—offered incentives to act inappropriately. Practitioners vary in the weight they assign to the cognitive and the behavioral explanations, and thus they tailor their treatment.

Cognitive-behavioral therapy seems more adaptable than psychodynamic because it can accommodate a variety of goals: children with incurable disorders can be taught to manage them and so make a slightly better life, while those with small problems, or difficulty negotiating the challenges of development, might learn to cope and need no more than an occasional touch-up later on. There appears to be no disorder in the DSM to which either pure behaviorists or cognitive-behaviorists haven't turned their attention, sometimes working in concert with therapists from other orientations (though least often, of course, with the psychodynamic practitioners). Oddly enough, their work seems more compelling when it's part of a varied treatment plan for clients with big problems than when it aims to fix milder disorders all by itself, and it must struggle with the challenges of applying and maintaining what the child has learned in the world outside the clinic. But cognitive-behavioral therapists in private practice, of course, may tend toward eclecticism, without the requirement for purity laid on by a research setting.

Kendall's approach—which is as cognitive as behaviorists get—has been applied to a host of different problems. Since the utmost irrationality, one might argue, stems from anger, a natural emotion that's often mismanaged (and thus plays a little bit of havoc with all our lives and destroys some lives utterly), I was particularly intrigued by the work of Eva Feindler, Ph.D., an associate professor of clinical psychology at Long Island University and a clinician in private practice, and her former student, Randolph Ecton, M.A., now a psychologist at Sagamore Children's Psychiatric Center on Long Island, who have for more than a decade, first together and then individually, been developing cognitive-behavioral training therapy for anger control. Two colleagues of Ecton's at Sagamore, Deborah Kingsley and Dennis R. Dubey, collaborated on some of the early work.

This appeared to me to be the ideal test of what a cognitive-behavioral approach might do: after all, a substantial portion of anger comes from distorted thinking. An outburst of temper exemplifies all the errors in logic that Ellis, Beck, Mahoney, and Meichenbaum delineate, combined with what practitioners call "externalizing" behavior. Could a treatment that focused on Freud's "secondary process thinking"—which aims to ward off explosions by making clients more conscious of and rational about their actions—be effective? Could you reason away emotions? How far could therapy go without regarding anger, in the psychodynamic manner, as an expression of the primary aggressive drive, an archaeological challenge whose buried origins need to be excavated and redirected?

Back in the late seventies, when Feindler and various colleagues began work on a therapeutic training regime they called "The Art of Self-Control," they were mindful of the same problems Kendall had noticed as a graduate student: that traditional behavior modification programs were not working with aggressive adolescents, and that attempts to teach the missing skills by behavioral training were only partly successful—while the new skills appeared, the old behavior didn't abate. Some earlier forays into cognitive-behavioral strategies for anger control had shown promise but hadn't dealt with the most severely disturbed teenaged clients.

A recent book edited by Philip Kendall contains a chapter by Feindler on anger-control methods in which she sums up the cognitive-behavioral formulation of anger as a stress reaction with three components, the cognitive, the physiological, and the behavioral. The cognitive part embraces which situations provoke us and how we interpret them: we are more apt to lash out when we perceive we have been thwarted by someone who means ill. Feindler believes this component of anger is most significant in work with aggressive adolescents because it sparks a particularly dangerous combination of intense feelings and limited skills to deal with them. And she cites a study of six hundred subjects in which "early aggressiveness in school was found to be predictive of later serious antisocial behavior including criminal behavior, spouse abuse, traffic violations, and self-reported physical aggression." The distorted worldview leads to habitual patterns of aggression as children mature.

Angry, aggressive teenagers typically don't know how to keep themselves from flying off the handle: they lack the inhibiting "self-statements" that Meichenbaum describes, and in problem-solving exercises they are hard put to come up with alternative responses or anticipate the consequences of their behavior. Accordingly, Feindler and Ecton have incorporated five stages of problem-solving: defining the problem; brainstorming for alternative solutions; evaluating the desirable and undesirable results of each solution; choosing the best one; and deciding how well it worked.

Educated adults, whether or not they are successful in carrying out these steps, at least understand what they ought to be doing; for teenagers with a skills deficit, problem-solving is a novel activity.

One of the distorted perceptions characteristic of aggressive children (and adults too, presumably) is the tendency to assume that other people's intentions are hostile and require retaliation; therefore the therapist teaches them "forgiving" or "accidental" interpretations (such as, "He probably didn't mean it, he was just trying to get my attention," or, "He was just joking"). Feindler reports, among other literature, a corroborating study of this idea among a group of teenage delinquents in a state prison compared with two groups of high school students, one rated highly aggressive and one rated not very aggressive by their peers. Surprisingly, however, the juvenile delinquents were least likely to believe that victims get what they deserve; one researcher hypothesized the delinquents "have also frequently been victims themselves." Beliefs about aggression, it turned out, were related to gender, with the boys more inclined to assume hostility without checking their assumptions, and the girls more likely to blame victims.

But while the authors of this study succeeded in training the delinquents to modify beliefs and solve problems, the delinquents continued to violate parole at the same rate as before. Thus psychologists designing anger-control programs must wrestle with the issues of generalization and maintenance, the bête noir of all behaviorists.

Another perception that affects behavior is the way people anticipate the results of that behavior. Assorted studies suggest that aggressive children may believe striking back will remove some annoyance or restore their self-respect; the probability that unhappy consequences will accrue to them as well as to their victims depends on whether the aggression is provoked and on whether it is aimed at the same or the opposite sex. While research thus favors teaching children to ponder the consequences of striking back, it also emphasizes that penalties must be "short-term, practical, and highly probable" to be effective; one study proposes that threatened punishments work only when "potential aggressors are *not* very angry," when "they have relatively little to gain from aggressive behavior," when "the magnitude of punishment anticipated is great," and when "the probability that such unpleasant treatment will be delivered is high."

Feindler's program was designed for use on teenagers in a variety of settings, and it later proved helpful for more than four hundred conduct-disordered teenagers. In one study the authors tried it out on 21 teenage boys who were inpatients at Sagamore, as well as on a waiting-list control group.

The subjects had been hospitalized for around a year. Most had below-average intelligence; two-thirds were white, one was Latino, and the rest were African-American; and the majority had aggressive conduct disorders. The authors gave three standard tests and a videotaping of role-play exercises, as well as evaluation by staff, to measure results. These techniques are similar to those Kendall uses in the Anxiety Disorders Clinic: here the tapes recorded eleven classes of verbal and nonverbal behavior (inappropriate or hostile comments, hands in pockets, eye contact, and so forth).

The eight-week training program included deep breaths and relaxation, homework assignments like a daily "hassle sheet" for the boys to describe how they handled conflicts, discussions of situations that triggered anger, techniques for responding to aggression and cooling down conflict without forfeiting one's rights, self-statements for controlling anger ("Keep cool," "Chill out"), procedures for thinking about the unfavorable consequences of losing one's temper, and practice in rating one's own behavior.

At the end of the program, the participants made more appropriate requests and decreased their hostile comments and "negative physical contact" (presumably they hit other people less, but the jargon doesn't specify) compared with the way they had acted before, while controls got worse over the same period. Some other behavior that reflected social skills didn't change much. More important though, the treatment subjects showed lower rates of breaking ward rules, while once again the control group's behavior deteriorated. By most measures the training helped, and at a booster session two months later the boys had maintained their skills; at three-year follow-up, 18 out of 21 of the subjects had been discharged.

One day I went out to watch Ecton, an informally dressed man in his mid-thirties, lead a group at Sagamore, which is a state-run psychiatric hospital for children from six to eighteen. The group I was to see consisted of teenage girls who were variously conduct-disordered, oppositional, depressed, and suicidal; about half had been physically or sexually abused. A stay at Sagamore might range from two weeks to two years. "The psychiatric hospitals are the dumping ground in New York State," Ecton told me. "Sagamore deals with the most out-of-control kids in the state of New York."

Ecton had come to Sagamore for a practicum in 1980, worked with Feindler on the anger-control program, and a couple of years later was doing group work with all the patients in the hospital and individual therapy for those who were so out of control that they couldn't succeed in the groups. Since then he has trained seventy-five to a hundred kids a year, depending on the hospital's finances, and has also taught parents and staff.

The girls in the group would range in intelligence from mildly retarded to high-average, and unlike the research projects I'd been reading about, in which everyone started and finished together, the group would include intermediates with several sessions under their belts as well as new-comers Ecton hadn't met yet.

Among them was Keshia, a fourteen-year-old of barely normal intel-ligence who'd been in and out of the hospital for the past couple of years; she and her brother, also a patient, had been taken from an abusive family and were unable to remain in foster care because of their aggressive outbursts. Keshia was "somewhat psychotic" and would probably never live independently. Danielle, on the other hand, aged thirteen, was learning-disabled, had been physically abused, and was "here for opposi-tional defiance. She was in a day treatment program and was self-abusive, banging her head and biting herself and slashing her wrists. She's been here about five months, and I worked with her individually first. She has become a little more verbal in group. She comes from an intact family so she might go home."

Brigitte, the brightest, a fourteen-year-old, had "posttraumatic stress disorder. Most of these kids do. A good percentage of them have orders of protection. She's been sexually and physically abused, and she's very self-injurious, very acting-out—but she's a real workable kid." I realized Ecton talked like a warrior in the trenches, using the lingo of hospitals and courts as a shorthand and reckoning which of the damned had a glimmer of hope. We went down the list, reviewing girls like Jane, who had been on and off "one-to-one" and "close observation" for two or three months. "One-to-one is when staff is assigned particularly to that patient for the entire shift," Ecton explained. "Close observation is when staff is assigned to a patient who's not allowed out of their sight, but can also supervise other kids. She's been taking pencils and pens and erasers and mutilating her arms, rubbing her forehead on the carpet, head-banging." He was balancing the more and less "needy," the "verbal," and the "verbal-with-prompting."

A flip chart in Ecton's office had the "anger triggers" from the previous session, which included "Teachers think they have full control and can run your life"; "When people push you, when someone provokes you on purpose to get hit"; "Fat people smell and get in my face and make fun of you"; "When they talk about mothers"; "Injustice"; "People who lie"; "When I'm upset and someone tries to talk to me and I don't want to"; "When people fart and don't say excuse me"; "Don't give you respect"; and a host of others.

The anger-triggers part of the training was a miniature talking cure, as I discovered watching a session in which the girls, most of them pretty and provocatively dressed, had infinite suggestions for what got in their faces; during this there was a lot more poking and touching and louder laughter than one would see in, say, Huntington High, but Ecton kept the class rolling, leaving minute interventions to the staffers, who hung out on the fringe. But the comments seemed more pointed than those on the earlier chart—"when people use group to diss other people" for example—and Ecton said some of the triggers were actually direct missiles to others in the room. None of this sounded like a canned behaviorist research paper: the lesson plan seemed a skeleton on which unpredictable emotional flesh and different kinds of psychological messy clothing could easily be hung.

After the class Ecton allowed that there was no perfect control of anger, but he ran me through the course, which included a sequence of five prosaic-sounding steps, beginning with "stop and freeze"; after that came "calm down the body," "think positive thoughts," "listen for understanding," and finally "act positively." They sounded like Norman Vincent Peale until you thought at length and in great detail, at your own intellectual level (whatever that might be), about the trigger in question. If you did this in a group with a leader, you were getting training; if you did it individually with Ecton focusing on you, it was therapy. Perhaps the most difficult of the five steps was "listen for understanding," which also meant getting the adversary to clarify what he means, looking him in the eye, and nodding to present a nonthreatening demeanor. "One way to de-escalate anger is to comment on it," said Ecton. " 'You look angry,' or 'You sound angry.' "

This was hard enough for me, let alone for Keshia, Danielle, Brigitte, and Jane: as Ecton pointed out, "out-of-control anger is learned. We learn how to lose control by watching people in our life, by the instructions that are given to us and by the reactions we get throughout life." I couldn't imagine the girls navigating life successfully without learning some of these skills, and at the same time they didn't seem sufficient; indeed, Sagamore residents got all sorts of therapy, both individual and group, in addition to the anger-control classes. (How do psychiatric inpatients spend their time? They take a lot of meetings.)

While I was discovering that cognitive-behavioral therapy is far less cut-and-dried than its literature suggests, I still sought to learn how a research strategy for anger control played out in private practice. For this I talked with Eva Feindler, who works with less severely disturbed patients in conflict-ridden families. What I called "the cookbook approach," Feindler said, "can be a very effective educational piece, but many times these kids still need more traditional types of therapy."

Aggressive teenagers are often just depressed, Feindler told me: "They hate their lives, they hate their families, they don't look forward to their futures, they feel hopeless and helpless. More typically adolescent males act out on that depression, while adolescent females get into sadness and despair and internalize it. The anger-control training enables them to manage their environments so they can get through a day without fighting, but it doesn't necessarily answer the underlying things."

Historical background is important even to a behaviorist, Feindler said, in answer to my question: a child's trouble separating from mother at nursery school age may signal early anxiety, and "how the mother attended to that and reinforced dependency will actually predict later difficulties in her interaction with the child. It's a dance that gets established early on, and the child gets older but the dance many times stays the same. It isn't genetically driven, and therefore it's changeable. It's important to show parents they can dance differently."

Feindler says she is teaching kids about "choice, what it's reasonable to stay angry about and what doesn't make any sense to stay angry about. If your parents got divorced when you were five, and you've been angry about that for the past seven years and you're still angry at your father for leaving your mother, that's anger that you can maintain so it can grow and blossom and continue to fuel aggressive behavior during your future. Or you can recognize that as a negative thing your dad did, and you can leave that anger in the past and move on.

"The other message I give to kids is that it's okay to be angry, it's what you do with your anger. A lot of good things come out of anger. You can move mountains with anger: a lot of political change, a lot of social change comes out of anger, but it's channeled anger. It's not impulsive aggression, which is 'take this chair and throw it through the window.' That won't solve anything. You're mad at your mother because of what happened between her and your father; learn to tell her directly, 'I'm angry with you and I don't like what you did and I don't want to live with you anymore.' "

As an example, Feindler told me about thirteen-year-old Adam; her story had as rich a texture as one of, say, Sarnoff's or Thompson's, but it was woven somewhat differently. "He's highly aggressive at home toward his younger brother: he likes to punch him, push him around—he's rather unsuccessful in his social relationships, which is why he focuses more on his family. He doesn't have a set of friends that he hangs out with because he gets into fights and he's rejected, so he ends up spending a lot more time with his parents and his brother than the normal thirteen-year-old, and he's angry that he's not out there playing soccer or basketball. He's not particularly athletic either. So his mother will say, 'Clean up your room,' or 'You didn't feed the cat,' and he gets very aggressive toward her.

"A kid like that will need some socialization in a group setting, but he has to be willing to accept that, and typically the attitude is, 'I don't have any problems, stay out of my face, I'm not going to therapy.' These are parents who are both musicians, they're very dramatic, they have a creative flair. But they're also volatile and hot-tempered, and they often fight with each other. So he has grown up in an environment where he's witnessed a dramatic display of anger, father stalking out in the middle of the night—'That's it! I'm not coming back!'—only to be back later.

"They're intellectual parents, very verbal, but also somewhat frightened by this thirteen-year-old's aggressive style toward them. He really dominates the family. And he's got what we call a coercive interaction pattern going—if he makes enough of a tantrum and a stink, if he yells and screams and throws things, hits his head against the wall, they eventually give in. So they feel they don't have any power. They end up saying 'All right, we'll take you to the movies, we'll give you ten dollars, we'll buy you new lacrosse shorts.' So he's very persistent because he usually wins out. He wears them down.

"In this family it may have started with the parents trying to nip it in the bud by giving in to the child's aggressiveness. It's hard to ignore. It's hard to look the other way. We ignore a lot of inappropriate things kids do, and those things drop out of the repertoire. If you don't attend to cursing when they start at age three, they don't know what the words mean and they'll drop out. But these parents were very sensitive and attended to all his aggression—'Stop hitting your brother'—so he got his attention. And he'd lost his position as the only child, so he resented his little brother.

"He has a mild case of what's called obsessive-compulsive disorder, in which he becomes very obsessed around a topic: he wants to earn five dollars to buy something and he'll berate his parents: 'How can I earn the money? Tell me how I can earn it. I need the five dollars by Friday.' And he escalates to the point where they give him the money to avoid physical conflict. His OCD doesn't involve a behavioral ritual like washing, it just involves an internal obsessional quality where he gets locked into it and very anxious. He's been on medication and it's helped somewhat, but he's anxious about being out of control. That's what OCD is about, attempting to control things so you don't feel anxious, and with a preadolescent who's already in a control battle with his parents, you have a very volatile family situation."

So how was Feindler unsnarling all this?

"I teach the parents some discipline strategies for ignoring inappropriate behavior and setting up contingencies, so if he doesn't have tantrums on a particular day, then he's earned a certain portion of his allowance: that's the behavioral approach. Then I'm exploring with the parents their underlying cognitions, the ones of 'We don't have any control,' 'We're lousy parents,' 'We can't go on living like this.' As they think those things, their behavior toward Adam becomes more impulsive and inconsistent. There's a sort of divisiveness around it. Adam treats the mother poorly and his father gets involved, and she says, 'Leave me alone, I'll take care of this,' and they start to war. So I'm working to change their perspectives so they're still the parents, even though he's loud and obnoxious. I'm trying to change their perceptions of themselves as parents and at the same time give them actual intervention strategies."

I asked Feindler if she thought the parents had problems with each other and used Adam to express them. It was one hypothesis, she said. The parents did have "issues" of their own, but since Adam's aggressiveness was so consistent with peers and in school, she was not convinced it was just part of the family dysfunction. "I would never see the parents without the adolescent," she continued, "because it just breeds a paranoia that's typical of adolescents anyway. It ruins the therapeutic bond. So I'll see the whole family and then ask the parents to leave, and I'll spend the last part of the session with Adam.

"My focus with him is much more on gaining self-control, recognizing early on that he is feeling angry and what he is irritable about. Usually in the summertime it's, 'I'm bored, I don't have anybody to play with. Why don't I have any friends?' What that generates is a combination of anxiety and anger. He resents his so-called friends, he resents his neighbors, he resents his parents because they made him move to this neighborhood, and as he gets angry he begins to look for an outlet. I'm working with him on changing that negative tape he plays and replacing it with what I call a problem-solving tape. We go into some social-skills training, we do role-plays. We'll identify a possible friend and rehearse making a phone call. It's better to have a plan—'Do you want to go to the movies?' as opposed to, 'Do you want to hang out?' We go through all the nuances of socialization, and then he's given a homework assignment where he has to try it.

"I'm also teaching him to control his temper when he does feel himself begin to blow. He needs to stop and do what we call a kick-back, which is to move back from it for a few minutes, take some deep breaths, and sit by himself and think about what he wants to say to his parents instead of impulsively telling them off. I'm trying to get him to use words in a more appropriate way, to say, 'Look, I'm having a bad day. I'm bored, I have no one to play with. Could you guys help me out with some ideas?' It's a reasonable thing to ask.

"So it's a multifaceted approach, working on the overt behaviors of the conflict and the behavioral deficits of the lack of socialization, and then what's underneath it, the self-defeating thinking. He thinks he's no good, no one likes him. The parents are thinking, 'We have no control, we're ineffective parents.' Those negative thoughts will breed negative behavior patterns, so if you change them as well as the surface behaviors, you make some progress."

I asked Feindler how long all this would take, and she estimated "about six months, once a week, to make a dent."

Nowadays her work with actual delinquents is indirect, training teachers and staff in schools and hospitals who return to their institutions and run groups similar to Ecton's. Institutional work is tougher not only because the children are more troubled but because there is less opportunity to do the custom tailoring that is effective in private practice, the children have fewer supportive adults in their families and schools, and "they're living in a culture with their peers and there's a group mentality as well." But violence-prevention programs are beginning to spread in the schools, including, Feindler says, "how to negotiate your way through your life without violence and aggression. If it's in the schools, the community, the media, if it's all around, then we have a shot at it, giving kids an alternative way to solve their problems other than by the use of weapons."

Behaviorists, as we've seen, distinguish themselves from psychodynamic and family systems therapists by their effort to measure and quantify success; Feindler's research papers include the appropriate measurements of short-term effectiveness noted earlier. I asked her what she knew about how well the programs worked over the long term in diminishing aggressive behavior. "It's difficult to do follow-ups, even on institutional populations, because you lose them. And I think really it's suspect. What's the level of change, and what is significant change? In my view if people change ten percent on whatever variable you're measuring, it's better than no percent. So it's not as great as eighty percent but it's something. From a clinical basis, to me any change is significant. Also measurement of anger and aggressiveness in children, particularly adolescents, is difficult. They're not aggressive in front of adults—it's all private."

"They get arrested," I said.

"But eighty percent of the kids who are aggressive don't get arrested," Feindler said. "It's only the stupid ones that get caught. The best delinquents never get caught, so even police records are not good sources of program evaluation. How do we measure, how do we know that we've impacted them?"

"If they can keep a job or a relationship," I suggested.

"Those are good questions to ask, but even if you get the answers, you can't make the inference that it was due to your treatment or your lack of treatment. There are so many other things that influence people from the follow-up times to the next follow-up times, which is why it's important to have control groups."

Feindler considers herself "probably eclectic" in clinical practice because she works with families as well as individual children and on occasion uses play therapy with younger children; but the way she describes a problem is clearly cognitive-behavioral. Like Kendall, she doesn't dismiss the work of therapists in other orientations. But she faults them for failure to assess results scientifically. It's important to recognize that the behaviorists' efforts at assessment are very preliminary and limited; a meaningful decision on whether a therapy really "works" is elusive, and thus the attempts at measurement—however commendable—are not in themselves evidence that behavioral therapy is always more helpful than other approaches.

Nonetheless, I was intrigued by the behaviorists' insistence on taking nothing for granted, subjecting the most minute and obvious beliefs to empirical questioning. As I spent time among behavioral psychologists, I learned that some were less cognitive than Kendall, Feindler, and Ecton; at the same time there seems to be an implicit cognitive orientation even in more purely behavioral research, since the research is there to challenge what therapists think they know about the world. This idea seemed particularly compelling when I looked at the work of Sharon L. Foster, Ph.D., now a professor at the California School of Professional Psychology in San Diego. Foster is a researcher with no current clinical practice, and she has in recent years been occupied with discovering what makes kids popular and unpopular.

Lay people tend to assume that all psychologists and psychiatrists attribute mental health problems to some combination of biology and parenting, and to a large extent this is true. But the importance of friendships (in behaviorist jargon, peer relations) in life is attracting increasing interest: while loneliness and rejection may not be the cause of mental disorders, they certainly exacerbate them.

Research on what makes some people likeable and others lonely has been done for at least fifty years, but it seems to have gathered impetus in the past decade. Some of the conclusions of these studies appear very obvious—warm, outgoing, cheerful people tend to be popular, for example—but on closer examination it's not quite so simple.

Most of us, over the course of our lives, acquire ideas about what it takes to be socially successful, which we pass on to our children. They are part of what psychologists call our cognitive schema, which may vary tremendously from one person to another. The children, forming schemata of their own, accept some of our biases and reject others, and in most cases that works reasonably well. But some children, for whatever reason, have trouble making friends. They may become the clients of therapists and of social skills training programs, which are—unless the material has been researched—infused with the therapists' own cognitive biases. So what are the skills that ought to be taught, and how can such training be improved?

Before talking to Foster—a suitably pleasant, cheerful, and friendly woman who is a contemporary of Kendall and Feindler—I read a collection of her papers and gradually became drawn to an article called "Adolescent Friendships and Peer Acceptance: Implications for Social Skills Training," by Foster and a colleague with the memorable name of Heidi Inderbitzen-Pisaruk. The article is a literature survey, telling us what is known and not known by researchers and providing a good example of how these researchers work.

The texture of friendships changes in adolescence. Studies say teenagers attach more emphasis to loyalty and trust, and therefore, adolescents may need to learn different social skills from those required by children and adults. There are two classes of literature in this area, the authors report: one that studies behavior that attracts or repels, and one that deals with the nature of teenage friendships.

Studies of peer acceptance tend to follow either of two methods: the researchers have the kids rate particular peers they like or dislike and then answer questions about all the peers' behavior; or they ask subjects to rate the importance of particular kinds of behavior in the abstract. It is useful, Foster and her co-author point out, to distinguish between rejection and neglect.

Despite some fussiness over the quality of the studies, the authors stress one message: the criteria for acceptance and rejection are different and don't overlap, so kids need to learn both what to do and what not to do.

Adolescents set store by cooperativeness, good looks and grooming, "unsolicited gifts, loans, or favors," humor, compliance, and initiative in group games and activities. They particularly don't like aggressiveness, problems with temper control, disruptiveness (thus supporting Feindler and Ecton's work), "excessive help-seeking," and bossiness. Another bunch of mannerisms children might correct are not being able to take teasing, showing off, violating rules, talking too loudly or too softly, too quickly or too slowly, standing too close or too far away (these sound like a researcher's categories), being a poor sport, and tattling.

Some questions may occur to the lay reader: Do Mom and Dad know how to help with this stuff? Are they willing to face what their children do or don't do? Will their kids accept help from Mom and Dad if it's offered? Has a neutral adult a better chance of success than parents? Perhaps the perceptions that seem obvious about other people's children (and accordingly not worth the time or money involved in hiring a professional) elude us about our own; perhaps, after all, the lonely child would benefit from a lesson or two.

Studies of teenage friendship reflect both gender and age differences, with an overall bent toward loyalty, trust, and intimacy that exceeds that of children and adults. Boys and younger teen and preteen girls seem interested in having compliant friends, while middle- and late-adolescent girls seek something more substantial and sophisticated. The authors point out that different abilities are necessary for initiating and maintaining friendships. Since teenagers are drawn to each other because of shared interests, lonely adolescents must acquire the skills for identifying these and for disclosing thoughts and feelings, demonstrating loyalty, and maintaining trust. How one acts out these global qualities remains to be determined. Conversational training may help; "gradual, reciprocal self-disclosure, eventually confiding one's problems, may be a skill that underlies intimacy."

Current programs don't work well enough, the authors state. Most training programs focus on things like eye contact and voice tone, which are not the particular conversational skills that bring peer status, and teenagers are trained in twosomes when they need to learn to operate in a group. Moreover, friendship involves a sequence of behavior in a particular context, and skills should be taught that way. Assessment of whether a program works should be tied not to performance tests but to whether the subjects gain closer and more lasting friendships.

What this and Foster's other papers were doing was training a microscope on the obvious, and I found it sobering to look through the lens. I asked what had drawn her to research subjects that seemed intuitively evident. "Back in 1977 I was on an internship where they asked me to design a social skills training program. So I began thinking, 'What are we going to teach these kids?' I realized that everything I would think of teaching was from my own adult perspective. I had heard about a colleague who was trying to teach a ten-year-old boy how to make friends, and he taught the kid to walk up and say, 'How do you do? My name is So-and-so' and shake hands. Of course, I thought this was about the nerdiest thing you could ever do. It was not how fifth-grade kids would initiate conversations. But how *would* they? I really didn't know."

"As a parent you watch," I said. "I think they sniff each other."

"They do. As a parent *you* might watch, and so you anticipate a whole host of literature that exists on how kids enter groups. Now we have a research base, but we didn't before. And in fact the effective kids sniff around. It's kind of like how effective adults enter cocktail parties. If you want to join a conversation you go up, hang on the edges, listen to what they're talking about, kind of figure it out, and eventually start to mimic the behavior of others. You're not too intrusive, and you throw in a little comment. Kids do the same thing, only more with games and physical things than with verbal things.

"We also know that for most kids the first time they try to get into a group, they don't get in. You're going to be rebuffed, so you have to keep trying."

"What if your temperament is not to deal well with that or understand it?" I asked. "Then off you go and that's that and you're depressed."

"Or if your temperament is impulsive," Foster said, "and your first try doesn't work. Then you call all kinds of inappropriate attention to yourself to get them to pay attention to you as part of the group. If you're more appropriate then, you're kind of patient, and you hang out and wait your turn, and eventually with prosocial strategies you can get into the group. Or as with adults at a cocktail party, if that group doesn't want you, you move on to a group that does.

"There are a whole host of these strategies that are fairly complex, and the more I began to think about it, the more I came to realize that what I thought as an adult might really not be what is important to kids. In the early seventies there were a lot of intervention studies taking shy, withdrawn kids or kids who were having problems with their peers, to teach them to interact more frequently with other kids. Then the question became, 'Does frequency of interaction really mean anything, or is the quality of the interaction more important?' Again people began to question whether the things adults chose to teach kids were really important."

"If you had a kid from a very pleasant nurturing family," I asked, "and the kid was all right in other ways, could he still be in a neighborhood where the other kids picked on him? If a kid is all right, will he be all right in any neighborhood?"

"Not necessarily," Foster said. "We don't know the full story of how kids move into poor peer relations, but I think your point is important, that there hasn't been much emphasis on the peer group and its role in both adaptive and maladaptive socialization. As I was getting interested in all this, one doesn't exist in a vacuum and other people were getting interested from different vantage points. Mine was whether there's such a thing as a *generic* social skill. What kinds of things should we be teaching kids that are truly going to make an impact on their relationships with peers, and what's peripheral? My second question was, How do kids make judgments about who they like and who they don't like, and how does their social behavior play into that?

"Now it turns out there's quite a bit of literature to show that problems with one's peers at early ages, in elementary school, can predict a host of problems later on, such as bad-conduct discharges from the military, delinquency, dropout and absenteeism and school problems in teenage years, and contact with mental health services.

"The problem with longitudinal studies is it's hard to do good research, because for one thing nobody's going to fund you for over twenty years. Another way is you get the idea and look backward, but that's a problem because you're picking a select population. If you want to look prospectively, do longitudinal studies, even if you get the money, measurement, and methodology people will say today's state-of-the-art is pretty primitive twenty years from now."

When Foster talked about the difficulty of producing training programs that work, I said, "A civilian would argue, 'Some of us are popular and some of us are not, and why should all this energy and money be put into how to win friends and influence people?' I assume this is for the extreme ends of the spectrum."

"It is, and I would have several answers to that," Foster replied. "One is that we know that many kids who are disliked or rejected by their peers are at risk: many wind up in clinics diagnosed with AD/HD or conduct disorder. They are more likely to have future difficulties. Is this the result of their rejection, or the result of whatever it is that led them to be rejected? We don't know that, but we know peers to be at least an important marker that something might be going wrong with the kid. Furthermore, it's not a matter of popularity but a matter of critical socialization experiences. What is important to us as adults? Our relationship with our spouse, our friends, our children. Except for our children, the other ones are peer relations, and how do we learn the skills to manage those? If you believe in learning them at all, we learn them through our experiences in childhood. We can be taught some things by our parents, but a lot of our learning has to take place in the context of the conversations and experiences we share with kids our own age.

"We know the kids who are rejected tend to spend more time playing with younger kids. What kinds of socialization are these kids losing out on? And as they get older, they are excluded from other groups, so what do they seek? They seek other kids with poorer skills. And who goes into these groups? The kids who are impulsive, the kids who are aggressive, the kids who are losers, and together they form their own little group, supporting loser behaviors.

"Deviant peer groups," Foster said, "support a variety of deviant activities, and it's not only kids with poor peer skills who wind up in loser peer groups. Some of the kids who belong to gangs are highly skilled. It would be interesting to look at how these groups get structured and operate."

Foster told me she doesn't deal with questions of self-esteem and the consequences of rejection; the minuteness of specialization in her field is extraordinary. But she is interested in how a child's behavior accumulates over time until another child makes a judgment: at what point is the first child dismissed as weird or flaky or accepted as cool? Having learned some lessons from Kendall, Ecton, and Feindler, I suggested that I personally might have cognitive distortions: looking Foster up and down, I said, "I might think that all women who wear purple jackets are weird."

"My roots are more behavioral than cognitive, unlike Phil's," she said. "I'm much more out of a straight behavioral tradition where the environment is all. I'm willing to acknowledge that these cognitions may be important, and it seems to be very important to work with the distortions and thoughts and perceptions that a person brings to a situation, but my own view is that both the cognitive things and the skills training things have really forgotten the role of the environment. In this case it's the interpersonal environment, because our social skills will be maintained only if they're reinforced, if other people respond positively to them. Perhaps some of our skills training programs haven't worked as well as they might because we've forgotten to make sure the skills are supported in the natural environment."

"People like Kendall and Mahoney and Meichenbaum went cognitive partly because pure behaviorism didn't work," I asked Foster. "But has that got something to do with not choosing the right reinforcers?"

"It may be a variety of things," she said. "One is you get your analysis of the problem wrong, and then some people use very simpleminded reinforcers. I do believe that kids go out and hit and steal because they don't have other skills. The first question you ask is, What is this getting them? What's reinforcing it now? We all do things because they work. They work better at getting us what we want than some other things we have available to us. With a kid who's doing drugs and selling drugs, you may find out that taking drugs served to reduce depressed affect, or it served to get attention from people who would then help the kid, or perhaps it served to help the kid avoid unpleasant thoughts if he had been abused and memories were starting to surface. Or he has to do this to gain the esteem of peers, and if he doesn't, they ridicule him. Those are all behavioral formulations because they have to do with a function the behavior serves—reducing something negative and providing something positive. Those are clear consequences, and with each you get a very different treatment plan.

"So getting the analysis wrong is one reason behavioral programs don't work. In residential treatment another reason why they fail is that sometimes the staff just aren't very good at implementing them. If a kid is in a very chaotic family or in school surrounded by peers all involved in deviant behavior with a demoralized teaching staff, it's going to be very difficult to get the natural environment to do any of the things necessary to support adaptive behavior in the kids. There are not reinforcers for the kids to make changes. You need to start with what's going on with the children right now—what situations they have problems with, what thoughts or lack of thought contribute to their behavior, what alternative responses they try, what the kids' strengths are, and how the environment might be supporting maladaptive behavior or failing to support the more adaptive responses. And from looking at their past, what are they likely to do in future situations? How can we change the probability of their reacting in a certain way? I personally don't buy the notion that insight is sufficient to produce behavior change."

This almost-purely Skinnerian formulation is far more complex than lay people exposed solely to pop-psych notions of Skinner might expect. There is a certain idealism in Foster's work: she is trying to embrace a sprawling, mercurial problem that has vagueness built in. Not far from Foster's office Laura Schreibman, a professor of psychology at the University of California, San Diego, puts pure behaviorism to work on a narrowly focused, clearly defined problem. While the gains she offers her clients and their families are limited, she is able to effect modest but important changes in their lives, for which they are touchingly grateful. For her clientele, most professionals in the world of mental health would agree that therapy like hers is now the treatment of choice and represents the behavioral approach at its most successful.

Schreibman treats autistic children. Behavioral therapy like hers represents a substantial advance from the parent-blaming psychodynamic formulations of the past. Unlike the more showy, controversial, and widely covered new "facilitated communication" (in which the "facilitator" holds the autistic person's arm, thus purportedly enabling her to type out complex thoughts she has hitherto been unable to express), it has moved forward steadily and cautiously, supported by rigorous documentation. When I asked Schreibman about facilitated communication, she rolled her eyes; "FC" is controversial because it hasn't stood up to objective testing, but the furor is beyond the scope of a general book on child psychotherapy.

Because understanding of "infantile autism" (called "Autistic Disorder" in DSM-IV) has changed so in the past few decades, it is useful to start by summarizing what is now known about the condition. In a book chapter published in 1990 Schreibman and her co-authors describe the characteristics of autism—which, despite considerable public awareness, occurs in only one out of 2,500 children—as "severe withdrawal and lack of social behavior, severe language and attentional deficits, and the presence of bizarre, repetitive behavior." They point out that while there are many theories about the etiology of autism, "there is no consistent evidence in support of any one of them. Most professionals, however, now take the position that autism is of organic etiology and the disorder is probably present from birth."

When Schreibman and I talked, she elaborated on this idea, pointing out that autism is "a behaviorally defined syndrome. It's not like Down's syndrome, where you look at chromosomes and there it is. There probably isn't a single thing that's autism. There are probably subgroups that may have different etiologies that seem to cross at some place where the behaviors look similar. As a diagnostic category it's very heterogeneous. Some autistic people have structural problems in the brain—the absence of certain cells in the cerebellum. But the earliest magnetic resonance imaging studies were with adults, so we don't know whether the deficit is the origin or the result of autism. Now studies are being done with younger children, but we're far from coming up with specific causes or organically based cures." Behavior treatment has been most successful probably because it's based on systematic analyses of the behavior without relying much on either the child's verbal skills or any etiological theory.

Autistic infants, Schreibman and her colleagues report in the paper, "may lack attachment behavior and typically do not posturally conform to their parent's body when held. They may remain stiff and rigid or may 'go limp' when picked up. When older, they may seldom seek out their parents for comfort . . . lack eye-to-eye contact, [and] may actively avoid the social overtures of others."

Profound speech and language problems mark the disorder: the children don't use language to communicate, often display echolalia (repeating what others say) and pronoun reversal (*I* becomes *you* and vice versa), and exhibit speech that "tends to be inaccurate in pitch, rhythm, inflection, intonation, pace, and/or articulation."

The third common feature of autism is ritualistic behavior and insistence on sameness: autistic children "may repeatedly line up toys . . . or collect many objects of a special shape or texture . . . may become so attached to a specific object that they must have it at all times . . . [may] have unusual preoccupations with such things as numbers, geometric shapes, bus routes, and colors . . . and are extremely distressed by even a small change in their daily routines."

Autistic children often display what is called "self-stimulatory behavior" such as flapping their arms, rocking back and forth, and gazing at lights, and self-injurious behavior like head-banging.

Aside from all these symptoms, the children are usually healthy and vary in intelligence; three-fifths have IQs below 50 and one-fifth are above 70, with some showing "autistic savant" behavior. Autism is sometimes misdiagnosed as retardation, schizophrenia, environmental deprivation, and pervasive developmental disorder. (In DSM-III-R and DSM-IV the last diagnosis, a milder form of the disorder, is called "Pervasive Developmental Disorder Not Otherwise Specified." DSM-IV now groups this, along with "Autistic Disorder" and several other variants, under the general rubric of "Pervasive Developmental Disorders.") Schreibman and her colleagues lay out the differences between these diagnoses rather clearly.

During the forties, fifties, and sixties, some famous names in the psychiatric world propounded erroneous theories about the origins of autism that became part of the common misunderstanding, hindered effective treatment, and caused considerable needless grief. Leo Kanner thought an innate disorder was exacerbated by cold, detached intellectual parents; Bruno Bettelheim laid the condition right on the doorstep of hostile, rejecting mothers, to whom the child was adapting in his symptoms. The treatment, therefore, was acceptance of the bizarre behavior, removal of the child from his "toxic" environment, and a balance of gratification and frustration with a slow increase in the demands made on the child. But later researchers faulted the subjectivity of Bettelheim's descriptions and failed to find large numbers of "refrigerator" parents of autistic children. Theory reversed itself completely: if parental behavior was pathological, this was a reaction to the child's disorder, not the cause of it, and institutionalization might even make the condition worse. It was better to involve the family in the treatment and keep the child at home whenever possible.

"This is a joint research project between UC Santa Barbara, where my colleague, Bob Koegel, is in the Speech and Hearing Sciences Department, and UC San Diego here," Schreibman told me when I visited her clinic. "We've been working together since 1976. What we do is train the parents to work with the children. We also work with the children, and what we ask for in return—the treatment is free to the families—is to be able to collect data. This means we don't see as many families as an ordinary clinic, and what the parents get here is probably much more state-of-the-art than would be available in most places because this is where it starts.

"The child has to have an independent diagnosis of autism—because I could guarantee who's going to do well by diagnosing right—and has to be living at home where there are parents or grandparents or foster parents or somebody we can train, anybody that's taking care of the child. Right now we're looking at our most recent parent training package, called pivotal response training. It leads to much better generalization of treatment effects than the old-style behavior treatment, which was very structured and mechanical. Lovaas at UCLA developed that—'Look at me,' and you'd give the kid an M&M and have him repeat and imitate you."

M&Ms have a long history in the behavioral psychology world. "I keep thinking of the M&M company sending all these detail men to conventions," I said.

"I don't know when it started, M&Ms and autism being paired," Schreibman said. "But it was all quite artificial. In the early seventies the most common procedure was for children to go to some kind of school or clinic and receive treatment. So first we looked at training the parent to provide the same treatment. We knew from studies Lovaas had done that if you train a child at a clinic, you may get some very nice gains, but you don't get follow-up. But if you teach the parents how to do it, the gains will hold up.

"But up to that time parents hadn't really been incorporated into treatment, probably because of the old Bettelheim psychogenic hypothesis. If I think you caused autism in your kid, the last person I'm going to have work with him is you. So Bettelheim did what we call a 'parentectomy.' The other thing was that the psychodynamicists were saying, 'You can't use the parents to work with their kids. It's stressful, the parents will go crazy'—the ones that didn't think the parents were already crazy. 'They're going to get divorced—the gains won't be worth it.'

"So we set up to see if that was the case. We did a comparison study where we had families for whom we provided the treatment in a clinic setting versus another group where instead of working with the child, we trained the parents.

"Then we compared them in terms of changing the child's behavior and generalization, and we also looked at family variables like the MMPI [Minnesota Multiphasic Personality Inventory] personality assessment test to see if they went crazy. We did a marital adjustment test to see if they were arguing, and a family environment questionnaire to see if the family environment would become more disrupted. We also gave them a twenty-four-hour time activity diary. They would write down what they did during the day, how they budgeted their time, how much time they spent on recreation, time alone, child care, and the like, to see the effects of these two kinds of treatment on how they actually lived day to day.

"That's a very behavioral measure. What we found pretreatment was that parents of children with autism look very like the parents of infants in how they budget their time. Most of the time they spend in child care, with very little leisure or recreation.

"Then we did our training and compared the two groups, and we found that for child improvement, parent training was better. In terms of better generalization, both groups improved, but the children whose parents had been trained showed more generalization than the other children. That was great, but the bad news was, it didn't generalize beyond the parents. The parents had to be there. This one child in Santa Barbara who wanted some punch at a party—he takes his cup and starts waving it over the punch bowl, going 'Aaaaaah.' His mother heard this, she was in the other room and he couldn't see her—so she pops her head in and says, 'Johnny, you say it right!' and he says, 'Punch, please.' This is classic autism. The minute he saw her, boy, he snapped right to it!

"Looking at parents, we found that pretreatment, parents of children with autism were not different from parents of normal kids. We even used a southern California comparison group because some people would say in southern California everybody's a little crazy, so we took care of that by having a normative group from southern California. And neither the clinic group nor the parent-training group had the parents of autistic kids going crazy.

"The psychological and marital adjustment tests showed no difference between the two groups, the ones where the parents trained the child and the ones where we did. But the families where the parents had been trained actually showed an increase in cohesiveness and positive environment. And the biggie was the time-activity budget. These graphs just go *whsssht!* After parent training those parents showed significantly more time in recreational activities, leisure activities, child-training activities as opposed to custodial activities like feeding the child, dressing the child. We didn't see that change at all in the clinic group."

"Was it the opposite of what Lovaas said, that the parents were coping, they had an effective way to deal with the problem and therefore more time to do other things?" I asked.

"It could be that," Schreibman said, "or it could be that the improvement in the child's behavior allowed them to do these other things because the child wasn't out of control all the time.

"So parent training was okay, but we still had to work with generalization of the child's behavior beyond the parents. We spent some years just looking at the problems, and we weren't the only people who noticed problems in generalization with autism. And we asked parents who had had both kinds of treatment which one they liked better. Guess what? They liked the clinic treatment!

"We were saying, 'Wow, what's going on here?' Our objective data showed the kids were better, the parents were better, with parent training. Why did they like the clinic treatment? We got to thinking a couple of things. One is that if your TV set breaks, you don't want to learn how to fix TV sets, you just want to take it to someone and then get it back. Also, we asked them their expectations about their ability to teach their child and about their child's future functioning. The ones in parent training actually had to look at their children, and I think reality set in. They began to gain an appreciation of how handicapped their child was and how difficult working with them would be. The people in clinic treatment were just watching clinicians.

"So we wanted a treatment that would generalize better but also that would be more acceptable, and we came up with two of what we called 'pivotal behaviors,' because a change in either of them should lead to changes in a lot of other areas. Motivation, the first, is a classic problem with these kids. That's why therapists used to use food and escape-from-pain and everything, if you look at the early behavioral literature. Of course parent training doesn't generalize—because it's not the same environment. People aren't running around with M&Ms to pop in the kids' mouths every time they say something. So motivation was one pivotal behavior.

"The other was responsivity to multiple cues. This attentional pattern they have, which is 'overselective,' gets in the way of their being able to learn from their environment."

I had read about "overselectivity" in Schreibman's papers. The word refers to a child's failure to respond to all of the important cues in an educational setting. A simple example would be a teacher pointing to a picture of a dog and saying, "Dog." The autistic child will either see the picture or hear the spoken word, even though he has no hearing or visual impairment; thus he will not be able to connect the object with its name. An enormous amount of learning might flow from correcting this problem, both in class and in the child's social world. Research has shown that autistic children can be helped to respond to multiple cues, and this is the other "pivotal behavior."

"The old-style behavior training was what we call 'individual target behavior,'" Schreibman told me, "because you focus on one thing, like colors or pronouns or concept-of-time for X number of trials, and then you go to something else. Teaching pivotal behaviors should be more economical."

Pivotal response training, or PRT—which has indeed proved superior to the old style—ties responsiveness and motivation together by letting the child choose the materials he works with and using those materials as a reward—an idea that sounds incredibly simple but took years of research to develop. If he wants the red apple, he learns to ask for it and gets to eat it.

"Theoretically the children would be more motivated to talk about something they're interested in," Schreibman said. "Maybe they're not interested in red and blue blocks, but there's a car that's red and they're interested in that car. We have a bunch of toys and say, 'What do you want? Pick a toy,' so we know they're motivated to play with it, as opposed to something you've chosen which they may not care about. Then we reinforce them for reasonable attempts to respond, instead of strictly requiring a right answer."

"Do you reward at different levels? Is there a 'Nice try' and a 'Whoopee, you did it!'?" I asked.

"Probably some variation, but there's always some whoopee. If the child can say a word and goes, 'Yaaah,' that's not a reasonable attempt. A reasonable attempt means they're looking at you or the materials, and they're making something. So you reinforce them for trying, and that reinforces the rate of trying."

"That relates to life in general," I suggested. "If the kid tries to do something and doesn't quite make it and that's not enough, then the kid will stop trying."

"The term for that is 'learned helplessness,'" Schreibman said, "and we think that may have happened with these kids. They're not very good at anything so they fail a lot, and they stop trying.

"So the reinforcer we use is directly related to the task. The kid picks up the car. We say, '*Roll* the car,' and if he makes some attempt to say 'roll' or 'car,' we give him some access to the car, as opposed to putting food in his mouth, which has nothing to do with rolling the car. He picks up the car, we put our hand on his hand so he can't move the car, and we say, 'What do you want to do with the car?' If he says, 'Roll car,' we say, 'Good,' and he gets to roll the car. Another thing is, we take turns. It helps them with getting an idea of the social nature of language and also allows us to model language: 'I'm going to make the car roll this way. What are you going to do?'

"We also intersperse what we call maintenance tasks, which means things the child can already do well, to ensure a high rate of reinforcement so it's a whole positive experience. These kids love to come here because they get an hour and a half of pure attention, toys, goodies, whatever they want.

"If the child doesn't want a toy anymore, he can say, 'No more, put away,' and we take that toy away and give him another. A good therapist can tell if a child's bored with the toy. You see them looking around the room.

"The other thing that's neat is that it doesn't work like the old style where you got a table and two chairs and cleared everything out of the room and set aside part of the day to work on these things. It was artificial and difficult for the parents to incorporate into their lives. Now they can do it all the time. When you're doing the laundry, you say, 'Give me the blue shirt.' 'What do you want to do now—should we fold the laundry?' Cooking—anything you do, you incorporate. At first it's very awkward for the parents, but once they get the hang of it, they do it without thinking, and they like it a lot more.

"We took videotapes of parents doing the old training and the pivotal response training, and we showed them to college undergraduates and had them rate how enthusiastic, happy, and interested the parents seemed to be. We've been looking at whether regular folk could see the improvements. That sort of social validation is becoming more and more prevalent in behavior work now, because we need to be accountable to the consumer. It's typically used as an adjunct to more objective measures. If we can't make the kid acceptable to the community—"

"He's going to work in some mail room," I said. "They'll grow up and won't be with their parents forever. Is your goal to enable him to have a low-order job and live in a group setting?"

"It varies," Schreibman answered. "For some of these kids, that would be a high goal—to get them functioning in some kind of sheltered community. Other kids could actually go further, live by themselves, have a job. There's a tremendous range."

"Will any of them ever be able to show or feel affection?" I asked.

Schreibman paused, and then spoke carefully. "Yeah, to a degree. I was quoted in *Newsweek* as saying there's always something odd about these kids. I've been in this field for over twenty years, since I was a sophomore at UCLA. I have worked only in the area of autism—that's all I do. I've never seen a kid become completely normal."

"That's not what I'm asking you, though. I'm asking, Do they ever give Mommy a hug?"

"There are hugs and there are hugs," Schreibman continued in the same slow, deliberative tone. "What we call 'operant hugs' and regular hugs. A lot of these kids learn the same strategies other kids do. They've done something bad, they're going to get busted, they'll hug. Sometimes it seems like there's genuine affection, but much less frequently than you would see in other kids. You ask the parents, 'Do you think Johnny or Susie really needs you?' They almost always think about it a bit. Some say yes. Some say 'Probably not really. If someone else were giving him his food, it would probably be okay.' I don't know what they feel, but in situations where you would see normal kids really needing affection— they're hurt and they're scared and they go running to Mommy—these kids don't do that. Maybe they'll just sit there and cry—or maybe not. A parent leaves, they don't care, the parent comes back, they're not happy to see them. Many of them learn how, but they have to be taught. They want to fit in. They know there's something different about them, and they learn what to say, but they aren't supergood at it. So you may not notice right away, but probably you'd figure out there's something eccentric about this person.

"We feel the ultimate generalization is to teach the kids to manage their own behavior as normal kids do. That's something we're just starting now—self-management training. To reduce the stress on the family. That's what's neat about the behavior approach: you evaluate, see what you still need to do, and then focus on that. The treatment is evolving, with a more positive outlook for a child than we had ten or even five years ago. But anybody that tells you they can cure autism is lying."

When we arrived at the clinic, it was bustling with children, parents, and graduate students. I sat in a small control room with one-way mirrors and a sound system that gave on two rooms where training was going on. In one room, Reza, a handsome six-year-old Iranian boy with shaggy black hair and long eyelashes, was learning self-management. He was all alone in the room trying to get dressed, putting both legs in one pant. When he finally extricated himself, he took a little piece of cookie from a tray nearby that held cookie pieces, candy corn, and the famous M&Ms. His mother, in the control room, said she couldn't let him do that in the morning because there's not enough time.

Reza was learning to play "appropriately" by himself and to monitor his behavior. Except for a bit of hand-flapping, he looked almost normal. After eight minutes of playing, he could take a stamp, stamp a chart, and have a piece of candy. Nearby was a jar of soap-bubble mixture and a wand; when a graduate student came in, Reza said, "I want big bubble! Big bubble!" "Good asking, Reza," said the student. "Big bubble!" Reza said again. "*I want* big bubble," the student corrected him. "I want big bubble," he said. The play continued: "I want green block! Yellow candy!" "Do you want yellow candy?" "*I want* yellow candy." "*There* you go! Good asking, Reza!"

"He's getting food because he chose that, but he has to talk about it," Schreibman said. "She saw him looking over to the dish, and that was a cue that he was probably motivated for something else, so that's when she said, 'Do you want?' Give him the chance to choose, keep that motivation up, keep him always working for what he wants."

Reza's mother sat with us in the control room. "He's really speaking clearly," Schreibman said, reinforcing Mom as well. Schreibman glowed like a grandmother whenever Reza spoke up. "That's what we find so interesting. We don't select or reinforce clarity per se, but as they get better, the clarity seems to improve. A lot of the children when they start, it's almost incoherent."

"Isn't he going to be full of all that candy?" I asked. "It's tiny, tiny pieces," said Schreibman, "and he's also asked for the bubbles."

"At home," said Reza's mother, "I say you don't clean up, you're not going to get Nintendo. He has started to defend himself with other kids. He now hits back." Reza had had a year of training and was also part of a new project begun by Aubyn Stahmer, a graduate student, to teach the kids symbolic play—just a primitive version of the "make-believes" that are so important to psychodynamic therapists like Charles Sarnoff— which, according to a paper by Stahmer and Schreibman, "has been correlated, in both typical children and children who have autism, with language, social skills, and general cognitive functioning."

Stahmer and Reza were playing with a doctor kit. There was a stethoscope and a syringe and a blue box that Stahmer was trying to convince him was medicine. Reza put it to his lips cursorily; whenever he pretended, he got to play with realistic toys like the blood-pressure equipment as a reward. Stahmer tried unsuccessfully to get him to examine a doll—looking in Stahmer's ear was more fun. Symbolic play appeared to be an uphill fight: Reza wouldn't bang with a hammer on symbolic nails, and when asked to make the doll family eggs and pancakes, he went off and sulked. In the control room Reza's mother told us last week he had climbed up on her lap and hugged her, sitting there and playing for fifteen minutes. It was a major event.

I asked Schreibman at what point she writes up the project, and she told me, "We usually go at three-year intervals, four years this time because we're doing a longer follow-up. When you start to see clear results, you stop as soon as possible, because then you don't have to give somebody ineffective treatment." (Schreibman was referring to the fact that a treatment is always studied in comparison with some other treatment or no treatment. Once the study is completed, the children in the control group, or those that are receiving a treatment that is shown to be less effective, can be shifted to the treatment that works.)

As I packed up my tape recorder, nine-and-a-half-year-old Erik, a Swedish boy who had been nonverbal in two languages, was working with a graduate student, drawing. "Coo-kie," he said, sounding, alas, like a muppet. "Where is the cookie?" the student asked. "In my hand," Erik answered, pulling on his ear. "Very good! Yeah, Erik!" Erik looked in the mirror and flapped his hands. "Cookie, please." "Who has the cookie?" "Hand! I do!" Erik's father took over and tried to get him to play with a dinosaur puzzle, producing a quick tantrum. The father was an authoritative man, Schreibman told me, and was having a bit of trouble with the child-choice part. "These are different skills from what most parents would need," she pointed out.

After I left Schreibman, I thought of Kendall puzzling over the two tines of the fork—one tine being the child who is trained to adapt to the environment, the other the environment which can be modified to suit the child. At present Kendall's fork had only one tine and was thus a limited tool. The family therapists we will meet in Part IV are working with the other tine, and that (as we'll see) has its limits too. Schreibman, perhaps earlier than colleagues who deal with less severely disabled children, had been forced to use the whole fork.

NO CHILD IS AN ISLAND

Family Systems Therapy

CHAPTER 10

GETTING UNSTUCK

It is essential to understand the complexity of child rearing in order to judge its participants fairly. Parents cannot protect and guide without at the same time controlling and restricting. Children cannot grow and become individuated without rejecting and attacking. The process of socialization is inherently conflictual.

In joining operations, the therapist becomes an actor in the family play. In restructuring, he functions like the director as well as an actor. He creates scenarios, choreographs, highlights themes, and leads family members to improvise within the constraints of the family drama. But he also uses himself, entering into alliances and coalitions, creating, strengthening, or weakening boundaries.

—Salvador Minuchin,
Families and Family Therapy
(1974)

The individual psychotherapy patient comes to the therapist with an almost automatic deference, a sense of dependence and compliance. The role pattern is old and established: the dependent child seeking guidance from a parent figure. There is no such traditional image for the family, no established pattern in which an entire family submits to the guidance of an individual.

—Augustus Y. Napier with
Carl A. Whitaker,
The Family Crucible (1978)

BACK IN 1962, WHEN RICHARD CHASIN, M.D., was a second-year resident in adult psychiatry, he was assigned to the Outpatient Clinic at Massachusetts Mental Health Center. "We were given six interviews in which to dispose of a case," Chasin remembers. " 'Dispose' could mean 'have admitted to hospital,' 'bring about a cure,' or 'start in long-term therapy,' but we were a walk-in service, and we had just those six meetings to make a decision.

"Frequently the people were very disturbed, some of them mute or incomprehensible. Their families were in the waiting room. They were Boston- and Brookline-area residents who weren't using private services. I did what many of the social workers were doing, which was to talk with the family after talking with the patient. I developed a lot of information, but it sometimes didn't jibe with what the patient was telling me.

"So as a simple matter of expedience, whomever the patient came with, I would just bring them in too. It was obvious to me that anybody who brought someone to a walk-in center was very concerned. So suddenly they were all in the room, and I would say, 'What's the story?' The group activity was highly mobilized by this context. They might yell and scream at each other and suddenly I was in the middle of a very hot drama. Instead of trying to pull something that made sense out of somebody who was mute or psychotic and then get another version from the family, I was able to make sense out of what was going on and even think of something to do very quickly.

"What struck me about it was the efficiency. There was a great willingness, partly because they were in crisis, to try something new and different. These cases made sense to me so much faster than the ones where I was alone with the identified patient and the social worker saw the families. It seemed only natural to continue doing this. My turnover was very rapid. Six meetings were much too long. I was working from no theory, just common sense. I was a naif. I knew there was a thing called family therapy, and that it was bad. There were two people in our hospital who were doing it, and they were considered wild."

The next year Chasin was chief resident and worked intensively with one of the two wild people. "I must have interviewed a hundred and twenty families and learned something about how to survive such an interview, how much you could get done, and some of the dangers. It got so I could no longer tolerate not knowing all the players and what they were like with each other. Sitting in a room with one person was a tremendous handicap, like wearing blinders. I was pulling them out of context."

While Alan Kazdin in his book *Child Psychotherapy: Developing and Identifying Effective Treatments* cites a 1977 study reporting that 94 percent of psychiatrists and psychologists see children concurrently with their parents at some time during therapy, concurrent sessions are not necessarily the same as family systems therapy, which is marked by the way it defines the patient. No one person has the problem; no other person caused it; the family is in a knot and must unravel it together. The notion of linear causality is anathema to family systems people. "The idea that A causes B which causes C is a very limiting way to think about causal chains and mutual influences," Chasin says.

Indeed, for parents family systems is the most collaborative of the therapies. As Chasin explains, "I'm trying to step back from the pathologizing of an individual. Let's say there is a twelve-year-old girl who one day says she really doesn't see the point of living out her life. Mother hits the panic button. Father says all twelve-year-old girls are like that. I start to talk with the mother, and it turns out one of her parents committed suicide. Now Father is really worried about this girl, but he is much more frightened that his wife will go off the deep end hearing this stuff, so he doesn't say quite honestly how he's feeling.

"The girl doesn't understand why he's so unconcerned with her. Do you see how complicated this is? One of the reasons she feels so depressed is that every time she brings up a problem, her mother goes off the deep end with terror and her father pooh-poohs it, so she doesn't get an honest down-the-middle response from anybody. Any one of these people in a different context could look very good. If the daughter had acute leukemia and the mother said, 'I have to drop everything and deal with this kid,' you'd say, 'What else do you expect this woman to do?' If the father played a sort of jolly role, people might say, 'Somebody's got to keep some balance in this horrible picture.' But here they are all *stuck* in a problematic behavior where the girl is facing life feeling abandoned by two people who are being relatively useless to her.

"It's not that I don't believe there are problems that inhere in people— there are genetic problems, developmental problems. But people are different in different contexts. If somebody is the same way in every context, then it becomes increasingly interesting to look at the kid's biology or maybe certain intrapsychic things. I would still think of the other people in the system as being potentially of value to the kid, but he may also need something more—a drug or individual therapy. That can go on side by side with family therapy, or after it or before." What family therapy doesn't do, barring cases of outright abuse, is blame the parents for the child's problem (although it does suggest the familiar bumper sticker that says, "Insanity is hereditary—you get it from your kids").

While family systems therapy has been in existence since the fifties (drawing on research done even earlier), it's gathered considerable steam since the sixties; like the behaviorists, the people in the field and the way they practice have a flavor of egalitarian rebellion. Lee Combrinck-Graham, M.D.—a peppery woman in her fifties who has published widely on family issues, directed the Institute for Juvenile Research in Chicago, and is a child and adolescent psychiatrist in Stamford, Connecticut (and went through seven years of analysis herself)—says, "I don't tend to use psychodynamic formulations, while I love to read about them. That's because I believe it's a kind of patronizing process. The theorist has the theory about someone else's internal workings. I believe people's internal workings are basically their own business, not mine. When a child goes into analysis, you as therapist urge the child to form a deep, abiding, and secret relationship with you. Unless you plan to adopt the child and the family is willing to give the child up, I think that's outrageous."

Psychodynamic therapists revere the towering figures in the history of psychoanalysis, most of them dead; cognitive-behaviorists and biological psychiatrists revere controlled double-blind clinical trials; family systems therapists revere the live geniuses who are constantly dreaming up new metaphors for framing the family's problems. The counterpart to the behaviorists' apology, "There's no hard data, but . . . ," in the family systems world is, "The field has evolved away from that." A family undergoing systems therapy may encounter a therapist who does elaborate genograms of grand- and great-grandparents, or one who doesn't; a therapist who tries to mix into the family drama as it unfolds, or one who stays carefully removed; therapists who perceive the family in terms of structure, boundaries, belief systems, or intergenerational loyalties. Yet however particular therapists may vary in technique (which may even be different from what the same therapist did last year), their common ground is the systemic approach.

Because of the focus on social context, it's not surprising that many family systems therapists are M.S.W.s, another factor that feeds into the field's disdain for "elitist" credentials and pecking orders. Richard Chasin's establishment credentials (Yale undergraduate, Harvard Medical School, Boston Psychoanalytic Institute, associate clinical professor of psychiatry at Harvard Medical School) give him credibility in the outside psychiatric and medical worlds, which on the whole tend to be uninformed and nervous about family systems therapy.

Chasin practices at an office in his home and also at the Family Institute of Cambridge, a training facility of which he is co-director. The most arresting feature of both sites is the abundance and elaborateness of television equipment. The control room at the institute might well be part of NBC News, with screens hooked up to four different cameras. There are viewing rooms in which twenty people, stationed behind a one-way mirror, can watch one family; another fifty people can watch the family on TV monitors in a large classroom. Every office at the institute has a one-way mirror into some other office, "so we can look at each other's work." There are rooms with stages for psychodrama. Chasin's home office is a smaller version of the studio setup.

Clearly, privacy is not the crux of this practice. "The whole atmosphere in family therapy is more open and comes much less from an expert position than many other therapies," Chasin says. "When you are learning family therapy, there's someone behind a one-way screen who's watching and calling in suggestions. Tapes are shown to supervisors. Consultation is frequent. 'Needing a consult' means only that we need an infusion of new ideas from a therapist who probably himself or herself would get stuck at points along the way and ask for consultation. It's in the culture of family therapy to work in the open."

"It's offered to people as an opportunity," says Sallyann Roth, M.S.W., Chasin's co-director at the Family Institute and a frequent collaborator both in writing and in therapy, "to have more people thinking about their case, more people focusing on what they need." Among the variations one might see in a course of family therapy are Mom and Dad watching children and therapist through one-way mirror; therapist watching consultant and family; consultant watching therapist and family; team of consultants watching family and therapist; family watching team of consultants discuss their case.

On the other hand, nobody *has* to be watched by anybody, and the watching is only occasional, by economic necessity: since the family generally pays for one practitioner per session, the others are donating time for their own professional development. In addition, good therapists work with a strict set of rules that might state that any family member may "pass" on a particular question, and that parts of the family can discuss certain things with the therapist in private. (Chasin will agree to keep a child's comments confidential if it's "safe" for the parents not to know; the older the child gets, the broader the definition of safety.) Just as individual therapists often talk with a child's parents, family therapists sometimes see individual members alone, but the focus of therapy is always on the individual in a family context.

Chasin's office reflects not only his therapeutic culture but Chasin himself: the counterpart of Sarnoff's pregnant symbolic artwork and Kendall's "grown-up" furniture is a waiting room filled with blow-ups of Steig and Feiffer cartoons on psychiatric subjects. Chasin, born in 1936, has shaggy, grizzled hair and looks as if he started the day neat and proper until life interfered. His most memorable mannerism is a belly-laugh that racks his frame and seems to express unending wonder at the varieties of human behavior: "What a piece of work is man," it says, or less elegantly, "Get this!" I watched a number of tapes with Chasin sitting by to provide play-by-play commentary; while he presumably sees these tapes repeatedly in the course of training and writing, he seemed as astounded by what was going on as if he were watching them for the first time.

Both the adult consulting room and the theater/playroom in Chasin's office are stocked with psychodynamic therapy's usual array of puppets and rag dolls. "Without psychodynamic and behavioral techniques, I'd be helpless," Chasin says. Chasin uses play not to unravel symbols but to help children act out what they haven't the courage or skill to tell him directly: the puppet king and queen say the same things Mommy and Daddy say. At the same time, I saw him ask some questions that duplicated those of the cognitive-behaviorists at Temple. Chasin remembers an old case of a teenage boy with "horrible self-esteem problems. I asked the family to name the things they liked about him, and almost everybody cited his terrific sense of humor. It then became a source of interest— How did he get this sense of humor? What might it mean for him if he grew up and had such a charming sense of humor? As we're talking about this, you can see the boy's face changing, and then he would say something clever, and I would say, 'Is that an example of what they're talking about?' and he'd say, 'Not a very good one.' I'd say, 'They're *even* better than *that*?' You can just see how the mood would move. It's highly behavioral, on-the-spot conditioning, eliciting the behavior, shaping it and rewarding it."

Chasin calls himself a technician, which means he doesn't come up with theories and test them out in practice; his greatest skill lies in the therapeutic interview, in which the way he pulls information out of people becomes therapy in itself. In the questioning and other interventions he draws on whatever theories seem useful, particularly one that says, "A problem is almost always associated with the family having very little variety on a certain issue, so that when they are in a particular context, they always do the same damn frustrating thing. If you ask the family, 'How would you do *this*?' and they honestly say 'There are eleven different ways we could do this that would be satisfactory,' it's unlikely that's going to be an area of trouble. But if you say to a teenager, 'When you're going out at night, what happens in the family?' and it's always the same thing, it's like a little flashing mark. Then the question would be, 'And the way you always do things, does it work?' If they say, 'It usually doesn't,' and I say 'Do you try other ways?' and they say no, I know that's a problem."

In two-thirds of Chasin's family cases in which there are children, one child is the lead problem, and in the third (warring couples, for example), "there's another problem, but I see the children." Like Kendall and Sarnoff, Chasin will order neurological and educational tests when he feels it's appropriate, but if a purportedly hyperactive child comes out normal, he won't leave it there. "I'm probably going to say if the family perceives there is a problem, there is a problem, even though it may not go by the name they advance. How is the family dealing with the fact that there's such variation in itself?

"I saw a woman this morning who said she had this intense kid who does everything at a fast pace. He rushes the family along, and she finds herself getting explosive about it. I suggested she tell the child it's wonderful he can do things so speedily, that probably makes him very good in school and a terrific soccer player. It's unfortunate he has to live with people who aren't so fast, and she must apologize. Then I talked with the kid about his mother's thoroughness. 'What a wonderful thing when the two of you do something, you provide the speed and she provides the thoroughness—you must make a great team!' That's called *reframing*, and it's a whole lot better than saying to this kid, 'What's with you? Why are you pushing everybody all the time?' " Chasin willingly accepts that some family therapy just involves encouraging tact (which is a form of child guidance). Most of his work, however, is more complex.

Family therapy begins with a process usually called "joining," which involves forming a new system composed of the therapist and family. (Chasin is free of the besetting sin of doctors and psychologists: he starts off saying "My name is Dr. Chasin. You may call me Dick if you would like to," and then he asks family members to introduce themselves by the names they prefer to be called.) Chasin seldom starts by asking what the problem is: he feels that's a bad beginning, and he usually has individuals describe their strong points. Then he asks the family members their goals. "I'm not interested in finding out how bad things are to the last little detail. I want to know where they want to go and how they're going to get there. If you ask how people are stuck first of all, you won't find out very much, and then it tends to aggravate the stuckness. You will discover the problem soon enough."

The efficiency Chasin describes is evident on tapes of sessions he's held: a surprising amount of work gets done in a few hours of family therapy with a skilled practitioner. I watched the second and third sessions he held with the Tyler family. Jane Tyler, an elementary school teacher, was a patient of Chasin's wife, Laura, a psychiatric social worker. (Both Chasins do adult therapy and sometimes work as a team leading psychodrama weekends for individuals and couples.) "It's common for an individual therapist to call in a family person when she feels the whole family needs work," Chasin says. "She doesn't want to change her relationship with her patient. My therapy with the Tylers was mostly separate from Jane Tyler's therapy."

Jane and Peter Tyler and their three sons had, however, started family therapy by meeting with both Chasins. The obviously symptomatic Tyler (the IP, or identified patient, in family systems lingo), four-year-old Bobby, was encopretic—in the nontechnical language used by the boys, he pooped in his pants. But as the Tylers' story unfolded, they proved to be a good illustration of the systemic point of view. Jane now remembers, "I was locked into a bitter struggle around Bobby's bowel training, and I couldn't distance myself from the intensity of our conflict. I was extremely angry and scared, and I wasn't getting much support or understanding from anyone else in the family."

Chasin found other problems. "The oldest boy, Ted, who was thirteen, was moving into adolescence a little too fast. I had the sense he was being disaffected and trashing things too much, precociously trying to put his family behind him. It would be okay for him not to abandon childhood so rapidly. On the other hand Andrew, the middle kid, who was nine, was superclean, overorganized, compulsive. One boy was too bad and the other too good, and in opposite ways each was unable to deal with his impulses." Lapsing into family systems jargon, Chasin says, "The whole male subsystem was so poorly bonded. The kids were not supported by each other, and the mother was dealing separately with each of them and with her husband. The concept was to find links, bonds."

As session two begins, Chasin and the boys are sprawled comfortably on the floor, nestled in pillows and cradling batakas, the large soft bats he offers to patients who are feeling angry. The older boys are talking maturely; Bobby is giggling, making faces, bopping Chasin with a bataka, and saying things like, "I'd like to pee inside your hair." Chasin, acting unflappable, gets the story from Andrew:

A: He has to have medicine to make him do it in the toilet.
RC: Have you ever told him how you feel about him pooping in his pants? Have you talked about it?
A: Yep. We tell him it's disgusting. I told him that only babies do poops in their pants.
RC: I see. And that doesn't seem to help very much?
A: I tell him it's really disgusting.
RC: I see. You tell him it's disgusting, and what do you do for him when he stops doing that, when he does it in the toilet?
A: Well, we used to give him a prize, but now everyone just starts cheering.
RC: I see.
A: And my mother does a jig dance.
RC: Well, why should he bother to grow up? Why will it be good for him to grow up?
A: It's fun to play with him when he's bigger.
RC: You like him better when he's bigger, huh? It's important for him to know why he should grow up, because otherwise he'll just keep on pooping and stay a baby. What would be a good reason for him to grow up, besides what Andrew mentioned?
A: So we can communicate with him better.

RC: You want him to go to the bathroom like a big boy, and you want to talk
        with him like a big boy, and you want to play with him like a big boy. So
        you want him to be part of your club, huh? You have a big boys' club in
        your house.

The "boys' club" is one of the themes of this session, and the other is
"control," which Chasin has introduced by asking the boys about their
mother's explosions of temper; summarizing their account of it, he says,
"So this anger of hers used to be more frightening. Now there's more
control."

Andrew also says Bobby bites and pinches, and he wishes he would
stop. Meanwhile Bobby, who has been soaking up what his brothers are
saying about him, continues to carry on. Chasin, growing sterner, finally
says, "I can see how the silliness is used to get attention." But when he
asks the older boys how *their* relationship could improve, he learns that
Andrew wants Ted to play with him more, and that Ted is getting punched
by Andrew as well as Bobby. "People get attention for the wrong things,
being silly or hitting," Chasin says.

Now he asks Bobby to stand on a chair and show him how tall he would
like to be. The brothers seem pleased when Bobby climbs up, and Chasin
says: "Now, let's make believe you're very big, okay? And see what
happens." Chasin, Andrew, and Ted all kneel down. "You're the biggest
one right now," Chasin continues. "Now, let's turn it upside down. Let's
make believe that Andrew's the baby." Andrew and Ted are having a
wonderful time regressing, rolling on the floor and hitting each other with
pillows. "Okay," Chasin says, "now look at those babies, look how they're
carrying on! *You can tell them to stop because you're bigger.*" ("I was really
laying on the double entendres," Chasin told me later, with a belly-laugh
or two.)

"Stop! Stop!" Bobby says, and the older boys' compliance is instan-
taneous. Now Chasin, ever the magus, asks Andrew, the overcontrolled
middle brother, to pretend he's pooping in his pants, and Bobby to tell him
what to do. "Do it inside the toilet!" Bobby shouts commandingly, and
Andrew immediately pretends to obey. Bobby orders the boys to do
peepee in the toilet, and the boys, laughing wildly, perform, till Bobby
says, "Hold it, hold it!" and they stop. Chasin is standing next to Bobby,
coaching him gently, and says, "You're a terrific grown-up."

Bobby tells Andrew not to hit Ted, and Chasin says, "They're getting good at holding it. Are you going to sing to them?" The game continues with Bobby getting to stay up later than Andrew and Ted. The brothers are clearly enjoying each other.

Now Chasin introduces "a very strange game called Poops. Everyone is a poop in this game." The boys get into this, with Ted yelling, "Someone's flushing me!" and Chasin saying, "We're all poops. What happens after we go down the toilet?" "We drown. Aaaah!" shouts Andrew, and all the boys jump off the chairs. Now everyone, including the therapist, is rolling on the floor, and the boys are laughing wildly. Chasin says, "Now we're swimming in the sewer somewhere. We're going into the ocean. Did you ever swim in the ocean?" There's lots of squealing, giggling, and roughhousing—"Look out!" "Get off me, you poop!"—and Chasin says, "I bet you didn't know your poops had this much fun after they left the toilet. I want to interview each of these poops." The interview goes this way:

RC: Now, did you go into a toilet?

A: Yep, I almost drowned.

RC: You almost drowned, but what happened? You seem to be quite alive right now. Did you go into the ocean?

A: No, I think I was resting in the sewer drain for about fifty years. I'm almost faded, you see?

RC: I see, you don't look quite a good color. Now, what about you?

T: I'm an old hand, I've been in the sewer for about thirty years. Sixty years!

RC: All right, and are you a poop over here? Did you go into that toilet, poop?

B: Yes, I just went down a big tube, yesterday.

RC: And what's at the bottom of the tube?

B: Poops! [The boys all pile on top of each other].

RC: All his brother poops. A whole family of poops.

By the end of the session, the boys seem much more of a unit. Chasin observes that he was drawing on psychoanalytic ideas—"Many kids are afraid their body parts are slipping down the toilet"—and playing symbolically, but the psychodramatic techniques were much different from those Sarnoff might use: instead of taking his cues from Bobby, Chasin directed the play himself. "Bobby was getting attention by being a baby. I wanted to see if he could develop an image of himself as big and have it fortified by his brothers, so I turned everything around. The other kids were given an enormous license to be childish. Each kid learned something about stopping impulses. For Bobby it was highly rewarding to replace this fearsome lavatory where you drop your parts with the idea of a romp with his brothers—a whole family of poops taking a trip."

The encopresis stopped soon after this session. Chasin's next—and last—move with the Tylers was a "bash" for Dad, Andrew, and Bobby, in which Peter Tyler and his two sons joined in picking up batakas and having at the people who needed bashing in each of their lives, represented successively by a giant soft-sculpture doll. Dad, a management consultant, wanted the boys to help him bash "clients that don't let me come home on time"; Andrew had a couple of teachers he wasn't fond of, and Bobby offered up some bullying playmates. The Tylers also got to bash each other (for specified reasons) and the absent Mom and Ted, who were going to look at the tape afterward, but the family-bashing was followed by a countervailing ritual in which each Tyler thanked the others for one good thing. The striking feature of the bash was its good humor. It was designed not to smoke out deep resentments but to build empathy.

Jane Tyler was pleased with the results. "I think the issue was to get me out of this problem completely and try to give it some lightness. The boys formed a sympathetic bond with Bobby in a way they couldn't at home because I was so uptight about it. I had been very down on myself because I couldn't deal with the problem alone. But then I thought, if Dick doesn't see it as such a horrendous thing, maybe I'm not such a terrible person."

While Jane, outnumbered by the men in her family, said she still needed individual therapy to deal with her own angry feelings, the Tylers decided after the family sessions that Bobby and each of his brothers would benefit by particular shared activities. He and Andrew started karate classes together, and "little by little we began to look more diligently for ways to involve Bobby in the life of the other boys." After three sessions Chasin felt his work with the Tylers was finished. "When the ice breaks, things begin to flow, and the therapist gets out of the way," he says.

I asked Chasin whether he felt Bobby's infantile behavior had served some buried family purpose, a notion that various family systems theorists have propagated over the years. "They were just stuck," Chasin says. "I don't know why, but unless I see a family resolutely rewarding symptomatic behavior and undermining my therapy, I give them the benefit of the doubt. I assume that solutions that once worked for them may no longer be useful, and they have simply developed some crummy habits for the next stage of life. They want to move on but don't know how."

Sometimes probing the problem is necessary. The most dramatic feature of Chasin's sessions is the amount of information he can draw out in a short time, and his ability to keep control of the session so that family members' outpourings don't get out of hand. I saw a compelling illustration of this in the tape of his conversation with Nicole, a fetching school-phobic seven-year-old with short curly black hair and blue eyes. It also showed how imaginatively family therapists use videotape, and how collegial consultations proceed.

Some years ago, Chasin and Sallyann Roth were attending a teaching conference in another city, at which visiting firemen and homegrown talent all demonstrated their techniques. As one of the panels was beginning, Harry Kling (a pseudonym for a well-known therapist based in that city, used here to further disguise his patient) got an emergency call from Nicole's mother, Joni. She told Kling, who had been working with the family, that Nicole's behavior had gotten out of control and that Joni, who had been abused in childhood, didn't trust herself. "Harry said, 'We have a visitor in town who has a lot of experience working with children. Maybe we should take advantage and get a consultation.' I asked him, 'Why is she so freaked out that the kid's not going to school?' and Harry said, 'Because she's been not going to school a lot in the last three weeks.' When a mother with a history of abuse says she's going to lose control, you stop everything and help her. You don't wait."

As Chasin was loading the cassette, he said, "I love this tape. I think child therapists are a little crazy about kids on the whole. The work is messier. You have to get down on the floor. Paints spoil your clothes. When you want them to sit still and talk with you, they might run around the room, and during a day you have a headache, they can be a real pain."

The tape came on, showing Kling, Sallyann Roth, Joni, Nicole and Chasin, who suggests a modus operandi: he and Nicki will talk in the interview room, while Joni will go with Kling and Roth behind a one-way mirror, "where you could have a conversation but also at times hear what was happening in here." If Nicki should ask to turn off the speaker and Chasin agreed, they would do so. ("I'm talking about privacy now," he told me as we watched. "I don't like to give the kids too much power—that's crazy. Whether her mother hears something or not, at her age she's not necessarily the best judge. If the kid is sixteen, though, it's murkier. Still, if it's not safe, there's a public policy issue." Chasin was referring to state requirements that mandate reporting by therapists to authorities when a minor appears to be the victim of parental abuse.) More procedures are set down and reviewed, and Nicki examines the room and equipment: "Explicit contracting is a very important part of family therapy," Chasin told me. "I'm assuming Harry's got a phone between the two rooms: that technology is in our culture. I want to show the girl where her mother is going to be."

Now Chasin is alone with Nicki and starts to join. "Well, let me tell you what I know. There are four people in your family, right? And another thing I know is that you've gone to Africa, right? And is there anything else amazing about you that I should know?"

N: I do all grade two math. And I'm in grade one.
RC: Wow! Is that because you're really smart?
N: Mm-hm. But I'm not really smart in this kind of stuff.
RC: And which kind of stuff is this kind of stuff?
N: Temper tantrums.
RC: Oh, you think you're not smart enough in temper tantrums. So are you in kindergarten in temper tantrums?
N: Yeah.

The joining done, Chasin now sets out to get the story, asking Nicki if she always hates school or only sometimes; Nicki replies she didn't "at the starting of it." Chasin launches the enactment of a typical day, with Nicki lying on his jacket as her bed. In order to engage her in the scene, he asks her if she had a good dream last night, but this doesn't prove fruitful, and they go on to how the day starts, in detail: who has breakfast together, where is every member of the family, and how does her brother Chad get to school.

RC: Let's be Chad for a little bit. Are you willing to be Chad? Hello, Chad, how old are you?
N   (LAUGHING): Almost ten.
RC: Are you going to school this morning?
N: Yeah.

RC: You don't have any doubt about it, do you?
N: No.
RC: When was the last time you had a tantrum? . . . It's been a long time, huh?
N: Yeah.

"I could just as easily have said, 'Does your brother have tantrums? Does he have problems getting to school?' " Chasin said to me. "This is the action equivalent. With her it would have been just as easy." But Nicki is throwing herself into it: she acts Chad with gusto, her voice dropping, her hands in her pockets, her walk cool and boyish. She is the last word in adorable. Chasin gets her to act how relaxed and happy Chad feels walking to school with his best friend, and then he asks her to become Nicole again.

RC: Now, Nicole, as you're eating breakfast, does it come into your mind that this could be one of those mornings that it'll be so easy for you to go to school, you won't think about it at all? You won't even remember that you ever had a tantrum?
N: No.
RC: You think about it while you're eating breakfast. So let's hear how your thoughts go as you think about not going to school. What's on your mind?
N: Do you want me to show you what it looks like when I go to school and when I don't go, and I try not to go?
RC: Have you shown anybody else that?
N: No.
RC (VERY ENTHUSIASTICALLY): Well, I'd love to see it then. It's very important. Show me how you go to school.

Chasin said to me, "She got the idea that I'd really like her to show me things. 'This is how we do business with this guy.' The kid is very adaptable. If I were a sitting-and-talking therapist, she'd say, 'Do you want me to *tell* you?' I'm guessing that the technique I happen to use is not the only one."

They start with what Nicki calls the "good way," when, like Chad, she walks over to a friend's house, bouncing along and humming. Chasin plays the friend, glad to see her and grateful to have smart Nicki there to help her get under way. Then Chasin asks, "When you arrive at school, is there anybody who's happy to see you at school?"

The plot thickens. "My boyfriend, David," says Nicki, "and my two best friends." Playing David, Nicki doesn't look that happy to see his girlfriend, but the friends are cheerful. "So this is the way it works when it's good," Chasin says. "Do you get a star? Or an award or anything? Do you put anything up on your refrigerator when you come home?" Chasin wants to find out whether the family is using any behavior-mod techniques (no) and then writes on the blackboard Nicki's name for the good days: "friendly day." Then they begin the enactment of a "sad day." "We're going to go very slowly," he tells her, and they run through waking up, getting washed and getting dressed to find out when Nicki first decides the day will be sad.

The sadness begins when Nicki is having breakfast. "I have one idea," she says, "that my friends will not let me play with David."

Chasin is listing all this on the blackboard. "Now, does that idea make it a sad day right away? Or you can have that idea and still have a friendly day?"

"Yeah," Nicki says. "I go, 'Oh, that won't happen.' "

But when it becomes a sad day, Nicki is doing her math problems at the breakfast table. "Well, then I think David will beat me up."

In a calm, journalistic tone, Chasin gets a repeat: "That David will beat you up?" "Beat me up," Nicki says firmly.

"So here we are, very interesting," Chasin continues, writing on the blackboard, reviewing the last two items Nicki has told him. "Now, has David ever beaten you up?"

"Yeah. And he's wrecked my skipping rope once. Both ends." With two more of those flat repetitive questions that therapists are known for, Chasin elicits that "he started playing tug of war with it with his friends, then both of the end parts fell off."

As we watched this, Chasin told me, "What I don't know at the time is that when Mother hears this about David beating her up, Mother is just riveted to the mirror because Mother was an abused child. She's not heard anything about this before. Nobody knows—they've basically said it's a mystery why this kid isn't in school. And here she is laying it all out. But I didn't know that most of these details were unknown to Mother."

With these thoughts in her head at breakfast, Nicki says, she tells her mom she didn't do all her math problems. "Are you telling your mother the truth?" Chasin asks. "Did you not do all your math problems, or are you telling her that because that's a good reason not to go to school?"

"Yeah," Nicki says. Chasin, watching the tape, produced one of his belly-laughs. "You've gotta be onto kids," he said.

RC: So you tell your mother something that isn't exactly true . . . and . . . does she check to see whether you've done them?

N: No.

RC: Does she start to get mad at you because she thinks, uh-oh, it's gonna be a—what does your mother call these mornings? She doesn't call them sad.

N: Mad days. (RC continues to write on the blackboard.) And then my mom drags me to school.

RC: How do you feel about being dragged to school on a sad day?

N: Bad.

RC: Do you have a tantrum?

N: I do cry. But I don't have a tantrum.

RC: I see. Have you told your mom about these fears you have about David?

N: Unh-unh.

RC (STILL WRITING ON THE BLACKBOARD): So she doesn't know that you have all these sad thoughts on your mind. . . .

N: But just wait. . . . Then I'm holding on to my mom . . . and then my teacher pulls me away. Then I start crying more, and then he pulls me into the class and then I like, cry my heart out.

RC: Oh, I see. So your teacher pulls you in the class crying your heart out, and of course all the other kids see it?

N: Uh-huh, and there's nineteen other kids.

RC: Are you really embarrassed a lot? Because they don't have any idea of what's happened, do they?

Chasin is hitting pay dirt. Nicki is sure her classmates think she's a baby: Chasin says, "It's just awful when you come into that class. It's one of the worst parts of it, isn't it?" Then he asks her to play David. She wants to play him outside, because that's where he beats her up.

Chasin is getting all the details of who gets beaten up (just Nicki) and who gets kissed (various other girls) in the school yard. The relationship between the children is intricate, and Chasin tries to sort out the details and dynamics of it all: David beats her up because she doesn't come near him, and she doesn't come near him because he beats her up. Chasin was still thinking about this sequence when we watched it: "Is this not the Hedda and Steinberg thing [alluding to a criminal abuse story then making the headlines] at seven years old? It's just mind-blowing, that this sweet-looking kid, she's obviously very intelligent, and she's in this sick relationship. Can you imagine what her mother is going through? If you viewed this, and you were abused, and your daughter is the one who is being beaten up on a systematic basis? She might as well know the information."

There is a long enactment of the children's games, with Chasin playing Nicki, trying to imagine her feelings and saying, "Tell me if I'm making any mistakes"; he's not. Finally after eliciting detailed information from Nicki about what David might think and what she thinks, he says, "Why don't you come over here and help me be you? I know he's my boyfriend, but on the other hand, he beats me up, so maybe I should just totally stay away from him. What would be wrong with that? What would be *wrong* with that?"

They do a bit of problem-solving: Who can get David to stop beating Nicki up? She is afraid to tell the teacher—David will deny it and claim she's lying. So Chasin enacts what the teacher might say to David: "I'm not interested in whether they're lies or not lies. I'm interested in what you do from now on. You have to not do it in the future. If you can't, we'll have to talk with your parents, and we may even have to find some way of punishing you." Chasin later told me he didn't really expect Nicole to run to the teacher, but Nicki's mother was watching and was likely to act on what she heard. Nicki simply needed to know there were effective ways to deal with the situation.

David might respond to that threat, Chasin says on the tape, if Nicki doesn't tease him. But there is more to the situation: Nicki's two best girlfriends are competing for "special time" with David at Nicki's expense, and they still won't let her play with him, and that makes her sad at breakfast. Chasin said to me, "Look at her standing in this social community. It's not good news. This looks like individual therapy, but there's this poor mother watching this thing, and the more it unfolds, the worse the news is for her." On tape he says to Nicki mournfully, "So it's really sad when you can't see him, and it's really sad when you do see him, and he beats you up." Nicki is totally forthcoming, and the intricacy of the detail and the spontaneity of her reactions are absolutely credible.

The phone rings. That is a familiar event in family systems sessions.

Joni and Harry have called to tell Chasin that even before the past three weeks, when David became a problem, Nicole sometimes had difficulties going to school. He asks her about this, about other sad thoughts that might have made her want to stay home before she got involved with David. This is harder to pull out, but off and on she has worried that "everybody's going to laugh at me because they think I'm like a baby."

"I can see how this happens," Chasin tells Nicole. "If you have any kind of thought that makes you feel like you can't go to school, then you may find yourself being dragged to school, you come in all teary, and when you show up in front of your class, you look like a baby and you hate that. I think I understand about these sad thoughts and how strong they are."

An obvious problem is Nicki's sad thoughts. And Chasin begins to attack it. "Now," he says, "there's going to be a perfectly wonderful girl here, and we're going to put her in this chair, and we're going to call her Nicole. And she's terrific. She's been to Africa, and she's very smart in math, she's a whole grade ahead of herself. We're going to make believe."

"Okay," Nicole says giggling. "But she doesn't have black hair and she doesn't have a mother named Joni."

"Now," Chasin says, "I want you to come over here, and I want you to be kind of a sad thought monster."

N: What's a sad thought monster?

RC: A sad thought monster isn't very nice. You see, these are the tissues that people cry into when they're sad, and you have a lot of tissues, and you can give anybody a sad thought if you want to.

N: Okay, that'll be fun.

RC: Here's a girl you could give a sad thought to. Her name is Nicki. Which sad thought are you going to give her now?

N: David's going to beat you up today!

RC: Drop the tissue [pointing to the imaginary girl's head], because that's a sad thought. Very good. Give her another sad thought.

N: And the friends aren't going to let you play!

RC: Terrific! Keep going.

N: Everybody's going to laugh at you today!

Other sad thoughts come out: that her brother will beat her up, that she will be lonely because her mother won't spend time with her, that her father will lock her in the bedroom because she's bothering her brother. I said to Chasin, "It all keeps coming."

"I just met her forty minutes ago," he said. "It's amazing what's coming out. Her therapy must be very good. As a consultant, I'm assuming Harry Kling is doing a wonderful job. See the high level of trust when a stranger comes in the room and talks with her!"

"But she hasn't told this to Harry Kling," I said.

"No," Chasin answered, "the therapy has a problem, but it's not a disaster scene, because if it was, she wouldn't trust me."

On tape, Chasin is saying to Nicki, "So you're quite a thing, sad monster. Do you enjoy doing this to her?"

"Yeah," says Nicki.

RC: Okay, now, do you know what I'm going to do? I'm going to be your sad monster. You sit over there in your sad chair.

N: *You're* going to put everything on *me*?

RC: You don't have to like it. And you don't even have to accept it if you want. I'm going to try to put this sad thought in your head, and let's see what you do. Her friends won't let her play with David! You can struggle against me if you want to.

N: How do I struggle against you?

RC: I'm trying to think of some way, because once this thought lands in your head, you're going to have to think about it. [Nicki swats away the next tissue.] Hey—you threw away my sad thought! Oh, it doesn't matter, I've got another one! Aha, David's gonna beat you up! [Nicki is giggling with glee.] I want it on your head! Your father's gonna lock you in your room! I've got a great one now: All the kids except maybe a few friends are going to laugh at you because you're such a ba-bee!

Chasin and Nicki are having a wild Kleenex fight, Chasin throwing the tissues—each a sad thought—at Nicki, who is laughing wildly and hurling them back at him. She is having as much fun as the Tyler boys impersonating poops in the sewer. It is all of a piece.

Then Chasin, continuing to be the sad thoughts monster, turns gloomy. "I'm doing very badly. I'm beginning to feel sad about my work. Maybe I won't be able to put sad thoughts in your head anymore."

"You will die," says Nicki, and she and Chasin both laugh exuberantly. "Are you going to kill me?" he asks. "Yeah. And I'm going to put a sad thought in *your* head!" she answers.

Chasin is writing on the blackboard, a list of sad thoughts Nicki suggests to give the monster. "You will go to jail because you did all those bad things to people! Your mother will stab you because you hurted everyone in our heart!"

Chasin suggests that when Nicki wakes up in the morning, she thinks about ways to fight off the sad monster by giving him some thoughts. He told me, "I'm about to suggest solutions for a problem the cause of which I really don't know very well, at the deepest level. I don't know how she found herself in this unique position in her social system."

"Behaviorists would model social skills with her?" I asked, evoking Sharon Foster in San Diego.

"Absolutely, and they would also have this forward-looking attitude. Who the hell knows how this happened, but there's obviously a lot of work to be done."

Nicki is supposed to be prepared with sad-thought tissues for the monster anytime he may strike. And now everyone agrees it's time for Joni, Harry Kling, and Sallyann Roth to come in. Up till now, it has looked like individual therapy, but Joni, as she reports, "was listening pretty closely. I'm very glad I know that now."

It has moved into a sort of brainstorming session, in which Joni says, "I wonder if this sad thought process works whenever she leaves the house to do anything, because we don't do swimming lessons anymore, we don't do dancing lessons anymore, we rarely go to other people's houses, but we have children into our house." Chasin asks Joni if Nicole tells her about the sad thoughts, and Joni says, "No, no, that just blew me. . . . I had no idea that that's what goes on in the morning for her."

But it also comes out that Nicki doesn't want to tell her mom about the sad thoughts, because then the events she fears will actually happen. They do a bit of acting out monster scenes, and Chasin introduces the idea that just maybe the sad thought *won't* happen *because* Nicki tells Mom. He says, "She seems to be eager to tell of ways she wants to attack this source of sadness."

At this point another voice is heard from: Roth has been wondering "what other people in the family do when the sad monster comes to put sad thoughts in their heads."

The rest of the family, it turns out, is fairly open: when Chad has a nightmare, he crawls in bed with Mom and Dad and they take him back, tuck him in, and stay with him till he tells about the dream. If he's nervous about something, he tells Mom, who tends to say, "I know what that's like,

I remember when I was your age." When Mom and Dad have an argument, they will talk it through in front of the kids. But Mom, who is sometimes harried, says about Nicole, "It's not offered from the *source*, whereas the other sources will offer, so I can't keep guessing. I don't know how to draw out what goes on." "The son goes to her," Chasin said to me. "Apparently Nicole doesn't. It's fascinating that Nicole who's so forthcoming here doesn't tell her mother these things. Maybe there's something special about a girl to her mother. It may be very easy for her to listen to the boy and not the girl." Then the conversation takes another dramatic turn:

> RC: Nicki, would you like to not hear about or hear more about sad thoughts your mother had when she was your age?
> N: *Not* hear.
> RC: Do you think you know what some of them are? [No response.] By not hearing about them, are you protecting yourself from getting sad, or are you protecting your mother from getting sad?
> N: Protecting *me* from getting sad.
> RC: Are there times when your mother's sad stories make you sad?
> N: Uh-huh.
> RC: Have you felt sad for her a number of times?
> N: Uh-huh.
> RC: Have you always told her that you felt sad for her?
> N: Unh-uh.

"Look at that!" Chasin said to me. "Here's the mother, doing what the mental health book says, saying, 'I used to feel terrible, have nightmares, and kids did this and that to me,' and the poor girl is feeling that way. How would you know?"

There follows a bit of what family therapists call "circular questioning," in which Chasin asks what would change in the family if Nicki's mother knew how sympathetic Nicki was. Would it be all right with her father, her brother, her mother? "When you introduce a new idea into the system," Chasin told me, "you check around, will anybody mind this? Will the brother be jealous that she's right there where he used to be? If it's all right all around, then it becomes a dyadic matter, between the two of them."

Joni is now able to make a suggestion: "What would happen if there was some kind of game that took place, and the game might have something to do with making up sad thoughts, some of which were real and some of which were completely make-believe, and nobody would know which were which." Chasin's addition is that Nicki tries saying to her mother, "I am sorry that you feel sad sometimes," and Joni, instead of seeming sad, says, 'I'm relieved to have such a good daughter.' "

Here Chasin told me, "I'm trying to open this pattern. This very natural thing on the child's part, to be sympathetic with her mother, has become something that jams things up. She gets the idea that 'if I tell her, it's going to remind her of all the horrible things that happened to her, so I'm gonna keep these things to myself.' " This way of reacting could play out in Nicki's relationships in the future: she might never be able to ask anyone to help her, as she was unable to talk to the teacher or to her mother.

Kling suggests that *Mother* pretend to be the sad monster, and Chasin wraps up that when Nicki gets a sad thought—she makes it into a tissue and drops it on her mother. "Mother *is* the sad thoughts monster in a way," Chasin told me. "Harry is so clever, I wouldn't be surprised if he were conscious of that: not until this minute did it occur to me. But by *pretending*, it takes on a different meaning. Instead of *involuntarily* being it, she takes it on voluntarily, and the child can give her hell for being a sad monster instead of feeling awful."

Everyone likes Kling's idea and refines it, and Nicki decides that a special box of colored tissues must be bought for this ritual. The group agrees that the teacher must be told to stop the other kids from laughing.

"This brainstorming is almost unique to family therapy," Chasin says. "I wanted to reinforce the process by which the daughter tells the mother the sad thoughts so the daughter could talk to the mother. She has to tell her mother where her sad thoughts are in order to play the game in which she rejects them. Both Sallyann and the mother have an appreciation for ritual, and when you bring them into the process, their creative juices flow." Chasin gave out a big laugh. "This is a bonding ritual between mother and daughter with Kleenexes!

"It is really very complicated," he went on. "The child can disclose sad thoughts to her mother but in a highly ritualized way. She has a lot of control over the way she tells them. My guess was that before, she picked up that her mother wasn't just saying, 'I know how you feel,' she was talking about very heavy stuff. The mother really resonated, and the kid picked it up as a no-no."

Chasin addressed me. "You want to be underlining differences among therapies, here it is. Because of our collaborative attitude, Mother's really using her intelligence: 'We need your thoughts' is the message to her, and that activates her creativity, which is what we want ultimately. We want these people to be able to go out and have something that *works*."

While the style of this tape was pure Chasin, the idea of the monster was not: the day before we watched this session, he gave me a 1984 paper called "Fear Busting and Monster Taming" by Michael White, an Australian therapist who represents the cutting edge of family systems work. White's core is a notion called "externalizing" in which the therapist portrays an internal problem as an exterior force against which the family struggles; this, White believes, will mobilize them into action. In response to my own questions, Chasin emphasized that this is not a form of "victim psychology." "Do you see how unthreatening it is for Nicki to be thinking this way, that she is not a kid who is *generating* sad thoughts? It doesn't matter whether it's true or not." While one might assume that "externalizing" problems makes children less responsible, in fact they learn to see themselves as combating an oppressor, an action they have chosen to take.

Much of White's work has been with children; he suggests there's a cycle in which children's fearfulness leads parents to become more protective, which invites the children to be even more dependent. "Monster taming" tries to establish a "virtuous cycle" in which the family gets together to combat the fear-monster. The child starts by drawing the monster, the first step toward capturing and taming it; then he is taught the Fourth Rule of Monsters: "Since monsters grow more fearsome with night-practice and more funny with day-practice, if children want to have a funny time, then they should stop their monsters from having night-practice." The family participates in an elaborate ritual in which the drawing of the monster is locked up in a steel box, tied with rope, taken into the garden, and tied to a tree so "the monsters' fury will not disturb the household. Whenever possible, the rope should be tied such that the box is suspended. This is because fears are less troublesome if they cannot get their feet on the ground." Every night the child puts his sneakers under his pillow so he can chase the fears if they escape during the night, and "the fears are to be let out every morning for day-practice to make them funny."

Fear-busting had a particular resonance with my research: I was becoming ever more curious to find out how Chasin would treat Freud's Little Hans. Later on, therefore, I gave him a call to discuss the case. It was many, many years since Chasin had read the story—although a number of family therapists, like theorists in other orientations, had found it amusing to recast Freud's original effort. I read Chasin my own summary of the paper to refresh his memory and found him questioning me in such detail that I felt like a colleague coming for a consult.

He was particularly eager to piece together the time sequence of Mother's threats to have Hans's widdler cut off, to beat Hans, and to leave him. He sought to weave this into the progression of Hans's curiosity, Hanna's birth, Hans's fears, and the giraffe dream. First he said to me, thoughtfully, "We know nothing about the marriage." "Except that it finally broke up," I answered. A three-year-old boy's curiosity about widdlers, Chasin observed, "is absolutely not notable. It would have been standard even before the age of three, but his father was probably not so careful an observer as he might have been."

Chasin was the first therapist I encountered to tie Hans's fears to the boy's own life and to contemporary culture; it had seemed obvious to me that Viennese childrearing practices were much to blame for Hans's symptoms, but Chasin put my cultural notions in context. "The idea of something being cut off is perhaps much more plausible to Hans than it might be to other Viennese children who heard such empty threats, because, unlike Hans, they weren't treated to seeing basins of blood all over the place with a screaming mother. The idea of the mutilation of private parts is in his mind a very plausible business. And he may fear that the kind of thing that happened to his mother will happen to him.

"So he develops a number of fears and gets pretty clingy, for many reasons. He has also a fear of losing mother and father. He had the idea that his mother was going to die in this horrible birth at home, for which, of course, he was not prepared. It's not that home is horrible, but *no one told him anything.*

"The mother's letting him into bed when he is wistful or sad or frightened could mean absolutely nothing except she felt badly for the boy. I don't want to make a federal case out of that. From this little boy's point of view, Mother is quite a mixed story. Father in a way is opposed but succumbs to the child's method for seeking reassurance. His fear of losing his parents doesn't strike me as such an extraordinary idea, given that his mother has threatened to leave and if she could leave, Father could leave too. Here's a boy who has a lot of fears, and on some subjects his father is absolutely no good for reassurance. Father is at the same time very interested in these subjects, but he won't disclose to the boy what he is finding out.

"Do we know if the boy is assured his penis will not actually be cut off? Does anyone *tell him straight out*? When the father asks the boy about masturbation, the boy sounds to me very clever but also evasive. If he has not been reassured, he would be completely crazy to confess to this crime, because he would pay a hideous punishment. The boy's denial means to me no one has ever squared with him.

"For the first time," Chasin said, "I'm having a family therapy thought. How does the father feel about Mother's threats?" It sounded, I told him, like what people said in *Alt Wien*, and while you could expect in those days that people might say masturbation is a sin, to threaten to cut his penis off is a whole other ball game; I was shocked.

"It may be another ball game if his mother is really very angry—angry at Father, angry about her life. A lot has to do with the tone in which she says things. If she says, 'Oh, I'll cut it off, ha ha,' that's one thing. But if she's under stress her threats may be really terrifying. Again, Hans probably was not directly brutalized more than other people, but once again, the quality of the 'beatings' is not in the story. We don't know whether Mother beat the children in a perfunctory way, like, 'I have to do this because they were bad,' or whether she was in a flaming rage."

Now that Chasin asked me these questions, it seemed clear that a lot of the texture of this case was not in Freud's account; Chasin said, "That's not the theory he's interested in. He's interested in sexual theory." Subsequent writers in other orientations were interested in proving Freud wrong. Chasin was trying to look at the real case.

"This is a very fearful boy, and my question is, What is he afraid of? He's clearly not afraid of horses, he's never been injured by a horse, it's some kind of displacement. Can he get a straight answer from his parents about what he's really afraid of? I suspect the answer is no. He doesn't get confirmation that in fact his penis will not be cut off, or that what happened to his mother was not some kind of horrible mutilating experience, and he does not get confirmation that she won't in fact leave. I question the tone these statements are made in and the reassurances available to him. If the child were in therapy with me, I would invite him to play the mother saying this and hear exactly how he hears it. He may exaggerate, but if he does, the mother might say, 'I don't say it that way,' and the father might say, 'My God, she doesn't say it *that* way,' and then I'd have the idea that there's some other source for the fear.

"We have a complete absence of information about the sexual relationship of Mother and Father. Father has a kind of interesting sexual relationship with the boy in that he's documenting the boy's sexuality. Mother has what may be in those days a standard relationship with the boy sexually in that she's trying to prevent his masturbation but also comforts him when he's fearful. But we have nothing about the parents' relationship to each other, and no analogue in the dimension that I feel seems more important in this case than sexuality, which is the dimension of bitterness, anger, and violence.

"It may be my culture, but I am at a loss to find this boy's sexuality so extraordinary. He might be very interested in this thing he might lose any day. It may seem like a lot of childhood sexuality to Freud because he, after all, was the very person who put the normality of childhood sexuality on the map, and maybe when they first documented this, it seemed like a lot of sexuality."

When I continued to press Chasin on secrecy, he told me that it was not secrecy per se, but secrecy about *a charged issue* that causes problems. "What seems in the 1990s like the most obvious thing is that this boy has been threatened and beaten and had scenes with a good deal more blood in them than most little kids see, and that he's fearful. I have some other questions: Does Mother want to cut off Father's penis in effect? What happened in the marriage after Hans was born? What happened later after Hanna was born? Was there a difference? How does Father feel about all this stuff?"

So Chasin would start with a session for just Mother and Father, and "I would do quite a lot of inquiry, not only into their observations but into their relationship. I probably would ask when they fight with each other, how they fight, and in this day and age I would say, 'How often does it become physical?' And if somebody says never I would say, 'How do you restrain yourself from doing that?' They might say, 'It's just not in my nature,' or, 'I have to count to ten.' I would basically normalize the questions, but I would want to know. You can't always be sure there is no domestic violence when you're talking with a husband and wife together. You might be able to pick up clues that would lead you to talk to the mother separately, though she may still be afraid to tell you. But I think it's unlikely that there is violence in this family.

"I am going to go at the subject of fear in a different way. I don't know why the boy is afraid, but I believe he has a good deal to learn from his parents on the subject, and by getting it out as an issue that everybody has to deal with, the world is normalized, and he has opportunities for identification with them.

"Here is a family therapy session at which Hans is present. The subject of the session is 'people and their fears.' I would ask Father and Mother what they remembered being afraid of, and what made it worse and what made it better, and how each managed to conquer these various fears they had, and who was reassuring to them and gave them reassuring information, and who aggravated the fears. I would have Hans not be the subject but the bystander of his parents' addressing the same issues that he is struggling with. Also in the process of doing that, the family, instead of being told what he's going through, will get what the interview is about, being able to give him a useful legacy for profiting from their experience and wisdom. No family will be mystified—they'll immediately see the relevance. It's a pain in the neck for them to deal with the kid—he says he can't go to the park, et cetera.

"And I would ask the father if he recalls his own masturbation as a very young child. Does he remember whether his mother ever told him his penis would be removed for masturbating? If he doesn't remember, does he imagine that she did or didn't tell him that? Where did the mother learn this? Was it in her family of origin that children were told that? And what does she say to girls who are masturbating? And on and on, but basically getting all this information out in a way that doesn't identify the boy so much as the troubled one, but *fear* as the troubling feeling."

In this exercise Chasin seemed less interested than psychodynamic or behavioral therapists in either forming or rejecting a theory of how Hans arrived at his fear. But theory is strong in family therapy: Chasin has, indeed, taken thirty years of inventive theorizing within his tribe and integrated it with his own exuberant clinical style. Sometimes when I questioned him, I found myself being mischievously drawn into a role-playing exercise, at the end of which the question was answered. Much of the theorizing in family therapy, it seemed to me, has to do with technique: it involves new ways to achieve the pragmatic goal of helping the family get unstuck. To discuss how the ideas have evolved and how Chasin as a clinician has evolved with them, I paid him a second series of visits sometime after the first. The next chapter focuses on what I learned.

CHAPTER 11

"BEING TOM IS DIFFERENT FROM BEING A WAGNER"

Like all therapists, the family therapist challenges people's perceptions of reality. . . . He erodes each family member's certainty of the validity of his experience. This is not a confrontation technique. Rather, the therapist supports the family members, but suggests that there is something beyond what they have perceived.

—Salvador Minuchin,
Families and Family Therapy
(1974)

Insight is often a feeble tool in the face of life's pressing urgency. All the major new therapeutic approaches in recent years have arisen out of a basic dissatisfaction among therapists with long-term, individual, insight-oriented therapy, the basic derivative of psychoanalysis. We know all too well . . . the patient who is interminably in therapy, understands a great deal about himself, and doesn't change.

—Augustus Y. Napier with
Carl A. Whitaker,
The Family Crucible (1978)

WHEN CHASIN, SALLYANN ROTH, AND HARRY KLING put their heads together with Nicole and Joni to tame the sad thoughts monster, they sought to evoke an atmosphere of family, friends, and neighbors working out a solution around the kitchen table. It was, then, apropos for Chasin to park me at his own large kitchen table, an ideal spot for spreading out cassettes and papers. And from the look of the kitchen—spacious and comfortable but rather plain vanilla, without the battery of trendy equipment and ingredients one might expect in a prime Cambridge neighbor-hood—I guessed that kitchen table had held more audiocassettes than apple pies. It gave on a den that housed the television and VCR, so Chasin could illustrate his comments from an extensive library of his own and his colleagues' sessions. Like Sarnoff's art-laden pied-à-terre and Kendall's bustling academic office, it was—down to the notes on the refrigerator—emblematic of Chasin's tribal mores, which cultivate un-pretentiousness.

I had boned up on the origins of family systems therapy, which—unlike psychoanalysis and behaviorism—represents a braiding of many disparate strands. The strands range from various historical traditions of therapy and counseling to ideas that were exciting and hip in several other fields in the middle of the twentieth century: family systems was—and continues to be—a marriage of down-home practice and the most abstrusely cerebral philosophy.

There was the psychoanalytically based child-guidance movement, founded in Chicago in 1909 to treat juvenile offenders, which had viewed delinquency as rooted in family tensions (and blamed mothers for their children's disorders). For years, child-guidance clinics used social workers to help the parents while psychiatrists saw the children; in accordance with psychoanalytic beliefs, however, the social workers and the psychiatrists often didn't discuss the cases, and *interpersonal relationships* (as opposed to *object relations*) got short shrift. (The first child-guidance clinic in America, now the Institute for Juvenile Research in Chicago, has become one of today's leading centers of family systems therapy in the contemporary style.) There was a grand tradition of mother-bashing in the psychoanalytic world from the forties on: as we saw in Chapter 1, the child psychiatrist Stella Chess found it nearly impossible to get accurate information from parents laid low by *"mal de mère."* But some psychodynamic therapists were beginning to move from an emphasis on maternal pathology to an interactive or "goodness-of-fit" view like that espoused by Chess and her husband and collaborator, Alexander Thomas.

In the early fifties another psychoanalyst, Nathan Ackerman, had begun treating the family as a whole when one member showed symptoms. Since the 1920s psychologists and sociologists had studied group dynamics, and while families have less in common with other groups than one might think, there was interest in the idea that shaking up a group is the best way to get individual members to change. Another strand was the social work tradition of family casework, which goes back to the late nineteenth century and often included home visits, providing these practitioners with insight and knowledge that the loftier psychoanalysts blocked out (and to their discredit still disdain). Marriage counseling, another type of therapy that grew up outside the psychiatric establishment, also fed into what became family systems therapy. And rebellion against psychoanalysis played an important part in the origins of family systems therapy, just as it did in behaviorism.

Finally, the Project for the Study of Schizophrenia, led by the anthropologist Gregory Bateson in Palo Alto, contributed ideas, theorists, and practitioners that helped the field to coalesce. In 1952, Bateson had received a grant from the Rockefeller Foundation to study family communication patterns; his research group and its clinical offshoots studied the role of disordered communication in psychosis and contributed a number of ideas that for several decades were basic to the way family systems therapists viewed other problems as well.

Since Bateson himself had been an anthropologist, his group was aware of the "participant observer" method that then dominated ethnographic studies: one joined a culture to learn how a particular custom served the group's need for survival. Symptoms, the Bateson people believed, also provide some protective function in a family's culture, and the "symptom-bearer," the identified patient, sometimes unwittingly sacrifices his or her needs for the good of the family.

The California group was also inspired by the cybernetics theories of Norbert Wiener—particularly influential in the nascent world of computer science—in which a system, seeking equilibrium or homeostasis, corrects its behavior according to information—feedback—from the environment. A third influence was the general system theory of the biologist Ludwig von Bertalanffy, who held that, just as a pile of different-colored mosaic chips acquire new power and meaning when they are arranged in a pattern, a system is more than the sum of its parts, and it is fruitful to study the pattern instead of focusing on each chip separately. But Bertalanffy studied living organisms, which, he said, do not seek homeostasis: they evolve constantly through interaction with their environment.

Schizophrenia is no longer considered the *result* of dysfunctional family communication, and as we will see, the notion that *all* symptoms serve a protective familial purpose has also been challenged and modified. But the rich intellectual stew of anthropology, engineering, and biology produced a number of chewy therapeutic ideas that launched the family systems field and even penetrated popular culture. Among the best-known and most misunderstood of these ideas is Bateson's famous *double bind*, in which a family member, usually a child, is repeatedly trapped by the duty to obey conflicting orders, with implied penalties for disregarding each. For example, the parents' first order might be a negative injunction such as, "Don't use swear words." The second order competes with the first but is indirect and often nonverbal: when the child actually uses the swear words, the parents laugh, suggesting they don't really want the child to obey the first order. For a pair of conflicting messages to qualify as a genuine double bind, there has to be no release from the obligation to obey both, no permission to point out that the orders conflict with each other, and no escape from the relationship.

While contemporary family therapists do not any longer believe, as did the authors of the original theory, that double-bind communication can cause hysterias, phobias, and obsessive-compulsive disorders, it clearly creates a stressful situation that many parents and children will recognize with a shudder of familiarity. (Another example that is perhaps more resonant, from a different author, sets up the requirement that the child "do exactly as we say, but on your own initiative.") Bateson also pointed out that family communications occur on two levels: a stated level, in which the parent tells the child to wash her hands, and the "metacommunication" of the same message, which lets the child know that the parent is boss. These ideas raise issues of power and control, which fascinated some members of the Bateson group and its descendants.

All these strands had been braided, more or less, by the early sixties when Chasin was a medical resident and caught the family therapy bug. And so as I arranged my gear on his kitchen table nearly thirty years later, I began enthusiastically. "You're ideal for discussing this," I said, "because when you were young and audacious, the field was too, and you have evolved in this evolving and almost churning field, and you are now old enough to be mature but . . . not yet stagnant."

"I can tell you," he said, "when the field was audacious, I was embarrassed by its audaciousness. I love the field, but I thought it made things almost unbearable. I am by inclination a kind of peacemaker. I have always felt a mission for that." (Chasin was active during the eighties in an organization called International Physicians for the Prevention of Nuclear War; as we spoke, Laura Chasin was on the road for another endeavor, the Public Conversations Project, which has engaged pro-choice and prolife activists in "respectful dialogue" under the aegis of a team of family therapists that included the Chasins and Sallyann Roth.) "When I was aware in the early sixties," he went on, "that many of the people devoted to family therapy were bad-mouthing psychoanalysts and getting bad-mouthed by psychoanalysts, I did not want to participate. I never got into a problem with the analysts and even became one. There's got to be room for both of these things."

Chasin's supervisor at Massachusetts General Hospital was Norman Paul, a pioneer in family therapy who was devoting his life to studying a particular set of theories: Paul was interested in the effects of a family's unresolved mourning on subsequent generations. "He had a very simple but important idea about the transmission down the generations of cata-strophic happenings with which a family cannot deal adequately," Chasin said. "He even told his own story publicly, where there had been a murder and suicide in his family of origin and it profoundly influenced his upbringing because anytime he did something off the mark, his mother would get very agitated. She would not necessarily understand why she was so anxious; or she might just not have told him; so he thought there must have been something wrong with him, which was really almost the only thing to conclude. He had not understood that she was worried that people would turn out to be as disturbed as the relative who had commit-ted the murder and the suicide." Paul was, in a sense, ahead of his time: later on the field became increasingly interested in how families transmit beliefs over several generations.

"He supervised a day hospital, a very active treatment center to which people with acute psychosis came during the day and left in the late afternoon in lieu of full hospitalization. We tried to do that in the early sixties because we had a strong belief that putting people in hospital beds was more stigmatizing than sending them home at night. In order for a day hospital like that to work, the family had to be fully engaged, so we began every hospitalization with a family meeting." While Paul's ears perked up when he heard of an unresolved loss, however, he seemed less interested in the technical details of running a family meeting, and so Chasin, as chief resident, honed his skills of necessity.

"I was very pragmatic, very goal-directed, interested in what the problem was, what interfered with the families' solving it themselves, and what we could do to help them get over the hurdle. By then I knew a bit of psychoanalytic theory and was also pretty familiar with the drugs that were emerging at that time. It's an important coincidence that in the early sixties the antipsychotic and antidepressant drugs were first widely available. Psychological theories of schizophrenia began to lose some of their utterly compelling nature because there were drugs that seemed to affect the most difficult symptomatology."

At this point I was puzzled: if schizophrenia was—as researchers were beginning to understand—a disorder of profoundly biological origins, there seemed little point to pursuing formulations of faulty family communication patterns. But Chasin explained, "I always had the attitude that until we have really hard data, we have no business making any presumptions about etiology. We're obligated to learn a great deal and apply common sense to what we know. So it was possible that somebody had a genetic predisposition for schizophrenia, and unless they were handled *just so*, it would emerge. The kind of child who would later be schizophrenic could look quite ordinary or could already be very disturbed. Whether the communications pattern in the family—which was definitely different from that in other families—evolved because at least one parent shared the gene or because with a child like that you may have to develop unusual communication patterns or some combination of the two, we just don't know.

"But not knowing either etiology or the precise mechanisms of therapeutic agents doesn't mean we are helpless. Penicillin worked for many years quite effectively before its mechanism of action was understood."

One of Chasin's favorite teachers, he told me, had made the point "that there were at the time about twelve perfectly plausible theories about behavior, and he thought being able to use each one was a great idea, and I totally agree." I was pleased to hear this, since it verified the impressions I was forming in the course of research. It is an important idea for lay readers to understand, because of the freedom of choice it implies for patients as well.

Chasin—who describes himself as "an intellectual omnivore, never driven by the overarching theory"—accepted that certain drugs were effective in relieving some symptoms of schizophrenia and making the patients' behavior more tolerable to themselves and their families, and also that people with schizophrenic symptoms had trouble communicating with their families in part because it was hard for them to make sense of things. He was drawn to simple, direct measures that made people feel better, and in this connection he made one more intriguing comment about etiology that seemed to reflect not only Chasin himself but family therapists in general. "I was tolerant rather than fascinated with exploring how things came to pass," he said. "But the degree to which people *need* stories of etiology varies from family to family, and when the human need for stories is so great, if I were to treat that disrespectfully, I would have failed in my pragmatic approach. That's one way I feel behavioral therapists run risks, by saying 'I don't know why, I'm just doing this.' A good behavioral therapist knows that most people need a narrative."

Family therapy books and papers, indeed, often read like novels. One could almost curl up with them, a refreshing relief from the social-science jargon of the behaviorists and the more convoluted speculations of psychodynamic theorists. I felt I was in a world where life is high drama; perhaps being part of this exciting family saga would be a compensation for the actual pain of living it, and this adventure must be one of the attractions of family therapy. Chasin was almost tame compared with some of the flamboyant celebrities of his tribe. And the tapes of his work seemed to show geological strata: they reflect many of the theories—therapeutic tools, as he described them—that have captured family therapists' imaginations over the years.

Early on Chasin was smitten by Virginia Satir, an alumna of the Bateson group who focused on clarifying communications among family members. "It seemed when you helped people talk in a clearer way that the terror and the symptomatology diminished," he said. "I was fairly committed to the idea that if people communicated more effectively, if they listened more carefully, they would work things out." This part of Satir's theories, along with some of Norman Paul's ideas, dominated his work until he encountered Salvador Minuchin.

Each orientation has its parental figure, the personage of stature who becomes the public's template of a therapeutic school. To the public

Minuchin is the personification of family systems therapy. Like Freud and Skinner, he is revered, controversial, and misunderstood, and he is the only family systems therapist many lay people have ever heard of. The book I read, *Families and Family Therapy,* came out in 1974, when Minuchin had been influential for nearly a decade. It is easy to understand both the reverence and the controversy: the book combines enormous basic wisdom with some fairly chilling examples of how that wisdom is carried out. It is difficult to read Minuchin without repeatedly invoking the deity. Sometimes one says, "Thank God"; other times one says, "Good God."

Minuchin, an Argentine-born psychiatrist, devised his "structural" methods in treating families of delinquents at the Wiltwyck School for Boys in New York State; later he became head of the Philadelphia Child Guidance Clinic. His work reflects cybernetics and the anthropological influences of the Bateson group. He called the method "structural" because it aimed to alter the relative position of each member within the family and thereby transform the individuals' experiences. Minuchin looked at the family the way our high school social studies teachers regarded the map of Europe before World War I, as a web of alliances, spheres of influence, and lines of power. At the end of therapy, the map would look different, to the benefit of each player.

Traditional therapy, he pointed out, had drawn "an artificial 'boundary' between the individual and his social context." While therapists knew the boundary was artificial, the process of examining the patient with a magnifying glass maintained the view that pathology resided in the individual. Family therapy was a zoom lens, permitting both a close-up and a broad focus. It brought three basic assumptions forward from the therapeutic shadows out to center stage: "that context affects inner processes, that changes in context produce changes in the individual, and that the therapist's behavior is significant in change." Moreover, structural family therapy was "a therapy of action," which aimed "to modify the present, not to explore and interpret the past."

Minuchin starts his explanation with models of normalcy, a currently unpopular idea that is surely useful to any family that seeks to place its own problems on the spectrum of disorder—which real clients want to do, whether or not therapists approve. He talks with the Wagners, a couple who have answered a newspaper ad seeking a normal family to be interviewed for a fee before a large audience of family therapists. The couple, who have gone to a marriage counselor in the past, now see themselves and their three-year-old son Tom as a normal family that has struggled through difficulties; "The family, having labeled itself normal from the start, will be confirmed and supported in this belief by the interview."

Minuchin asks the Wagners detailed questions about the habits of family life—he learns, for example, that on Saturday they do things together and on Sunday they go their separate ways. "Moral and emotional components accompany contractual transactional patterns, even those whose origins and reasons have been lost." He asks the Wagners about their relationship with their "families of origin." Young couples need to negotiate rules for dealing with the in-laws, and they also bring expectations based on how things were done at home. In Emily Wagner's family, for example, "parental authority was split, and each parent attacked the other spouse through their daughter," while in Mark's, where the father was peripheral, "the children experienced their mother as representing their father's authority."

As the Wagners describe their early adjustment problems, Minuchin does a kind of summarizing that removes both nuance and prettification and forces people to call a spade a spade. For example, when the Wagners describe how, as newlyweds, they had moved in with Emily's parents, and Mark had stayed neutral when Emily fought with her mother, Minuchin says to Emily, "Look, if he didn't take sides, he was taking sides. . . . If he did not attack your mother when you attacked her, then he was siding with your mother, even if he didn't do anything." And in the end he tells them young couples "come from different cultures with different ideas. . . . They need to create boundaries around themselves . . . and they struggle and they blunder and they have bloody noses, right? All of us have. And you know, some marriages survive, and some don't."

Unlike most psychodynamic theorists (with the notable exception of Erik Erikson), Minuchin defines the basic human tasks of separation and individuation in context: everyone's identity is influenced by a sense of membership in a particular family, but each member derives individuality from being part of a number of distinct subgroups: the children or the parents, the sons or the daughters, the men or the women in the family, the eighth-graders, the woodwind section of the school orchestra, and so forth. And as the child and family get older, they grant him "areas of autonomy that he experiences as separateness. . . . Being Tom is different from being a Wagner."

As individuals need to be placed in a family context, so must families be set in the larger society. Minuchin—in this twenty-year-old book— notes that the family is a target of political contention in an era of social change, with different groups seeking to hurry or slow down movement toward a new order: "Today the American family, like American society, is in a transitional period." He then offers a compelling and prescient explanation of current social problems (many clinicians I met who were working with deeply troubled teenagers told me the same thing, but Minuchin said this in 1974): "The family is relinquishing the socialization of children earlier and earlier. The school, mass media, and the peer group are taking over the guidance and education of older children. But society has not developed adequate extrafamilial sources of socialization and support." The outside world is full of stress, and this impinges on modern families: we tend to cherish a dated ideal of normal family life (though perhaps less than at the time Minuchin wrote the book) and to label "many situations that are clearly transitional as pathological and pathogenic."

The pattern of daily family transactions establishes a family's hier-archy, and deviations from the rules result in "calls to family loyalty and guilt-inducing maneuvers" as the system seeks equilibrium. Minuchin describes a number of family structures and ways of interacting, and says that no structure or style is inherently pathological. A family's "subsystems"—conventionally, two parents with authority over several children, but sometimes, as Minuchin points out, a single parent with either a grandmother or an oldest child holding sway over younger children, and innumerable other variations he hasn't thought of in this book—need clear boundaries to function well. In terms that became basic to family systems jargon, Minuchin characterizes families' interac-tional styles as *enmeshed* or *disengaged:* only the extremes of these patterns are pathological, when "the enmeshed family responds to any variation from the accustomed with excessive speed and intensity. The disengaged family tends not to respond when a response is necessary."

It is, incidentally, an important and misunderstood part of Minuchin's structural approach that he *does* see parents separately from children: "If in these sessions they continue to discuss parenting instead of husband-wife transactions, the therapist would do well to point out that they are crossing a boundary."

It is important for therapists to distinguish between "average families in transitional situations, suffering the pain of accommodation to new circumstances," and pathological families, who "in the face of stress increase the rigidity of their transactional patterns and boundaries and avoid or resist any explanation of alternatives." With the former the therapist can count on "the motivation of family resources as a pathway to transformation." But when the family is pathological, "the therapist needs to become an actor in the family drama, entering into transitional coalitions in order to skew the system and develop a different level of homeostasis," the equilibrium (drawn from cybernetic theory) that the family will always seek.

After describing the ideas that underlie structural family therapy, Minuchin demonstrates how they affect the therapist's behavior. In making a diagnosis, for example, the structural family therapist wants to know who is the family spokesman and who chose him: that is, if it's the father, is he speaking as the executive head of the family, or is mother really the boss but, by deferring to him, temporarily yielding to cultural notions of who should exert power? When the father talks, does the mother support him or disagree with him? Does the family's behavior in session reflect what its main speaker (father or mother) is saying? The therapist must respond, observe, and form hypotheses about patterns in the family, beginning, in Minuchin's phrase, to draw a "family map"—an organizational scheme of the family.

Minuchin emphasizes the difference between the family therapist's behavior and that of the psychodynamic practitioner:

> To join a family system, the therapist must accept the family's organization and style and blend with them. He must experience the family's transactional patterns and the strength of those patterns. That is, he should feel a family member's pain at being excluded or scapegoated, and his pleasure at being loved, depended on, or otherwise confirmed within the family.

Minuchin draws clear parallels with the way anthropologists work, citing Claude Lévi-Strauss's description of participant observation. The therapist, like the anthropologist, oscillates between letting himself be absorbed by the society—the family—and attempting to disengage in order to analyze it. (Contemporary therapists are skeptical of the notion that one can ever be really disengaged from a system in which one participates, and in that respect early Minuchin is as out of fashion in the family systems world as Lévi-Strauss is among anthropologists.)

The therapist practices such accommodation techniques as "maintenance," which means following the family's rules and addressing his first questions to its designated spokesman, and complimenting members on their insights or their clothing (a criterion for choosing a family systems therapist should certainly be the therapist's ability to "join" with the children on their level); "tracking," which is asking questions that clarify without challenging; and "mimesis," which is adapting the family's style ("In a jovial family he becomes jovial and expansive. In a family with a restricted style, his communications become sparse."). Chasin, the eclectic from whom no geological layer disappears, can be seen doing all these things.

Another essential difference between the family therapist and the psychoanalyst, Minuchin points out, is the "use of self." Psychoanalytic therapy posits that patients change by re-experiencing feelings they repressed in the past, and that they can do this only through a symbolic, transference relationship with the therapist; accordingly, the therapist has to muzzle his own personal responses to avoid acting out his counter-transference. In structural family therapy the therapist's personal responses are used to help him to join the family, probe and observe it, and ultimately change its patterns.

Minuchin says flat out that the different ways two therapists behave to achieve even similar goals result from their own varied life experiences. His own childhood in an enmeshed family of numerous aunts, uncles, and cousins in a small town in rural Argentina led him "to empathize with children and to blame their parents" until he had children of his own; then, having worked with different ethnic cultures in Israel and the United States, he became sensitive both to cultural differences and to universal similarities. It is notable that while psychodynamic therapists are trained to understand their personal biases, they don't give the patients a clue as to what these might be. In their greater willingness to be self-revelatory and to acknowledge their subjectivity, family therapists seem a bit humbler and more respectful of the patient.

The goal of therapy, Minuchin avows, is not the independence of each family member but a "flexible interchange between autonomy and interdependency that will best promote the psychosocial growth of its members. . . . The derogatory connotation of the notion of dependence in individual psychodynamic theory is not carried over into family therapy, which recognizes the interdependence of all systems."

After all this good theoretical common sense, Minuchin gets down to cases, and here he sometimes seems dicey. A family therapist is, he says, "an expert in experimental social manipulation." How might a structural therapist feel free to intervene? In one family a mother and children were assessed to be in coalition against the father, who had just come out of jail. Among the reasonable options for the therapist in this transitional situation were: "the therapist may affiliate with the father. . . . He may block the mother-children transactions, perhaps by conducting therapy with them alone or by blocking the mother's movements in the session. . . . He can join the mother and father in a coalition against the children, attacking them for disobedience, or he can use the tactic of pointing up the parents' incompetence with the children. Either technique makes the parents join to form an effective parental unit." To the lay reader, this sounds a bit like ganging up in the schoolyard.

In another case, treated by a colleague of Minuchin's, the "identified patient" was an anorectic fourteen-year-old girl whose father and maternal grandmother, the therapist judged, were in league to isolate the mother, who had therefore invested all her self-esteem in her relationship with the girl. The therapist's goal was to "create distance between the mother and daughter, and to define a boundary around the spouse subsystem that will make it possible to free the girl and the mother from their deviant positions." (While I am reluctant to jump the gun, I am flagging this formulation as an example of what caused a feminist rebellion in the family therapy world later on: the mother is held responsible for redefining the spousal boundary, while nothing is labeled "deviant" in the father's relationship with his mother-in-law.) At one point in this case, the therapist "whispers to the girl, 'Tell your mother she doesn't love you enough, and that is why you look like a scarecrow.' The girl, seeking the therapist's support, obeys . . . the family therapist is encouraging the girl to be openly aggressive toward her mother, on whom she is pathologically dependent."

Minuchin lays out a bunch of reasons why an individually oriented therapist would "question this intervention." It would make the girl feel guilty later; it makes the girl parrot the therapist; it blames the mother, minimizing the girl's responsibility and reinforcing the dependence of mother and daughter; and it's unfair to the mother, "who is undercut by her husband and her own mother." To this list of criticisms—which sound on the mark to me—I would add that it reflects, like many of the cases in the book, a belief that the ends justify the means. Indeed, Minuchin says it's all in the service of separating mother and daughter so that Mother is forced to increase her demands on Father.

While acknowledging that structural family therapy may sometimes seem unfair to individual family members, a good therapist, Minuchin says, keeps a firm hand on the tiller, always balancing the roughness with support tactics. He points out that families who don't accept the therapist's tactics will simply dig in their heels (or vote with their feet). He emphasizes how difficult it is to achieve change in family therapy, in which the clients are formidable opponents. I was not completely sold by this argument; but at other times in my research, I did see good therapists use harsh tactics in cases that had not yielded to greater delicacy. An incompetent therapist can, of course, make things worse, but that risk applies to all orientations; no approach seemed to me (or has been proven) more idiot-proof than others. Anorexia nervosa is a potentially life-threatening disorder, and one thing Minuchin didn't include here is the weight of the girl and her therapeutic history.

When I asked Chasin about this, he looked uneasy. "I am very activist," he said. "I am comfortable being directive. I think what Minuchin called for was a higher level of directiveness, managing and manipulating the situation, and I was comfortable doing that. But it's hard for me to do his style of therapy. I've never been comfortable forcing a crisis—not that I haven't done it. Minuchin had what I consider nerves of steel.

"In many cases of anorexia nervosa, there was pretty good evidence of almost a cross-generational coalition between the girl and one parent, the other parent was disempowered, and the girl in some ways was made too powerful. He decided that if the parents were joined with each other rather than split by the child, they would be more effective, so one of the ways he tried to get them unified was to say, 'Make her eat.' He thought this was foolproof because if she did eat, they would see how effective they were working together, and if she didn't, he would say they were joined in defeat. The girl was suddenly isolated, she didn't have a power person on her side. From these forced crises, sometimes wonderful things happen very quickly. Not everyone has the stomach to do what he did. Some of his films are horrible. They're trying to ram a frankfurter down her throat, she's weighing seventy pounds. It's almost unbearable to watch and you know how desperate the parents are—she's going to die—and you know how she feels too. But isn't it better than IVs? It personally would be very hard for me to work like that. I *would* do it if I didn't feel I had something that worked as well."

In other ways, however, Minuchin had been an epiphany for Chasin, who could no longer believe that improved communication and insight were enough to bring about change: "People could never talk straight to each other because it would be horribly disloyal to a particular coalition to be straight with the person they decided was the enemy." Minuchin's map of the family, based on the power structure, the alliances, and the boundaries between subsystems, "would suggest to you many different things to do. Through three different types of building blocks you could construct a map that would be absolutely unique for every case."

So in putting some of Minuchin's ideas to work in his own style, Chasin got interested in families' strengths. "It was hard to imagine two parents of a teenager who had never gotten together effectively on *anything*. What could be accomplished by strong, persuasive structural moves could also be accomplished by finding out when in their lives they had worked together, helping them remember it, and then doing what Minuchin very often did himself—seeing that teamwork happen in the room and saying, 'Look at that,' in a straight Skinnerian behavior-modification way. Minuchin asked for the behavior; I felt that one did not have to ask, it was going to happen, and you just put a frame around the picture. 'Look at the two of you right now. You're figuring out the unbelievably complex thing of getting all the family here, when you tell me you've never worked together. You've done the logistics of an army general right in front of my face. What is this about?"

Chasin's hesitation about copying Minuchin's style moved him toward the psychodrama for which he is known: "It occurred to me that asking people to do things as themselves was more manipulative than asking people to engage in a fantasy that didn't necessarily count. There was an opportunity to show people how well they could do things, and that much directiveness was not harmful." A good example of Chasin's adapting Minuchin is the "poops" tape in Chapter 10, which Chasin later showed to Minuchin with some trepidation because it involved only symbolic play and focused only on the "sibling subsystem." But the great man, to Chasin's relief, was enthusiastic.

Another of family therapy's flamboyant early gurus was Carl A. Whitaker, a psychiatrist who began treating families together back in the forties. Like many of the field's founders, he first worked with schizophrenics, and he pioneered in the use of co-therapists and observation through one-way mirrors. Whitaker, who recently stopped practicing, has impressive academic credentials: he was chair of psychiatry at Emory University and later moved to the University of Wisconsin. His style of therapy, described in a renowned 1978 book called *The Family Crucible,* written with the psychologist Augustus Napier, his co-therapist and Boswell, is called "symbolic-experiential": the book has the flavor of its decade, demonstrating an approach that critics today might dub "warm and fuzzy" or "touchy-feely." While experiential techniques might not please everyone, the book is a fascinating in-depth account of the family therapy process, which in this case is complex, intricate, and difficult to summarize without oversimplifying.

The Family Crucible is actually one long case history of a fictionalized composite family called the Brices, whose "identified patient" is Claudia, a troubled teenager whose constant fighting with her parents and running away has strained everyone. Claudia complains of mysterious aches and writes frightening poetry about death; her unsuccessful previous therapists (not family systems practitioners) have diagnosed her disorder as probable schizophrenia. The rest of the family consists of Carolyn and David, the parents; eleven-year-old Don; and six-year-old Laura.

Whitaker and Napier are the ultimate participant observers, and their personal backgrounds are a leitmotiv in the book. After Don fails to show up for the first session—"through a very complicated unconscious process he got *elected* by the family to be the one to stay home," Whitaker tells the Brices—Napier describes the relationship between the team and the family:

We were engaged in a subtle, often predictable, and very important contest with the family about who was going to be present at the meetings. Carl and I had revealed some of what our relationship had to offer: a good-humored liking for each other, an ability to cooperate, and an insistence on remaining ourselves. . . . Carl had intuitively modeled some of the process of therapy for the family. By sharing insight into his own personality, he was saying by demonstration, "It's important to search for your own unconscious agenda."

This is more self-revelation than I saw in the rest of my research on family systems therapy, and the thought of Charles Sarnoff talking this way boggles the mind. In the course of the book, we learn that Whitaker himself has been in therapy five times and Napier two; we find out something about the texture of life in their families of origin and their marriages; and we hear Whitaker tell Don he does therapy " 'because it pushes *me* to grow. I'm here for me, not for you guys. This is just part of my plot to try to be a more alive person. You didn't think it was for charity, did you?' " Don says, " 'I thought it was for money,' " and Whitaker answers, " 'Touché, but only partly true. I would have made more money if I had stuck to being a real doctor, delivering babies and stuff.' "

As Napier describes symbolic-experiential family therapy, it is "a symbolic parenting experience"—a sort of group transference—and "the most significant breakthroughs will occur in moments of peak experience. These moments may or may not take place during the therapy hour." Peak moments are those in which the family risks either greater anger and divergence or greater intimacy, toward the goal of becoming "more real, more direct, more alive."

In the course of the book, Napier takes a number of diversions to discuss therapy in general. He has some valuable and incisive comments on Freud, who comes in through the team's irritation with Claudia's former therapists: Freud's "elaboration of the defenses, the fancy footwork that the mind must perform as it steps delicately between innate desire and social conformity, remains perhaps his most brilliant achievement." But Napier also says that Freud "looked deep *inside* the person; he hardly looked at all at the social environment." This and Napier's accusation of "naiveté" about people's interaction seem rather a bum rap; Minuchin's assessment—that psychoanalysts knowingly drew an artificial boundary between the patient and his environment that ultimately came to skew their definition of the problem—sounds more cogent. But Napier's remark that doctrinaire therapists, ignoring the obvious underlying family problems, "betrayed Freud's sense of quest and inquiry by following his example so slavishly, for so long, and with so little question" is a telling strike.

Like Minuchin, Napier points out the pressures of social change on family life. And while Whitaker and Napier are less brutal in idiom, they also view the family in terms of its coalitions and use the same restructuring ploys of shifting alliances from one family member to the next. The Brice family conforms to the traditional American stereotype:

> Fathers usually *are* the outsiders in the modern family, and often they find coming into family therapy very uncomfortable. This father was typical in attempting to shift the focus away from himself. . . . Most of the time, the mother is the psychological center of the family, and our moving quickly to her would have given the father an excuse to feel himself more and more removed, until he had become as isolated and alone in the therapy as he felt in the family. . . . Women are more sophisticated about the interpersonal world, the world of feeling, and we were trying to compensate for this kind of cultural inadequacy in men.

This description, and Whitaker's general belief that troubled families are emotionally constricted and overpolite (" 'If you could break out of this dreary reasonableness,' " he tells the Brices at one point), suggests a white-bread view of America that later theorists noted doesn't apply to everyone: some families are pumpernickel, cornbread, pita, tortilla, or nan in their structure, their values, and their mode of expression.

It turns out, as Whitaker tells the Brices, that "the most serious problem seems to have been the slow, quiet drifting away of the parents from each other and the gradual cooling of the marriage. . . . Claudia's crisis may be a way the family has evolved of trying to deal with this bigger problem of the coolness." So Dad aligns with Claudia, Mom gets jealous and angry, Mom and Claudia slug it out, and the battle escalates until the parents have to unite to deal with Claudia. In family therapy jargon, Claudia is being *triangulated*—brought in by her parents to deflect attention from their own emotional pain.

Napier describes Carolyn, the mother, as "wrapped in sadness." Some of the tension between mother and daughter is a replay of Carolyn's relationship with her own harsh and controlling mother. In the course of therapy, everyone gets confronted and badgered. But Napier says, "You can't only be warm and benign with people, because it isn't honest and it isn't respected. . . . You must push them, sometimes very hard indeed. But you can't only push—you have to be caring too."

The role of Laura, the six-year-old, in the therapy is controversial, since she herself is not the identified patient. Whitaker draws her in and gently asks her some highly sophisticated questions, worming out her fear that Claudia will leave and Mom and Dad will divorce. Napier asks Laura if she worries that Claudia will kill herself, and Laura bursts into tears. But Napier feels Laura's reactions soften the atmosphere, and he allows the child to "expose her painful fantasies and cry about them."

It's not a surprise in a book on the benefits of family therapy that ultimately the parents work out their problems (although a year after they finish, Claudia reports some backsliding) and the children do fine. For several months after termination of the family work, the mother remains in individual therapy with Napier, and in proper seventies style she goes back to college and gets involved with the women's movement. Summing up, Napier, in an attractive demonstration of eclecticism, says,

> At the end of therapy the family should have resolved their major relationship conflicts, and the individuals should really *be* individuals in a psychological sense. The conflicts that remain are then of an intrapsychic nature, remnants of past experience that continue to trouble the person.

I had asked Chasin if he encountered much countertransference, and he said, "In a highly technical sense and in the ordinary sense, yes. Because I engage with people in such an intense way, I'm full of feeling for them." This evoked a request from me to compare his work with Whitaker's, and he said, "A lot of people think Whitaker becomes a family member—a kind of very well-intended maverick grandfather who actually has a right to talk about what's happening, and if it's a little irreverent or salacious, that's the family's tough luck. They're just going to have to tolerate him. Whitaker takes these very fixed patterns, and he blows them to smithereens."

As to some of the more radical moves, Chasin feels Whitaker's knowledge, confidence, and feeling for the family make them "probably all right." He adds that "many of us are fully as idiosyncratic, we're just not as dramatic and startling and iconoclastic in the way we do it. Some of the moves I make might also seem very strong: 'Let's play a game in which we all fall down the toilet and land in the sewer.' A lot of people look at that and say, 'Oh, God, this is so out of control. You think they're all pieces of shit.' I'm confident that what I'm doing is done out of caring in a medium I'm comfortable with."

Is all of family therapy hot-blooded and confrontational? No: that is to say that even the most flamboyant practitioners, then and certainly now, pass many hours in humdrum routine. (Nor are family therapists unique in this respect: psychoanalytic sessions, as we learned from Sarnoff and Falcone in Chapter 3, also include lots of filler.) Would a family in search of a cool, detached therapist ever find satisfaction? It would if the therapist were a disciple of the late Murray Bowen, whose approach, the antithesis of Whitaker's, displays the variety that exists in the field. Bowen, like most of the founders of family therapy, was a psychiatrist treating schizo-phrenics back in the mid-fifties when he too concluded that the problem resided in the family as a whole. But when he brought families together to talk things over, they became engulfed by emotion, and he had to take care not to be sucked into the vortex, which he called an "undifferenti-ated ego mass." He assumed the stance of the calm, neutral observer, describing to the family what he'd learned about their interactions.

Bowen, like the Palo Alto group, at first believed that dysfunctional communication patterns cause schizophrenia, but later on he discovered the same patterns operating, to different degrees, in all families. He found it more useful to see parents without their symptomatic children, and Bowenian therapists still follow this procedure.

Couples in Bowenian therapy talk to each other indirectly through the therapist (the opposite of Minuchin's rules). The goal is to be rational at all times, constantly distinguishing thoughts from feelings, to avoid *fusing* them and to keep them *differentiated*. Therapists, to remain *"de-triangled,"* coach their clients to talk directly one-on-one with other family members and not to gossip about those who are absent. Unlike Minuchin, the therapist avoids taking sides, even temporarily.

After a crisis in his own family of origin, Bowen evolved procedures that aimed to duplicate his own successful differentiation. Clients, guided by their therapists, begin by working out differentiated relationships with each parent through visits, letters, and telephone calls, but refusing to be drawn into their quarrels; they learn to keep thoughts and feelings differentiated and in balance in the presence of their siblings and other relatives. The best time to do this is in the context of important family occasions like weddings, births, and funerals or, failing these, at holiday gatherings-of-the-clan.

Bowenian therapists draw *genograms* of the family, diagrams in which marriages, births, divorces, deaths, geographic separations, and other events (alcoholism, suicide, mental illness) are laid out. The genogram is a medium for helping clients to learn about and discuss family history and trace the origins of problems. As Freudians are trained by undergoing psychoanalysis, Bowenians must go through the differentiation process with their own families; when it is completed, an individual can discuss formerly explosive issues calmly and directly, without either getting hysterical or changing the subject.

I surmised, correctly, that Chasin was not drawn to Bowen. But this, he said, was a matter of his own personality: some of Bowen's ideas had been useful. "Two brothers are in a big issue with each other," he said. "Each complains to the father. The father listens to the complaint from one and then says, 'Your brother thinks you're a son of a bitch,' and the other one says, 'How can he say that about me?' and meanwhile the brothers won't talk directly with each other. There is a triangle. If they really talked to each other and left everybody else out of it, that father would have two very important relationships in terrible jeopardy. He is being the *'switchboard.'* The grief they have with *him* is always avoided. They crab about the old man with each other. There's always two people gossiping about a third one. To sit down and hold a conversation with someone in which you do not refer to anybody else, just talk about your relationship with that person, is very hard to do, and failing to do it means a tremendous lost opportunity. It wouldn't be me to coach like Bowen, to be as cool and removed, but there are times I feel nothing new will happen until these two folks level with each other."

By the mid-seventies, Minuchin, Whitaker, and Bowen had been among the leaders in family therapy for several decades. The field had become an established mode that was no longer fighting for respectability, and as we saw in *The Family Crucible*, it was in tune with the Zeitgeist. But as should be expected, the techniques and philosophies of the early masters raised some questions, and family therapists were ripe for a new guru. In discussing Bowen I noted that he, like Chasin's old supervisor, was going back through generations to find family problems. "Everybody is," Chasin says. "If the quick and dirty or the quick and clean doesn't do it, there's a very good chance that you're dealing with strong influences so deeply embedded in the culture of the family that the people don't recognize them."

"How often does that happen with you?" I asked.

"It happens very often."

There now appeared on the family therapy scene a theorist who combined cybernetic and general system theory perspectives, the historical interest and cool, cerebral objectivity of Murray Bowen, and the authoritative demeanor of Salvador Minuchin, with an extra *qualche cosa* of glamour and theatrics. Word of a new team approach to treating families was beginning to travel across the Atlantic in papers that appeared in *Family Process*, the field's leading professional journal, and shortly afterward in a book, *Paradox and Counterparadox*, published in the United States in 1978. The authors—Mara Selvini Palazzoli, the leader, and her colleagues Luigi Boscolo, Gianfranco Cecchin and Giuliana Prata, all psychoanalysts at the Centro per lo Studio della Famiglia in Milan—were highly original. At around the same time that hip Americans were learning to cook from Marcella Hazan and buying originals or knockoffs of Armani suits and furniture by Ettore Sottsass, family therapists were also succumbing to Milan fever: like Milanese in other fields, Selvini Palazzoli and her colleagues offered a combination of intellect, elegance, and earthiness that exerted a powerful magnetism. At the same time the Milanese presented an alternative to the bluntly coercive style of the American family systems pioneers. All psychotherapy faces the dilemma of whether it is more effective to change behavior directly or to examine its meaning: in family systems the pendulum was starting to swing from the former to the latter. Some American family therapists were also beginning to ponder the influences deeply embedded in the culture of each family and indeed in society itself.

Chasin assigned me two papers from *Family Process* to capture the essence of the Milanese approach. The first, "Family Rituals: A Powerful Tool in Family Therapy," which ran in 1977, reads like the treatment for a 1948 Rossellini film, updated. A compelling illustration of the way myths can dominate a clan, it tells the story of the Casantis, farmers in Tuscany, and begins, "During the 1930's, in the Tuscan Maremma areas, the patriarchal family was still isolated and was considered by its members as their only assurance of survival and dignity. To leave the family meant tearing up roots and emigration without any financial means or preparation."

In this family the father and sons were fortunate: they labored in the fields, and the daughters-in-law worked obediently in both the fields and the house. The sons were encouraged to marry young and bring in wives to help out, subject to a chain of command in which the patriarch ranked highest, the husband second, the brothers-in-law third, the mother-in-law fourth, and the older sisters-in-law fifth. But after World War II the family was less isolated and the chain of authority began to break up. Siro, the youngest son, brought home a city wife, Pia. The other daughters-in-law were no longer willing to be chattels; they sought more personal freedom. The sons joined their parents in trying to control their wives; rivalry among the children was forbidden.

"Thus was born the family myth of 'one for all and all for one,'" the authors recount, "a myth also shared by whoever had contact with the family . . . everybody loves one another . . . no fighting, no bickering."

Pia, the city wife, helped to build the myth, and her parents-in-law thought her saintly: she was wise, helpful, and impartial. But when sons were prized, poor Pia had two daughters, for whom she never showed any preference over her nephews and nieces, and she always served her own last. Still, sometimes her daughters found her crying in her room.

The authors cite the characteristics of a family myth, as described by one scholar: that in the first generation, that of the patriarch and his wife, it is realistic and it works. In the next generation, when times change, tension appears. Of the brothers, the authors observe, "Their strength was always the old one—to work hard and to be united. To stay together, they had to create a myth, a collective product whose very existence and persistence would . . . reinforce the homeostasis of the group against any disruptive influences. . . . Like all myths . . . this one imposed on its adherents certain limitations that ended in gross distortions of reality."

Allora. The grandparents died, and the sons abandoned the farm, moving to the city where they formed a successful family construction business. While they were part of a more competitive society, they lived in a sort of commune and rigidly perpetuated the family myth, which "did not permit any gesture or comment whatever that could be said to be motivated by jealousy, envy, or competition."

The elder of Siro and Pia's two daughters, Zita, was a good student and a tomboy: she had been anorectic for a few months when she was sixteen, but she recovered. The younger daughter, Nora, had no interest in studies and spent her time hanging out with her plain-looking cousin Luciana. Then suddenly, as will happen, Nora, thirteen, burst into gorgeous bloom: she was the beauty of the family, and her father was very proud of her (although Nora got edgy whenever she was complimented). By age fourteen, she had become severely anorectic, a frightening skeleton. In 1971, when the family—Siro, 50, Pia, 43, and Zita, 22, as well as the identified patient—finally made the long trip to the clinic in Milan, Nora was fifteen, five feet nine and seventy pounds, and showing symptoms of psychosis. She kept saying, "You should make me put on weight without making me eat."

The family therapy team contracted for twenty sessions, to be held every three weeks. During the first half of the therapy, they inquired into relations between the nuclear family and the clan; they found the myth and attacked it forcefully, with "naive prescriptions intended to force the family to open rebellion against the myth." This proved to be an uphill fight: whenever a family member allied with the therapists and criticized the clan, another member disqualified what was being said or diverted the discussion.

Still, from the fourth session on Nora began to abandon her anorexia, and by the sixth, she was physically thriving. The team, suspicious of this all-too-rapid improvement, decided to verify it by halting treatment; if her rally was just a false move to perpetuate the system, there would be eleven sessions left to continue the job. And sure enough, after therapy stopped, Nora became reclusive; Siro, the father, was ambivalent about resuming. But then Nora took an overdose of alcohol and barbiturates and landed in the critical ward of the hospital. She did this after returning from a dance at which she met her homely cousin, Luciana.

The family confessed to the team that the clan had opposed their return to therapy. First Zita said Nora had felt persecuted by Luciana for years, and then she tried to nullify this idea. The family defended Luciana and criticized Nora.

The team halted the session and went out of the room to discuss the case. (Leaving the family to stew alone is a hallmark of Milan-style therapy.) They realized that "going against such an iron-clad myth had only served to strengthen it." Meanwhile, Nora was assailed by self-doubt: "How could she dare think that Aunt Emma and Luciana didn't love her? Perhaps she perceived Luciana as being a hypocrite, envious and evil, only because she, Nora, was all of these things."

So the team decided to say nothing more but to propose a ritual. The ritual reflected a technique called "prescribing the symptom" that was not original with the Milan team: it went back to Bateson's Palo Alto group, particularly to its master strategist, Jay Haley, and his colleague, Paul Watzlawick, who had visited the Milan team several times. Chasin told me earlier, for example, that if a child's problem was getting into fights in school and you directed him to get into precisely six fights a day, no more and no less, the child was in a bind, because behavior intended to be rebellious had now become obedient: the point of this directive was not to wreak mischief for its own sake but to change the meaning of the behavior and thus cause the patient to re-examine the whole structure of his beliefs.

In this case the "pathology" the Milan team was prescribing was "fidelity to the myth." Chasin agreed that this type of assignment could fairly be considered a benign double bind. While it fits into a therapeutic category called *paradoxical interventions* that crop up in other therapeutic orientations as well, it is now somewhat out of style in the family systems world, which has turned away from "anything that smacks of outsmarting the patient." Chasin does believe, however, that patients usually saw through the paradox and understood they were supposed to emerge from the assignment having learned something new. It was, he said, "like sweating out a fever."

The therapists told the family they were worried about its emerging hostility to the clan, which endangered the well-being of the larger group. Thus it was important to follow the team's prescription. Here is the ritual the team dreamed up:

Every other night, after dinner, the family was to lock and bolt the front door. The four members of the family were to sit round the dining room table, which would be cleared of all objects except for an alarm clock . . . in its center. Each member . . . starting with the eldest, would have fifteen minutes to talk, expressing his own feelings, impressions, and observations about the behavior of the other members of the clan. Whoever had nothing to say would have to remain silent for his assigned fifteen minutes, while the rest of the family would also remain silent. If, instead, he were to speak, everyone would have to listen, refraining from making any comment, gesture, or interruption of any kind. It was absolutely forbidden to continue these discussions outside the fixed hours; everything was limited to these evening meetings, which were ritually structured. As for relations with members of the clan, a doubling of courtesy and helpfulness was prescribed.

The underlying purpose of this intervention, the authors say, was to define the nuclear family as distinct from the clan and allow it to speak clearly on forbidden subjects while preserving secrecy; to restore Nora's position as a member of the nuclear family; to bring the sisters closer together; and to establish the right of individual family members to express their ideas without being contradicted. Anyone who chose to dodge being forthright by remaining silent would face a very tense quarter-hour.

The most paradoxical aspect of this ritual lay in ordering reverence toward the clan, when the family was ready to accept the position that the clan was dangerous. Paradox, as Chasin pointed out to me, is a technique that dispels ambivalence and gives the family the sense that it has healed itself, instead of having a cure imposed upon it. What the Milanese added was the inherent power of ritual—a minutely detailed and often written out ritual that was "more apt than words to unite the participants in a powerful collective experience." The authors reported that two weeks with the ritual was sufficient to shatter the taboo against speaking ill of relatives, and Nora (who, of course, ultimately became a successful model) recognized the bullying of Luciana. The ritual was not portrayed as an instant solution to the family's problems, but it broke the logjam and freed them to deal with other issues honestly.

The second paper, "Hypothesizing-circularity-neutrality," which ran in *Family Process* in 1980, lays out techniques I'd seen Chasin use (particularly with Nicki, the school-phobic child in Chapter 10) and explains some fundamental differences between contemporary family systems therapy and psychodynamic practice: thus it merits a rundown here. The goal of this paper is to replace intangible attributes of therapists—intuition, charisma, concern, and so forth—with three principles that can be taught.

The authors remind us that a hypothesis as defined in experimental science is an "unproved suggestion tentatively accepted to provide a basis for further investigation." As we all learned in chem lab, even a false hypothesis is informative in ruling out some possibilities. In a family interview, however, the active tracking of a hypothesis helps to smoke out the pattern of a family's relationships. In a notably anti-Freudian statement, the authors say, "If the therapist were instead to behave in a passive manner, as an observer rather than a mover, it would be the family that, conforming to its own linear hypothesis, would impose its own script, dedicated exclusively to the designation of who is 'crazy' and who is 'guilty,' resulting in zero information for the therapist. The hypothesis of the therapist, however, introduces the powerful input of the unexpected and the improbable into the family system and for this reason acts to avoid derailment and disorder."

The most dreaded word in the family systems world is "linear"— applied, as Chasin noted in Chapter 10, to the notion that A directly causes B, which then directly causes C. And so the next tool, a highly powerful one, is circularity, the capacity of the therapist to use feedback and see everything in terms of relationships. This leads to circular questioning, which became a favorite style of Chasin's. Instead of asking the mother about her relationship with her daughter, it is richer and more fruitful to ask the son how *he* sees the relationship between his mother and his sister, which gives another informational twist of the wrist: we learn some facts, we learn the son's point of view, and we watch how the mother and daughter behave while the son is discussing them.

The questions always concern behavior, not traits; they often involve the ranking of family members by other members. (For example, when your brother goes away to school, who will be the most bereft, your mother, your sister, or your grandmother?) In their cadenced style, Selvini Palazzoli and her colleagues remark, "Thus the warp will pass through the woof, until the design will be clearly seen in the fabric, without the necessity of posing the most expected, and therefore the most feared and defended-against question, 'But Marina, how do you see the relationship between your mother and father?' " The authors say this approach, which is sometimes called "gossip in the presence of others," avoids "the tedious listing of symptomatic behavior."

Finally *neutrality*, as the Milanese define it, means the sum total of the therapist's behavior in the session, which appears to shift alliance from one member to the next, so that after the session, if someone asked the family members who the therapist sided with, they'd have no idea.

Richard Chasin was profoundly affected by the Milanese. "I had begun to have very little use for talk," he said, "and the thing that kept striking me about the Milan school was that the family could produce such an immense amount of fresh information in so short a time that it was impossible to go on holding narrow, pat theories. I wanted to talk with people just enough about what had to get done."

"You wanted to make the whole therapeutic experience shorter."

"Very short," he said.

"You wanted to see people three times."

"That would be fine."

I asked whether this shift had to do with economics, and Chasin said, "No, those were pretty palmy days. The insurance coverage was almost never an issue. What was driving me to be short-term was partly personal. I like to do intense, high-impact work, and I felt very alive when I was doing it, and it had the effect that I wasn't messing in the family unnecessarily. They would not get in the situation of 'What am I going to do if my therapist takes a sabbatical for six months? My life will come apart.' There are situations when you need that kind of relationship with somebody because it's healing, but to have them rely on themselves a lot and make good use of a small, intense encounter made them feel better about themselves."

In the field in general, Milan-style therapy made a strong contribution, much of which lasted, particularly the power of carefully constructed questions that reveal the circular process through which family members influence each other. (Often the actual answers to the questions were less important than the way they stimulated the family to see their problems differently and devise new solutions.) It is fair to say that via the Milanese, family therapy, despite its antipsychoanalytic origins, was at last moved to focus on the meaning of behavior as well as its social and historical context. Family therapists have done so ever since, however current approaches might differ from the original Milanese techniques. Those who found the style of American luminaries like Minuchin and Whitaker too aggressive and domineering were attracted to the Milanese spirit of intellectual curiosity and to their "neutral" stance, in which the therapist does not side with one person over another.

But there were concerns about the approach that ultimately brought on some disenchantment. In the manner of Bateson's group, it saw symptoms as serving a complex function and often viewed the family in terms of power struggles (Selvini Palazzoli even used the phrase "dirty games"), an attitude that American therapists were moving away from, believing it demeaned the family. There was a bit of lordliness assumed by the therapeutic team, which went off to whisper among themselves and then returned to deliver Delphic pronouncements. And the interventions were often the same for every family, when American practitioners were shifting toward more custom-tailoring and a collaborative stance between therapist and clients.

The past decade has brought about three developments in the family systems world that lay people should be aware of: I saw their effects both on Chasin's work and on that of other therapists. The first stems from a philosophical position called "social constructionism" and reflects parallel developments in philosophy and the other social sciences and indeed in the psychodynamic and cognitive-behavioral fields. It is strongly influenced by Michel Foucault. As we have noted in Chapters 5 and 8, all types of therapy are rooted in the nineteenth-century principle of induction, which held that a scientist is capable of—and should always pursue—objective observation. Now there has been a growing appreciation of the fact that no human being can be totally objective, that one sees the world through one's own personal prism.

The upshot of social constructionism was, necessarily, a new humility on the part of the family systems therapist. The only justification for bossing people around is the absolute certainty that you have their number and are doing what is right, and the most discerning therapists no longer feel that certainty. Accordingly, I have seen sessions like the one where Chasin, Harry Kling, and Sallyann Roth discussed their hypotheses about Nicki's school-phobia with Nicki and her mother and collaborated with them on prescribing a ritual, and I have seen therapists introduce formulations with the phrase "Do you suppose?"

These attitudes have penetrated the other therapeutic worlds, as is evident in comments made by Charles Sarnoff, representative of the most self-confident and old-fashioned orientation of all: that the analyst seeks to get an "aha reaction" and "is not going to be rewarded for getting the month right." As Daniel Stern, the psychodynamic revolutionary, points out (see Chapter 5), the therapist's job is to "search with the patient through his or her remembered history to find the potent life-experience that provides the key metaphor for understanding and changing the patient's life." Among behaviorists this is the "cognitive click."

Perhaps the most visible figure in contemporary family therapy is the Australian Michael White, the monster-tamer of whom we had a taste in Chapter 10. Underlying his work is the idea that efforts to alter behavior alone are ineffectual without altering what behaviors mean to people. First, as we saw, White "externalizes" the problem: while family therapists might not be happy with this comparison, it is less demoralizing to have a physical disease like diabetes, which has landed on you, than to have a mental disorder like depression, which brings with it guilt for your own weakness in being ill. (This is one attraction of the medical model of psychological problems.) So the family bands together to fight "the sad thoughts monster" or "depression" or "anorexia" and thereby feels some sense of dignity and power.

Then White, through his questioning, asks the family to attend to "unique outcomes"—that is, times when the problem could have defeated them but they won out over it. This is similar to but more systematic than Chasin's "working from strengths": the idea is that at *some* time the depressed boy called his friends up and went to a baseball game, or the parents got together and stood up to the in-laws. Direct questions find the unique outcome; other questions—quite intricate and sophisticated—are designed to fit it into a pattern that helps the family to reconstruct its view of itself and its ability to change. White emphasizes that "insofar as this practice alerts family members to, and encourages them to struggle to account for, contradictions, it is not suitably described as 'pointing out positives' . . . the therapist is not required to convince anyone of anything." He is simply calling their attention to information they have ignored. (A somewhat similar approach, devised by a group at the Brief Family Center in Milwaukee, is called "solution-focused therapy": it also uses ingenious questioning to get families thinking differently about their goals and strengths, and it is gaining wide acceptance.)

White's colleague, the New Zealander David Epston, takes externalizing one step further: after every session he writes the family a long enthusiastic letter describing their recent progress and posing new questions that continue the work of combating the problem between sessions. A letter Chasin read to me—it seemed to go on forever—contained sentences like "You told me that girls often bully you and I just wondered, knowing young girls and shy boys, is it their way to attract your attention, or if they admire you so much that they feel they have to bring you down to their level, all the better to get to know you? I don't know if I am right or not but could you keep an eye on this possibility?" With clients' permission, he may show the letters to other clients who have similar problems, showing that progress can be made in fighting the family's psychological dragon.

Epston often deals with patients who have suffered long and serious difficulties. Through exhaustive questioning he helps them appreciate that they have more choices than they might have realized and seems to smoke out any ambivalence to change. As Chasin illustrated:

> "What is the cost to you of being thin?"
>
> "I throw up four times a day."
>
> "So if you're thin and throw up four times a day, are you better off than if you're chunky and throw up no times a day?"
>
> "In some ways, yes."
>
> "There are some boys who would like you. What would life be like with somebody who didn't know you were throwing up and liked you for your thinness?"
>
> "I'd have to keep throwing up."
>
> "What would your life be like with somebody who liked you chunky?"
>
> "I wouldn't have to throw up."
>
> "Would that freedom bother you? Would there be any confusion, or would you enjoy that freedom? Think carefully about this, because you would not know whether to throw up or not if you were with somebody who liked you chunky, because you might not like yourself chunky. Then you could get into a fight with your husband because he would think you're fine and shouldn't throw up and you would think you're not fine and should throw up, and this could be a very serious problem."

The end of all this is "deconstruction," in which the therapist helps the client to "unpack" the beliefs, stories, and cultural practices that have shaped her behavior. It occurs to her that she could weigh 135 pounds and feel happy and loved. Chasin pointed out to me that "this is not an invitation to delusion. Where will you *put* your game leg? Where will you put your tendency to get demoralized when somebody omits you from a conversation? When you repack and reauthor, is this something you can omit, or will it have to be packed in somewhere? It's not a nicey-nice have-a-nice-day thing. It's a very serious endeavor."

It is, I thought, cognitive therapy with a bit of flash.

The second development was the influence of feminism on family therapy. As we've seen, many psychodynamic therapists tended to blame mothers for their children's symptoms. Family therapists like Minuchin believed mothers were enmeshed because fathers were detached—a slight improvement—but he still tended to "rescue" the children from overinvolved mothers by introducing large doses of strong, rational fathering. Feminists, on the other hand, saw mothers as imprisoned by the role imposed on them, and they brought the father in to fulfill *his* responsibility: the villain was the society, for ordaining unhealthy norms for men and women. In 1988, Marianne Walters, Betty Carter, Peggy Papp, and Olga Silverstein, four well-known therapists, published a book called *The Invisible Web* that explored new ways of looking at family problems. They had been exploring women's issues in family therapy for about a decade and were among the first theorists to do so. The book is a useful explanation of the feminist perspective. The essence of their argument is that

A major conceptual error is to assume that traits such as "autonomy" or "dependency" are intrinsic to the person of men or women rather than assigned to them by a patriarchal society on the basis of gender. Thus men are assigned "autonomy" with both the power and [the] emotional disconnectedness that goes with it, while women are assigned "dependency" with both the emotional connectedness and the powerlessness that goes with it. . . . The systemic view of male-female and intergenerational relationships is that they are *interdependent*. Ideally, maturity in this context would be defined as *autonomy with connectedness*. This ideal is in contrast to the patriarchal splitting of these attributes, assigning "autonomy" (actually separateness) to males, and assigning "connectedness" (actually dependency) to females. In effect, such splitting leads us to mistake separateness or disconnectedness for autonomy, a valued sign of maturity, while "connectedness" is equated with dependency, a sign of immaturity, and thus devalued.

While it is customary for some these days to dismiss these ideas as "politically correct," they are, on the contrary, commonsensical: socializing people to suppress half of their natures is a formula for disaster. The four authors of the book practice several different flavors of family therapy, all of which, as they illustrate, can easily absorb a view that is indeed more balanced than the attitude that preceded it. And as we saw in Chapter 5 with followers of Heinz Kohut, other orientations—and not just feminists—are also celebrating the balance between affiliation and independence; the need for "selfobjects," they say, is lifelong, and healthy adolescents learn to transform rather than break their ties with their parents.

As I finished my two-day conversation with Chasin, I thought that the family therapy school has one skill the other therapists would do well to learn: the best of them can extract and preserve the wisest essentials of early theorists, discard the chaff, and still move on. It is a long way from stagnation, and I can safely predict that if Chasin is still in practice twenty years from now, when he is in his late seventies, he will be bubbling over about some cutting-edge practitioner (in Antarctica?)—and interposing a bit of Minuchin. "If you reread the more brutal parts of Minuchin and Whitaker now," I asked, "would you be horrified?"

"I think there's no need to be as reckless as they were in breaking up family patterns, though there was a fundamental benignity in some of those more flamboyant therapists that actually made it safer to be in the situation than it might look from the outside. But it is a fairly high-risk way to bust up the patterns, and one can fracture the mold without endangering people so much. Mostly therapists don't take those risks any more.

"It's the same problem with any field. The great founders—Freud, Skinner, Minuchin—are the people folks read about, but almost every field gets more sophisticated, softens, gets more intricate, and has much greater variety. I don't think at the time they knew that there were twenty ways to interrupt the pattern of the system. But the fundamental idea to perturb it is still here."

CHAPTER 12

JOINING THE CULTURE

Every family is a miniature society, a social order with its own rules, structure, leadership, language, style of living, zeitgeist. The hidden rules, the subtle nuances of language, the private rituals and dances that define every family as a unique microculture may not be easy for an outsider to perceive at first glance, but they are there. The wife knows what it means when her husband looks at her that way, and he knows what that curling inflection in her voice signifies.

—Augustus Y. Napier with
Carl A. Whitaker,
The Family Crucible (1978)

Freud pointed out that therapy changes neurotic patterns into the normal miseries of life. His comment is just as true for family therapy.

—Salvador Minuchin,
Families and Family Therapy
(1974)

IT IS NOT SURPRISING THAT AN OBSERVER—more precisely, this observer—sitting behind a one-way mirror or in front of a VCR or reading accounts of therapeutic sessions should feel a particular affinity for some practitioners and a particular resonance with some patients. It was my job to ask myself, "Why this one and not that one?" and to put the answers into some useful perspective for the reader. Obviously, some therapists offered formulations that sounded more reasonable or showed greater skill than those of their colleagues, and some patients' suffering seemed especially poignant or unfair. Clearly, some therapists and patients were more charming than others. And various therapists themselves had confessed, from time to time, a greater empathy for one class of disorders and irritation with another. But there appeared to be one more dimension (or set of dimensions) to the therapeutic relationship, and when I raised it some practitioners got nervous—or even downright defensive. The only school that seemed to be dealing with the issue head-on was the family systems therapists, a logical circumstance because they consider the clinician's personal history a useful tool, and because they study their patients in context. This is the set of dimensions that starts with ethnicity.

While I was doing my research, I happened to read a book called *Number Our Days*, written by the late anthropologist Barbara Myerhoff in 1978. Myerhoff had studied a group of immigrant Jews who frequented a senior center in Venice, California; they dealt with the process of growing old by drawing on the values and customs they had learned in the shtetl. I am Jewish too. But although I had been reared more than a generation later by highly assimilated, nonreligious middle-class parents in New York City, I was surprised to find how many of my values were similar to those of Myerhoff's population; I was closer to the old world than I had ever imagined. Its culture ran deep in me, and I assume the same is true of other Americans, however far back their roots go to County Kerry, Ghana, or Shanghai.

It is hardly startling to observe that the immigrant drama is the basic American drama, and if—as family systems theorists have come increasingly to consider—beliefs are carried through over generations, those of us who were born here had better think carefully about our origins. And since some emotional problems arise from the poor fit or conflict between individuals, the requirements of their families, and the society they live in, therapists need to understand different cultural values: families choosing a therapist must be sure they're understood. Because this is a period of heavy immigration, all professionals who deal with children and their families should recognize the role of culture and cultural transition in mental health problems.

Monica McGoldrick, a psychologist and social worker who is director of the Family Institute of New Jersey in Metuchen, has been raising these issues in the family systems world since the early eighties. Before we met, she sent me a 1992 paper she co-authored, "Intergenerational Relationships Across Cultures." While it is aimed at professionals in the field of human services, it offers a useful broad view of ethnic influences and some insight into the problems therapists face and why they sometimes fail; the paper's multicultural attribution—to McGoldrick, Paulette Moore Hines, Nydia Garcia-Preto, Rhea Almeida, and Susan Weltman— further establishes its authority, rather in the manner of an old-fashioned New York City mayoral ticket.

The authors consider ethnicity a "critical but not sufficient" factor in understanding development, and they observe that cultural values, "often unconscious, influence . . . what we label as a problem, how we communicate, beliefs about the cause of a problem, whom we prefer as a helper, and what kind of solutions we prefer." The relations between parents and children over the years follow different rules in every culture; the roles played by each gender vary enormously; and ethnic culture affects what we consider normal, whether we are the patient or the therapist.

With the appropriate caveats about stereotyping, the paper describes some frequent issues for several ethnic groups; we now know enough about family systems thinking to understand that problems between adult family members or even problems left over from the parents' childhood affect the children. This subject is obviously a minefield, and the degree to which the authors pull—or don't pull—their punches seems to depend on how much an ethnic group is discriminated against.

African-Americans, they observe, are mindful of a shared heritage of slavery and oppression that transcends individual differences in educational, financial, and social status; thus they consider it particularly important not to forget one's origins. Strong and far-reaching extended-family ties affect therapy because relatives are a reliable resource in time of trouble (as in the oft-cited informal adoption network within African-American families) and because people the therapist hasn't met or heard much about may be very influential in a family's life. Deference to elders has traditionally been very important: children are not supposed to question parental edicts, and profanity is taboo except with one's peers. The upside of a complex and fluid multigenerational family style is flexibility to roll with the punches; the downside is that the household can be vulnerable to poorly defined lines of authority and what some family systems people call boundary problems.

Some common reasons for therapeutic failure with African-American families are the labeling of one family member as the villain (which may cause the others to stiffen and withdraw); perceived insensitivity to the effects of racism; and the suggestion that individuals focus on their own needs above those of other family members. The authors recommend that therapists addressing problems between single mothers and teenage sons enlist male relatives as mentors, not disciplinarians. (Family therapists from Minuchin on have made the point that there are functional and dysfunctional single-parent families; the aim of therapy is generally to make sure that there are clear lines of authority, the parent is accessible, and all the children's needs are met, whether the parent is working or on public assistance. This goal applies to families from all ethnic groups.)

"Hispanic" families (a controversial term nowadays, because Latin-Americans consider it an inaccurate descriptor) set great store by the duty of parents to children and children to parents throughout their lives. Gender issues are important: women suffer from *marianismo*—the obligation to emulate the Virgin Mary and endure whatever men inflict on them—and *hembrismo*, the need to be a superwoman at work. Relationships may be skewed, with children emotionally allied with mothers against authoritarian fathers. Acculturation may produce a systemic problem when parents find it difficult to adapt, take refuge in the old-world culture, and become rigid and overprotective, which makes the children even more rebellious. And parents may also feel beleaguered by conflicting demands of old-fashioned grandparents and Americanized children.

The paper seems unusually tough on the Irish, McGoldrick's own group, perhaps because they're the only one discussed that no longer worries about discrimination in the United States. Unlike African-Americans, Hispanics, and Italians, the Irish experience very little intimacy between generations: "[H]aving a problem is bad enough, but if your family finds out, you have two problems: the problem and your embarrassment in front of your family." So they suffer alone, and the need to keep up appearances results in many intergenerational secrets. Caretaking is the mother's responsibility, and while "the Irish sense of duty is a wonderful resource," Irish families stress conformity and obedience over expressiveness and creativity; not being sent to the principal's office is more important than being a star student, and "Irish parents tend to have a superficial sense of child psychology."

The authors describe the "sainted Irish mother" as sometimes "critical, distant, and lacking in affection." They do say that "such attitudes and behaviors make sense in a culture with such a long history of foreign domination, in which Irish mothers sought control over 'something' through whatever means were available to them and felt a need to keep their family in line to minimize the risk of members being singled out for further oppression." Irish fathers tend to be peripheral, perhaps because they are uncomfortable expressing their feelings: "Father-daughter relationships are distant, possibly because the father fears that closeness will be confused with trespass of sexual boundaries," and while fathers "may share sports, work, and jokes" with their sons, they may also inflict painful teasing. For clinicians dealing with Irish families, the authors recommend "therapy sessions that are not too frequent; letters, journals, or other forms of expression that allow a degree of control over expression; clear directions; and a gentle humor free of negative connotations that would feed their already guilty conscience."

A section on Asian Indian families discusses the importance of caste and karma, with the former prizing the "purity" of light skin over the "pollution" of dark skin and the latter valuing "passivity and tolerance, suffering and sacrifice" to assure a better afterlife. Efforts to alter karma may include fasting, head-shaving, and suicide; "therapists might suggest . . . less destructive 'solutions' such as limited fasting, praying, meditating, or even haircutting." The dyadic relationships that family therapists study so carefully are set up differently in Indian families: mother and son, rather than mother and father, are at the center of the family, with fathers responsible for their sons' education and their daughters' dowry and marriage but not expected to be emotionally connected. The women in the patrilineal extended family share child-care responsibilities, which means an immigrant mother cut off from her relatives may be under particular stress that plays out in relations with her children, not her husband. Highly acculturated Indian families may still follow old-world customs in marrying off their children. A fundamental clash between Western and Indian values involves privacy and individualism versus obedience, collectivity, and family-centeredness. Therapists, the authors say, should ask specifically about cultural beliefs since families will not volunteer this information otherwise, and they should recognize that the family is unlikely to talk about problems except when recounting its immigrant history.

Therapists who are not Jewish may find Jewish families mysteriously sensitive to perceived anti-Semitism, the authors say. And even among nonobservant Jews, ambivalence about assimilation, interfaith marriage, children finding Jewish peers to play with and later to date, and diversity of Jewish practice raise problems; the next generation may either be not religious enough or too religious. The Jewish focus on children is a mixed blessing: much is expected of Jewish kids, and relatives feel free to mix in. Teenagers and young adults may have problems separating from enmeshed families. The authors cite tensions among Jewish women of different generations: while women had traditionally exerted power in the home and ceded the workplace to men, many mothers had to work in the Great Depression. Their daughters became homemakers, and their granddaughters career women. As for men, younger fathers may prefer a modern, active parental role, which the extended family may criticize.

Jewish families value education, social consciousness, tradition, and discourse, and they respect expert opinions. Thus they are often receptive to therapy once the practitioner has passed the third degree, and they may gladly do assigned reading, but "families may need to be reminded that the goal of therapy is not to tell a good story or to be 'right' in the eyes of the therapist, but to resolve the conflict or assuage the pain." I found this encapsulation of Jewish family issues accurate, which increased my confidence in the authors' summaries of other groups. (Indeed, the discovery that Jewish guilt was not the only kind, that there are, in fact, an Irish, Latino, and African-American guilt, with a special texture for each, made me feel less, well, guilty.)

McGoldrick, a strawberry-blond-haired, fair-skinned woman born in 1943, is a Bowenian, of the school of family therapists that draws genograms, coaches clients to differentiate from the family of origin, and effects change by calming things down rather than stirring them up. I asked her for some examples of how ethnic characteristics played out in her practice, and she told me about an Irish family whose sixteen-year-old daughter was dealing drugs in her school and was about to get busted.

"The mother wanted to come in with the daughter but without the husband and the eighteen-year-old son. She didn't bring the son the first time, but she did bring the husband, who acted as if he had no idea of what was what. He was just totally embarrassed to be there, he didn't want to talk about it, and he just smiled.

"The mother too was a little bit unclear of her reaction about this drug-dealing—which seemed to me a very serious issue—and they hardly looked at each other," McGoldrick continued. "The kid was skipping school and staying out late, challenging them about abortion and various other things. The mother would go around the house shutting the windows so the neighbors wouldn't hear any fighting. The parents, who came from

Ireland and were a little bit older, were just freaked by the words the daughter would use and the things she would talk about, though they aren't that unusual for teenagers today. The kid was having no limits set on her. Whatever she did, the father would go down into the basement and try to get away from it while the mother would go around closing the windows.

"I tried to get the parents to set limits and put the father in charge of enforcing it because he had been too far removed, but when he came back the next time, he hadn't done it. I couldn't figure it out because usually the Irish will do what you say. But then it came out that the father was afraid he would lose control."

"He was afraid he was going to haul off and smack her?" I asked.

"Right," McGoldrick said. "He had no repertoire between zero and one hundred, and so he was afraid that if once he engaged her, he would lose it completely. He couldn't articulate his fear, but that seemed what the issue was. So then I realized I had to give them some specifics: if she doesn't do what, then we'll do what, and what are the consequences. Once I told them specifically what to do they did it, and I think that's what the kid wanted. She was screaming for some sort of limits, and they were petrified of her. Once they could see there was something they could do, she got better."

I asked McGoldrick if there was some common drama in each ethnic group for people who came into therapy, and she said, "I don't think you would get parents in a black family who would give no reaction, unless they were just too overwhelmed by their own issues to pay attention to the kid or just so disgusted with the kid. In a Wasp family they wouldn't be intimidated—they'd say, 'These are the rules, and that's the deal.' And in a Jewish family they would insist on talking about it—'What's the matter that you're skipping school?' In a black or Wasp or Jewish family, you wouldn't, out of embarrassment, not have a clue what to do with adolescent kids, but the Irish just hope for the best. With some Irish families you wouldn't get that because the mother comes on strong."

The father, McGoldrick said, was pretty cut off from his family of origin in Ireland, and she didn't get anywhere directly with those problems. But a year later, at follow-up, she learned that he had taken the daughter over for her first family visit, even though—in typically Irish style—"he couldn't acknowledge to me that anything I said got through to him, that he was too distant from his family, that his reconnecting would make a difference, and it also would be a way to connect with his daughter." She had about ten sessions in this admittedly simple case, and the daughter finished high school instead of dropping out and ended up working as a probation officer.

McGoldrick and I had talked about the different attitudes of various ethnic groups. Betty Karrer is another family therapist who places ethnic values in the context of several cultural dimensions in which practitioners and clients interact. Karrer is a psychologist with an M.A. who directs the Family Systems Program at the Institute for Juvenile Research in the Department of Psychiatry at the University of Illinois in Chicago.

The IJR has a distinguished history: it is the descendant of the first child guidance clinic in the United States. Since its catchment area is an inner-city neighborhood a mile west of the Loop, Karrer sees many poor immigrant families, and her experience is varied by private practice in the suburbs. She herself, as a soft Spanish accent testifies, emigrated here from Mexico; but since her family there was of Irish descent, she is one of those Latin-Americans who don't like to be called Hispanic. Accurate communication is a particular concern in working with immigrants, Karrer says: "What is the meaning of 'respect' or 'obedience'? You almost have to have them teach you their meaning."

"If somebody said, 'She has no respect for me,' what would you ask?" I asked.

"I'd ask 'How would you know that?'" Karrer said. "At times we may say to the teenager, 'What does your mother do that deserves your respect?' It's rare that the answer is 'Nothing,' and if we suspect that, we don't ask the question. Usually there's ambivalence. We ask the daughter to come up with some things she respects her mother and father for. We use a bit of the polarity: when they hear from the children about the good things, they can be far more trusting and give more, and then we can talk about 'your daughter wants more autonomy. Are you as trusting of her as she is of you?' You need to be very careful of your language and your metaphors, and you look for the commonalties."

The commonalties are the subject of an interesting and sophisticated chapter of Karrer's called "The Sound of Two Hands Clapping: Cultural Interactions of the Minority Family and the Therapist," which views the family's values in relation to the therapist's. Distinctions, family therapists currently point out, also serve to illuminate the person who makes them. (I was reminded of the famous split-screen sequence in the film *Annie Hall*.) Karrer quotes a highly articulate Colombian immigrant woman she once treated, who described cultural transition this way: "[I]t seems that the next difficult step was being seen by others in very different ways than I saw myself. It was as if all of a sudden I had become someone else. My identity and beliefs were all put through a different filter and came out unrecognizable, limited, and above all dissonant with my previous views of myself. . . . Was I this person I thought I was? Or the person they said I was?"

Karrer observes that early discussions of ethnic differences were monolithic and ignored variations within a culture. Current thinking considers other cultural dimensions that a therapist of a different origin may share with the family, thus bridging the gap between them. These dimensions, in addition to ethnicity, are economics, education, religion, gender, generation, race, minority status, regional background, and in the case of immigrants, cultural transition. They all interconnect: that is, poor, rich, and middle-class people vary according to their religion, ethnicity, regional background, and so forth. A rich Catholic from Milan looks at life differently from a poor Catholic from Sicily, and this affects how she relates to a therapist from Mexico City who is a Catholic professional woman.

In the course of my research among all the therapeutic tribes, I encountered discussions about the importance of "the therapist's personality" to the effectiveness of treatment: some practitioners thought this a valid criterion for choosing a therapist and some didn't, but most thought "personality" and "chemistry" elusive qualities you couldn't nail down. But much of what "can't be nailed down"—what is, more accurately, *uncomfortable* or *bad form* to nail down—has to do with Karrer's dimensions.

In illustration of overlapping "points of entry," Karrer writes of an Afghan family that fled to Iran after the Soviet invasion and finally emigrated to the United States during the Iran-Iraq war. When they came to therapy at IJR, they had been in the country for five years; the father was a doctor and the mother a housewife, and they had five daughters aged thirteen, twelve, ten, nine, and eight. The identified patient was the thirteen-year-old, who was suddenly doing poorly in school and had, the parents believed, withdrawn from close family relationships ever since the father, preparing to take medical boards, had himself become unavailable. He asked the therapist—an Italian woman who was a fellow in child psychiatry—to fix the family so he could get back to studying. Behind the one-way mirror sat a training team of three other child psychiatry fellows who hailed from Thailand, the Philippines, and Argentina, and their supervisor, Karrer: in all, four women and a man.

It was hard to find common ground with the father, and while the team was tempted just to deplore his patriarchal attitude, this focus would hardly help. To engage him, the team disclosed that they were all immigrants who had had to reestablish professional careers in the United States. Starting with the man on the team, each of the psychiatrists came in and discussed how he or she had got through studying for the medical boards. This joining technique succeeded in bringing the father into the therapy.

Ethnic patterns, Karrer says, are often so subtle that we are not aware of them. Families vary in the intensity of their ethnic affiliation, as do generations within a family. Ethnic loyalty seems to grow with feelings of loss of the native land: "Italians are more 'Italian' in this country than in Italy." And she observes that "ethnicity seems to have been described as a characteristic of the families we serve, but not of the therapist." Karrer says acculturation has three stages, and she describes a family with five children in which "the parents were Mexicans-in-America, the older children Mexican-Americans, and the younger children Americans of Mexican descent. The children sought independence, while the parents tried to hold on. Karrer and the therapist she was supervising, a young man who had just dealt with separating from his traditional Polish family, led the clients to discuss "the cost of leaving home in pursuit of dreams," a process that was fulfilled over three generations. The shared Catholic religion formed a useful bond among family, therapist, and supervisor.

Attitudes toward gender are a crucial dimension that interacts with all the others. First of all, the therapist's gender is bound to make a difference to the various family members; moreover, "if the family is traditional and the therapist contemporary, clarification of and respect for their difference should be acknowledged." In pondering ethnic issues, I had felt baffled by my perception—which the McGoldrick et al. article seemed to confirm—that all the old world cultures now considered so precious had in some way restricted, demeaned, or stereotyped women.

I had asked both McGoldrick and Karrer whether this presented a stalemate for therapists whose values were modern, and both thought there were ways around the issue. McGoldrick, in her Bowenian style, would lead a daughter to accept that the old values were a mixed bag, find other strands in the traditional culture that might bolster her ambitions, coach her in seeking the support of mother and aunt, and find models in her family who had somehow bent the traditions—all this in the interests of encouraging greater personal development without breaking with her family. Karrer's discussion of "the cost of leaving home to pursue your dreams" marked her approach, and when we talked, she emphasized the need to learn how far the family had moved in acculturation and whether they believed they had got what they were seeking in leaving home; families who feel bitter and failed would have different reactions from successful ones. Karrer's chapter illustrates successful efforts to move families into a more pragmatic view of gender roles: in telling one story, she comments, "Imagine, for example, a well-meaning therapist who, in an effort to be respectful of what she had either read or heard about Mexican families' traditional patriarchal structure, had either not seen, or [not] supported a change in the couple's relationship . . . cultural differences are neither static nor impenetrable."

Other dimensions that are particularly important (sometimes more than we might imagine) are what Karrer calls "generation," which means that family members and therapists can join or differ over contextual markers like World War II, the Kennedy assassination, and musical preferences; regional background (being urban, suburban, or rural and coming from hot or cold climate affects mood, style, and attitudes); and race (she tells an interesting story of a single white mother who had two children by an African-American father and two by a native American father, with neither father on the scene; the children all chose their fathers' racial identities, and the therapist had to "help the children explore their white part and see it as legitimate," which they finally learned to do at home, though not in public).

The goals Karrer states represent currently accepted objectives—motherhood and apple pie, that is to say—in the family therapy tribe. "The cultural values of the family need to be understood, validated and challenged," she writes. "This is easier if therapists conceptualize all cultures as sanctioning both stability and change." She states that therapist and family need to develop their own cultural context, the better to "transform . . . the world views of both the family and the therapist."

As I roamed the field, I found a particular problem in which those goals were more than empty motherhood-and-apple-pie phrases, a problem for which family therapy would have to be the treatment of choice. This was a situation in which the family, due to circumstances both inexorable and beyond its control, must arrive at some new view of itself or else suffer and break apart. And it was a situation in which the cultural values described by McGoldrick and Karrer played an important role. While it is possible to try to make a hyperactive child less hyperactive, families with gay children are faced with one choice only: they can either accept the children as they are or reject and lose them.

While there is still much to be learned on the complex causes of homosexuality, several recent genetic studies compellingly suggest there is some innate predisposition to be attracted to one's own sex. As we'll see in more detail in a later chapter, nature-nurture studies are often done on twins: if the identical twins in a study (who are genetically matched) show more of a trait than fraternal twins or ordinary siblings who share an environment and only some of their genetic makeup, the finding argues that something about the trait is inherited. In studies of male and female subjects, researchers found that more than half of the gay men's identical twin brothers were also gay, versus only 22 percent of their fraternal twins and 11 percent of their adoptive brothers, who, of course, had only environment in common; just under half of the lesbians' identical twins were lesbian, compared with 16 percent of their fraternal twins and only 6 per cent of their adoptive sisters.

Two later studies by different investigators also found identical twins more concordant for homosexuality than fraternal twins. And a researcher at the National Cancer Institute has tied male homosexuality to a small region of the X chromosome. Nobody yet knows how the gene or genes might act to produce homosexuality in an individual.

Other promising neuroendocrine and neuroanatomical research suggests the importance of biological factors. At the same time, since the twin studies haven't found absolute concordance, researchers believe there is also some environmental role. (This could still be biological, emanating from prenatal factors.) While these studies don't wrap up the answer to sexual orientation with a lavender ribbon, they do make a persuasive case that people don't decide to be gay.

Moreover, psychological research going back to the fifties has failed to distinguish the Rorschachs and other projective tests of homosexuals from those of heterosexuals except on one question, which showed a scene of two men in a bedroom. Since no psychological study has succeeded in defining homosexuality per se as pathological, it has not been listed as a disorder in the DSM since 1973. Gay therapists (and probably most straight ones these days) look at sexual orientation as rather like left- or right-handedness, and I shall proceed under that assumption here.

At the same time, it is hardly surprising that growing up as social pariahs takes a toll on gay teenagers in innumerable complex ways. Back in 1983 the late Drs. Emery S. Hetrick, a psychiatrist, and A. Damien Martin, an education professor, both at New York University, founded the Hetrick-Martin Institute for Gay and Lesbian Youth, a counseling and advocacy agency in New York City. A 1987 article by Hetrick and Martin called "Developmental Issues and Their Resolution for Gay and Lesbian Adolescents" draws on both adolescent developmental psychology and sociological research about outcast groups, in addition to data collected from teenagers who found their way to Hetrick-Martin during its first year. It is an eminently logical piece of work, and one cannot fail to be moved by it.

The chief task of an adolescent in our society, as we have seen, is to become an autonomous individual; different theoretical orientations may use different terminology and haggle about what constitutes the "sense of self" and how it grows, but they know it when they see it. Identity develops in a social context, and for the homosexual adolescent that context is one of stigma. The experience that Betty Karrer's Colombian immigrant client described—a feeling that what you think you are and what others think you are are drastically different—is pervasive for gay people, who must at the least endure disparaging rhetoric and sometimes, when their sexuality is known or suspected, suffer actual discrimination and violence. Most devastating, the authors say, is "the daily need to hide an important aspect of their personal and social identity."

African-American and Jewish children can be prepared for racism and anti-Semitism by loving parents who have faced the same ordeals. Gay adolescents, until they successfully come out to their parents, must put up with it all alone—indeed, they are often thrown out of the house by their parents.

The authors report the presenting problems of 329 teenagers who came to Hetrick-Martin in its first year; these clients tended to be over sixteen because younger kids who telephoned for counseling hadn't the freedom to come in. The ethnic and racial breakdown parallels that of the New York City public school system at the time: more than a third black, more than a third white, a quarter Hispanic. Nearly three-fourths were male, matching the ratio at most service agencies for kids in New York. Every known religion and sect in the city was represented.

The most common problem was isolation: social, emotional, and cognitive. The social isolation comes from being always on guard: "having no one to talk to, feeling alone within every social situation, including the family, peers, school, and church or synagogue." Many of the adolescents who became sexually involved with an adult said they'd done so more out of social need than sexual desire, and they had felt the adult was exploiting them. From this came a belief that "sex is the only bond possible with another homosexual person . . . and that they have no emotional or spiritual worth other than as sex objects."

At the same time they felt cut off from both their families and their straight peers, with whom they were afraid to make friends for fear of being either misunderstood or found out. The way the young gays coped with isolation differed by gender: the boys found places to pick up other gays and accordingly developed a social pattern in which they had sex with someone first, and (maybe) got to know them afterward, instead of the other way around. The girls, on the other hand, went to the other extreme: they would find a companion and hang on for dear life, thus being "deprived of important social learning during a critical developmental stage." Both girls and boys lacked information and suitable models to identify with.

The isolation led to truancy among boys, who fled the teasing of classmates; some lesbians hid by getting pregnant. The fear of giving themselves away (and thus the need to watch the way they dressed, spoke, and walked) limited the development of social skills, and the teenagers felt cut off from their religious faith insofar as it condemned homosexuality.

When I read this paper, the theorist who came quickly to mind and remained with me was B. F. Skinner: the way we as a society treat gay adolescents seems not only brutal but illogical, tailor-made to reinforce what is known in Skinner's world as maladaptive behaviors. Hetrick and Martin reported that a fifth of the agency's clients had either considered suicide or actually attempted it.

The risk of suicide for gays is a controversial question that researchers are only beginning to study; it's complicated by the fact that "psychological autopsies" don't necessarily uncover homosexuality. But among 137 fourteen-through-twenty-one-year-old gay and bisexual males in the Midwest and Pacific Northwest, surveyed in a 1991 article in *Pediatrics*, 41 reported they'd attempted suicide and half of those had made several tries. A third of the attempts occurred during the same year that subjects identified their sexuality, and most other attempts came shortly after. In this group suicide attempts were linked with "gender nonconformity and precocious psychosexual development. . . . For each year's delay in bisexual or homosexual self-labeling, the odds of a suicide attempt diminished by 80%." Thus the younger the kids were when they came out to themselves and to others, the less equipped they were to cope with isolation and stigma. In other ways, however, the suicide attempters resembled the profiles of heterosexual suicide victims, with "high levels of family dysfunction, personal substance abuse, and other antisocial behaviors." These factors, the authors say, "often complicate 'coming out' at an early age and may further contribute to the high rate of suicide in this group."

It is impossible for a reasonably compassionate person to read about the life of gay adolescents without feeling moved and angry. At the same time parents have dreams for their children, and often those dreams include weddings and grandchildren. They certainly don't dream of their sons or daughters living as outcasts; they are usually terrified of AIDS, and they may feel they are in some way guilty of causing their child to be gay. One is hard put to imagine even the most freethinking parent serenely accepting the news of a child's homosexuality. How do family therapists deal with this situation?

I talked to three gay therapists, a man and two women, and to a straight woman who specializes in working with the families of gays. I had guessed that the experience for a child and a family might be different for boys and girls; for one thing I had an informal impression that parents of boys are constantly nervous that some experience might cause their sons to end up gay, while it never dawns on parents of girls that their daughters could be anything but straight. This, the therapists said, was an accurate perception: boys' parents tend to worry more than girls' parents, although once the girl comes out, she has as many—although different—problems.

The therapists I saw also differed in the demographics of their clientele. John Patten, M.D., a lanky, gray-haired man with a trace of an accent from his native Australia, is associated with both New York Hospital–Cornell Medical Center and The Ackerman Institute for Family Therapy in New York City. Ackerman therapists are expensive, which means that terrified children generally can't afford to show up alone on his doorstep. He gets families of the middle class and above who either know or suspect their children are gay and are unlikely to throw them out of the house: they hope for some sort of modus vivendi, though perhaps not without strings attached.

I asked Patten to tell me at what age a child begins to discover that he or she is different from other family members and the mainstream culture and how this plays out in the family drama. "If you take retrospective histories of gay adults," he said, "they will talk about how they knew they were different when they were five or seven. They didn't have the language to describe it since there were no role models then. Now you hear the word *gay* in a presidential campaign, so with that you have the increasing possibility of somebody coming out." That is, today's children might be sophisticated enough to figure out that their being "different" means being gay, and they thus "come out"—at least to themselves—at an earlier age.

I pressed Patten on *how* a preadolescent boy knows he is different, and Patten said they are "not as interested in the stereotypic male-boy pursuits." Because there are heterosexual nerds, bookworms, and violinists, I countered that "one hears of very unathletic skirt-chasers." But it was hard for me to nail down just what sort of difference Patten meant, except that this was not the same as what a transsexual might feel: "It's different from feeling they're not male, it's much more that they're a different sort of male."

So I moved on to ask what happens next and when the difference becomes an issue with Mom and Dad. Here he was clearer. "Adolescents come out because of accidents or because they want to. Usually they need some peer group or another gay person they can communicate with outside the family, and perhaps they have some sort of sexual experience, so the person who stays exclusively within the family tends not to come out." He pointed out that gay teenagers must follow two developmental lines: one is the usual identity development that all adolescents experience, and the other is the parallel development of a gay or lesbian identity. The latter, Patten said, "must be pretty secure, or else they don't come out ever, or they may come out in their twenties or thirties. There's a difference between coming out to yourself and having integrated that enough to tell your family."

"Is the kid ever going to say, 'Mom' or 'Dad, I'm worried, I think I *might* be gay, but I don't know?' "

"Very unlikely," Patten said, "because of all the stigmas. By the time they've developed enough identity, they're also aware of what the attitudes are."

I imagined the millions of interactions a boy has with his father, playing baseball and doing male things, or exchanges with a girl in which parents are speaking quite innocently of her future boyfriends and weddings, and the way it would all ring phony; it seemed the kids must go through torture every single minute. Patten said, "One adolescent described it to me: 'It's like having a secret when you don't want to have a secret but you have to because there's nothing else,' and so the homophobia of society or of the family is internalized in gay people and becomes part of their identity."

The family, of course, may have other problems that have nothing to do with the child. "It's common for coming out to get confused in some other family dynamic and become the cause célèbre when it isn't really," Patten said. "Then you have the variations of religiosity—a very religious Orthodox Jewish family or a Catholic or fundamentalist family, or with certain ethnic groups. If you're black and blue-collar, it's very difficult for a gay adolescent to be out."

I asked Patten for a case history, and he told me about a seventeen-year-old Jewish boy whose parents called him because their son had told them he was gay; what should they do?

"With this particular family," Patten said, "I spoke to the kid and asked him if it would be okay to meet with the parents once and then meet with the three of them, because that's what the parents wanted, and he said it would be helpful. So what the parents needed was 'Homosexuality 101'—that it's not a mental disorder, that gay people can lead successful lives, have intimate relationships, and are not alcoholics, and that the parents are not to blame, that it's a complicated issue, you can look at every sort of family constellation and find a heterosexual child or a gay child. If you can get the parents over that sort of obsession with what caused it . . . and you usually can with the sort of family I'm talking about, then they go through a period of mourning.

"They feel like they've lost the child, that the child is an alien. If they're coming seeking advice, obviously they're not going to cut off the child, but what's common is that the child is cut off emotionally for a number of years. There's no place in the family for a person who's gay until you *make* a place for them, which takes quite a number of years of restructuring. We're talking here about fairly ideal situations, where there's not a real rigidity."

In the case Patten was describing, the boy wanted immediate acceptance from his parents; he was involved with activities at a gay center and was advanced in his gay identity. He went to private school, where he was not out except to a few good friends.

"So he lives this sort of second life," I said.

"Right. All gay people live in two contexts, and if you're black as well, you live in three. Gay people are masters at living within a family, the heterosexual family, and within the gay family, but it's much better for them if gradually those two families have more contact with one another." Patten confirmed that the ability to deal smoothly with one's family, as in any other problem, has much to do with the child's temperament.

The story would continue with the parents saying, "Wait and see. Maybe you aren't gay. Maybe you're bisexual. Maybe you're just experimenting." He emphasized that "when somebody reaches adolescence, it's not optional. I think a gay identity is formed much earlier. What usually happens, even in this city, is that the parents from the West Side [the progressive, relatively sophisticated upper-middle-class neighborhood in Manhattan] would then send the child to a psychotherapist, and even though they might be very liberal, there would be this whole push to keep the child away from gay people. This is the recruitment theory, the old homophobic theory that homosexuals are created by other homosexuals who recruit them to their ranks."

"And you could be on a desert island, actually, and sooner or later it would hit you?" I asked.

"Right," said Patten.

"It sounds to me, though, as if the mom and dad are coming in and announcing, 'Tom has told us this,' you sit down and give them the 101, they walk out fifty minutes later saying, 'Thank you, doctor,' and they may be in shock for a while but everything is really fine. What happens when it doesn't go so well?"

"You may get a father who refuses to accept it. I would meet with the father alone and describe the life course of a gay person who doesn't come out, in terms of the internalized homophobia. What I would do is go back to the father's own belief systems about this and see whether there's any flexibility." Patten does emphasize, though, that it is "a normative thing for an individual to come out, and the family's reaction to it is normal. It's a developmental node in a normal family's progression through life. I think in the next twenty years families will become more accepting."

Before leaving Patten I got him to give me a more difficult case history, which makes a good cautionary tale. "Two sixteen-year-old boys were caught having sex by one boy's mother," he remembered. "I had seen her years ago with some other kind of family problem, so she comes to see me alone. She wanted to know if this was a passing phase. I felt, since they were Catholic, that there was no way to bring the father into this right now. The mother felt—and I was inclined to agree with her—that bringing him in at this stage would explode the whole thing out of the water. So I had some meetings then with the boy and his mother, and he said he didn't know yet whether he was gay or straight.

"In about three sessions he was able to become much more connected to the mother, and they were able to talk about it. Usually the mother is very upset and confronts the boy, and he says, 'Well, I'm not gay,' and it becomes a bone of contention. If the father's brought in, the son has to say he isn't gay, so that particular part of his identity gets submerged for twenty years." Patten notes that according to Kinsey, many heterosexual people have had a homosexual experience. "It's better to try and understand it and to look at it in the long term rather than have to get the adolescent to fess up as to whether he's straight or gay." There is, he says, a difference between behavior and identity.

"Is there *frequent* gay behavior by heterosexuals?" I asked Patten.

"No," he said.

"So that still, if a parent has a kid who says, 'I am gay,' or even, 'I think I am gay,' then the chances are that the kid is gay."

"Right," said Patten.

Some parents who must learn to live with this complicated situation might feel intimidated by a gay therapist: indeed, when homosexuality is the issue, sexual orientation may be added to the points of entry that Betty Karrer, the ethnicity specialist in Chicago, describes in her paper. Rita Gazarik, a social worker at Gouverneur Hospital in New York City, was associated with Hetrick-Martin while its two founders were alive. "They felt the real world has everybody in it and everybody's got to talk about this together. Sure, there's a place for gay people to get together and feel comfortable and open, but they also have to join the heterosexual world and feel as comfortable as they can. So I was there to be identified with the family and to help the family. Families hated dealing with gay therapists on these issues!"

Gazarik happened into this specialty after her cousin announced he was gay. "I was very into analysis at that time, and I said, 'It's a passing fancy. Why don't you go see my analyst?' which he did, and it didn't work. But I reacted as a family member. I said, 'Omigod.' " Hetrick had been a colleague at Gouverneur, and the two talked at length about family reactions to gay issues; thus Gazarik ended up consulting for Hetrick-Martin.

"Two days before Emery Hetrick died, he dictated to me a whole list of questions and research hypotheses about families of gay kids. I had wanted to look at the families from a systemic point of view, to demonstrate why the kids are gay, that there was something wrong in the family system that led to their homosexual behavior. That was the wrong premise, though. Emery said, 'I'm not looking at family systems for that reason. Let's see what goes on in a family when one member is gay and comes out.' "

Gazarik often worked with Joyce Hunter, a lesbian therapist who was one of the founders of Hetrick-Martin. In the eighties the staff at Hetrick-Martin "were the only ones who were very realistic about dealing with kids' coming-out issues. One of the things they said very clearly was they don't encourage kids to do this in adolescence because they get kicked out of the house and they're not financially independent, they're not emotionally independent. Until they are, it's very dangerous to say, 'Hi, Mom, I'm gay,' over Christmas dinner. They have a whole process they take a kid through to make sure he's gay. Then they would coach these children about the timing of it and start with one parent. Who in your family would accept this most easily? they would ask. Who would have the most difficulty? They were doing Bowenian coaching without knowing it. I would work with the family after it leaked out or they were told, with the child present and the staff member who worked with the adolescent. We'd see the family together, so the kid had an ally and I was the ally of the family."

Like other therapists who deal with gay issues, Gazarik has found that ethnicity plays an important role in each case. She told me about a well-to-do but not highly educated Italian family in Brooklyn whose daughter, a college student living at home, had been thrown out of the house when she told them she was in love with a woman. "She was gorgeous, a smashing nineteen-year-old, and she was very, very close to her father. He was her favorite parent and she was his favorite child, and now they weren't talking. I would see her separately and I would see the parents, and then I brought them together, and then I'd see the mother and daughter together and the father and daughter together.

"The father blamed it on the woman who had seduced his daughter on the soccer team. The family was very much into sports, and one thing he worried about was, 'I shouldn't have introduced her to sports.' There was also an interesting family secret. The mother had had a child before this marriage and given it up for adoption, and her present husband came in like a white knight and saved her from humiliation. The daughter of course knew, but nobody talked about it.

"The mother was still quite troubled by this. When I did a genogram, there was a connection between the age at which she had this child and the age at which her daughter came out. Consciously it wasn't known. There is a theory I have, that kids sense what's going on in a family, and they will announce they're gay at a time to absorb a conflict because there's something else going on that the parents may not want to deal with."

"What happened in the sessions?" I asked.

"Once the father stormed out, then he stormed back in and threw the daughter out. I saw the daughter afterward alone, but she was very sad. I questioned whether he would still be upset about her getting married to a man, even though it would be socially acceptable; I thought he would. The sessions after that were separate, over a year. The father stopped coming. I coached the daughter to talk to her father on the phone and then meet him for lunch.

"They gradually let her back into the family, to come to big events like a christening. She got blamed for everything that was going on, but without talking about it they let her into the family. Sometimes that's okay. You don't have to talk about everything all the time—in some cultures you really don't."

We were back to cultural differences, and Gazarik said, "The Italian family rejects them—'Don't come home for Sunday spaghetti anymore. You've hurt your mother, she's upset, look at her. You can't tell your brothers, nobody is going to play football with them anymore.' The Jewish family would send the kid into analysis. What's interesting about Hispanic culture is that a lot of men are very sympathetic, the ones that aren't absolutely macho. They are fatalistic—'I love my son, I'm sorry.' Non-assimilated families, West Indians too, are concerned about how hard this kid's life is going to be, and they're terrified of the rejection and humiliation. In more sophisticated families it's guilt. Their own embarrassment is the least. When you have children, that's the least of your worries, you're so giving. They're more concerned about what they did wrong, which is the real reason for rejecting the kid."

I met once more with Gazarik and her old Hetrick-Martin colleague, Joyce Hunter, also a social worker who is now a research fellow at the HIV Center for Clinical and Behavioral Studies, a part of the New York State Psychiatric Institute at Columbia University. The center has a grant to study the coming-out process, and Hunter was planning to do an ethnographic substudy of twenty college kids with diverse backgrounds.

Hunter is a muscular woman with short, tightly curled dark hair. Like Patten, she told me that the gay kids she works with perceive they are different at an early age. "The younger they are, the less they have a hard time saying 'always.' "

Was the "difference" in the context of sex? "There's a heterosexual assumption," she said, "and your expectation as you grow up is that you're going to be heterosexual, and then all of a sudden you're not fitting in. They don't articulate it that way, but I would. A lot of times they don't get it until they see somebody they like, and then they understand."

"Like a flash?"

"No, it's not a flash," Hunter said. "Kids don't wake up one day and say, 'I've decided to be gay so I can aggravate my family and put myself at risk of being beaten up or murdered.' "

Once more I brought up the shy bookworms, but Hunter said it has nothing to do with shyness. "Going to a movie," she offered. "All your friends are carrying on about the star of the opposite sex, and you're thinking, 'Huh, what's all the commotion about?' You're feeling that way about the star of the same sex, and you know instinctively not to say anything. By the time they're having these feelings, especially coming into adolescence, they know. I knew, and I wasn't telling anybody anything."

Hunter says she has more questions than answers about coming out and that it's hard to get data in a community that's hiding; a lot of information is anecdotal. But a colleague at the New York State Psychiatric Institute had studied 100 heterosexuals and 100 homosexuals and asked whether, in their teens, they had ever been concerned about their homosexual behavior or their orientation. None of the heterosexuals, even those who had had gay experiences as adolescents, had been concerned about it, while all the gay people had been concerned. Hunter says it is "more common than you think" for straight people to have gay experiences.

"Over the years I've had kids come in and define themselves in a couple of ways. My experience with those kids who identify as bisexual first is six, seven months, a year down the road, they're gay or lesbian. But you will also have a kid who comes in and is confused, so you stay with that. You let the kid be confused, help them and support them in their confusion because that's okay. You're in a process of developing sexuality; who says you have to make choices here? I say, 'What you feel, you'll know. I can't tell you if you're gay, I can't tell you if you're straight. You will know, but let's talk about it.' A lot of times they know and they're afraid of rejection."

"Does anybody ever turn out not to be gay?" I asked.

"No," Hunter said, "or if they're not gay, you know it very early on. A lot of times the confusion has nothing to do with how they're feeling about

the person they're attracted to. It's the fear. I had a girl sit in my office—
'I'm gay. My father will kill me.' I ask them, 'What do you think you can
do that this won't happen?' and they say, 'Well, I don't have to tell him,'
and I'll say, 'That sounds good to me.' We never encourage them to come
out to their parents, because you cannot predict how a family is going to
respond."

"But unless the parents are monsters, sooner or later the child is going
to want to," I said.

"They do, and most of the kids really want to tell them, because they
love their parents and they want to share this information. It's not an
acting-out experience."

I asked what happens when the kids become active. "Boys are socialized to have their needs met," Hunter said, "and they know they can't be
sexually active in their neighborhood because they might be found out
and beaten up. So you have this kid who wants to meet people his own age
who are like him, he wants to have a relationship, he wants to have a
boyfriend. They're no different from their heterosexual counterparts in
that way, and lesbian kids are as romantic."

The lesbians, Hunter told me, "are not socialized to go out and have
their needs met," and they enter the kind of totally dependent relationships described in the Hetrick and Martin paper. Moreover, since coming
out involves sexual experimentation, lesbian girls may have sex with the
gay or bisexual boys they know; they too are therefore at risk for AIDS.

Hunter and Gazarik were discussing the Brooklyn case Gazarik had
described to me, in which they differed at first on whether the girl was
really gay. "I remember saying to you, 'Rita, this woman's a dyke, forget
it!' I'm very blunt. It was what she felt about herself and how she defined
her relationship to the woman she was living with. Someone walks
through the door and your heart will start to dance. The greatest-looking
guy could walk in this door now—dead meat! Forget it—nothing. If some
woman walked in the door, it might be different. And that's what I got from
her. It was about who she was and who she wanted to spend her life with
and make a home with. It was about love. It's the same thing as with
heterosexuals."

Hunter's therapeutic sequence was different from Patten's: both because Hetrick-Martin is free and because of its reputation among gay and
lesbian teenagers, it sees the kids first. By the time a family comes in, the
child knows he's gay. "He's out all night," Hunter says. "They don't

understand why he doesn't come home till early in the morning. Since these boys and girls can't socialize like their heterosexual counterparts in school, they try to get involved in the gay scene in the Village, where nothing begins till nine o'clock. They go to the bars and lie about their age.

"For the parents, there are a lot of conduct issues. I have to become a mediator. It's helping the parents and the child come to a compromise, so I say, 'How about weeknights nine thirty?' and the parents say, 'Eight,' and the kid says no. I've actually had counseling sessions around stuff like that. One of the big fears is that they're going to get hurt, that they might get involved in sexual situations they can't get out of with somebody older, they're going to be doing drugs."

"Those are not unreasonable worries," I said.

"No, they're not, and what helps is having somebody who is openly gay say to the kid, 'Look, that's legit.' "

"So I would assume you are trying to bring in an air of normalcy," I said.

"I try to get them back together and say, 'Look, there are no bad guys here.' And I tell the parents they have to understand why the kid wants to be out that late and also let the kid know that the parents have a legitimate concern. 'And if you're coming in at three or four o'clock in the morning, you are not going to school, and your *job* is to go to school. Let's talk turkey here.' I will work with the kid individually, and the kid will tell me, 'You say what my parents say,' and I say, 'Get out of here! What would you do if it was *your* kid, if you had somebody you cared about, and you know they're supposed to be going to school every day?' I usually bring it back to them and let them solve it. 'If they said you can't go out with your gay friends, I'd be all over their case, but this is a legitimate concern.' "

"I would not define myself as a psychotherapist," Hunter said as I was leaving. "I actually consider myself a very good clinician. I think I work well with youth, and their families also, but I consider myself a social worker who does good counseling. I did private practice for six months, and I hated it."

We have seen the evolution of family systems therapy from an emphasis on behavior to a focus on belief, from the directive to the collaborative, and from the absolute to the relative. And we have seen therapists in other orientations confronting the limits of treating individuals without carefully examining the context in which they live. Fair enough; but has family therapy its limits too? How profound are those restrictions? That is, can a practitioner accept the paradigm of "viewing in context" and still study the individual's inner workings in that frame? One family therapist who believes he has found a way is Richard Schwartz, Ph.D., a colleague of Betty Karrer's at the Institute for Juvenile Research in Chicago and co-author of a widely used family therapy textbook. Schwartz, a slightly built, soft-spoken man in his forties who is as low-key as Chasin is exuberant, has actually been raising the hood—looking inside his patients—and has evolved a technique, with theoretical underpinnings, for reconciling family systems work with individual therapy.

He began in 1983, inspired by his experience with a twenty-three-year-old bulimic and her family. As he later wrote in *The Family Therapy Networker* (a magazine aimed at professionals but written in lay English good enough to have received a recent National Magazine Award nomination), the relationships within Sally's family were now on track: they "had done everything we asked. She had given up her role of family protector and her parents had adapted well to this change. She had moved out of her parents' home into her own apartment and was performing well in a good job. For the first time she was making close friends." If the paradigm was working in the classic manner, Sally was supposed to stop bingeing and purging. But while the bulimic symptoms occurred less frequently and intensely, they didn't go away: as Schwartz put it, "Sally seemed unaware of her cure."

Schwartz finally decided it was time to start asking Sally what was happening internally before she went on a "binge and vomit spree." She described a clamor of voices arguing inside her head, and when the therapist asked her to characterize each one, he found she could do so readily. One voice was highly critical, telling her she was fat and lazy; another was defensive and parent-blaming; a third was sad and helpless; and a fourth just said, "Binge." The therapist was fascinated: what seemed to be going on inside Sally, and inside his other bulimic patients when he interviewed them about it, and come to think of it, inside Schwartz himself in times of angst, was a very familiar sort of family battle, with the same dynamics he was used to treating among relatives. Perhaps he could work with these inner voices in the same way he treated an actual family—that is, "try applying the concepts of systems thinking to the internal processes that direct thought and feeling."

Moreover, Schwartz was reading neurobiological and artificial intelligence research that depicted a brain composed of modules performing separate functions, and computer science literature in general emphasizing parallel over serial information-processing. As one psychoneurologist had written, "We are not a single person. We are many." Thus multiple personality disorder (which DSM-IV has renamed "Dissociative Identity Disorder"), Schwartz believed, "only represents an extremely disengaged and polarized version of the ordinary operation of our internal system."

There was even a useful, accessible lay person's language for this phenomenon: Sally would often describe ambivalence, as most of us do, by saying, "Part of me is afraid, but another part says, 'Go for it.' " Schwartz thought the parts were not temporary moods but actual subselves, each one "a discrete and autonomous mental system that has an idiosyncratic range of emotion, style of expression, and set of abilities, intentions, or functions."

In Sally's case, she had a part that focused on measuring her achievements and a part that watched whether other people approved of her. Both parts let out a barrage of criticism the minute someone appeared to deliver a slight. But when the assault got too heavy, it activated the "poor me" part, which overwhelmed her with sadness and even suicidal feelings. At this point the "eating machine" swung into action, cutting off Sally's despair by getting her to comfort herself by bingeing and repent by vomiting, which disgusted the self-critical voices and set them off again.

Schwartz believed that traditional family systems formulations missed the internal complexity of individuals, labeling them globally as needy children, controlling mothers, distant fathers. He felt people mistook the parts for the whole and thus became locked into rigid ways of relating with each other. This view, as readers will recognize, bears a certain resemblance to psychodynamic theories, from Freud's tripartite theory through Daniel Stern's conception of the four selves. "Everybody who's looked inside of people sees basically the same thing," he told me. "The observations are very similar. The interpretations are where the differences are." Schwartz felt many psychodynamic theories tended to pathologize the patient. As he continued to work with his prototype, he became more familiar with other therapeutic models—in particular the Gestalt and the Jungian—and also drew on these. But he still operated from the family therapists' assumption that people behave differently in different contexts.

In his work with Sally, he found she also had an observing intelligence, a *Self* that was able to rise above the parts and offer a mature perspective. He described this system as

> a kind of orchestra, in which the individual musicians are analogous to the parts and the conductor is the Self. A good conductor has a sense of the value of each instrument and the ability of every musician, and . . . can sense precisely the best point in a symphony to draw out one section and mute another. Indeed, it is often as important for a musician to be able to silence his or her instrument at the right time as it is to play the melody skillfully. Each musician . . . has enough respect for the conductor's judgment that he or she remains in the role of following the conductor yet playing as well as possible. This kind of a system is (literally) harmonious.

Cacophony or confusion results, Schwartz observed, when the conductor always favors one section over another, loses sight of the whole symphony, or just walks off the podium, or if one of the musicians tries to muscle in and take over.

So Schwartz aimed to get Sally's Self to lead effectively. He began by working with each part individually: first the critical parts would stop attacking; then the Self had to nurture the "poor me" part and turn off the eating machine. He also tied all of this to external relationships: parents who try to motivate by criticism develop highly self-critical parts in children (*introjects*, in psychodynamic language), who later use these techniques on their own children. Most important, he said, you can't change one part of the internal system without paying attention to its relations with the other parts.

I had two visits with Schwartz, the second three years after the first, by which time his model of "internal family systems" had evolved. He now believed we have a whole tribe inside us. "Clinically," he said, "it helps to think of them as people, with different ages, temperaments, and talents, and in their harmonious state the people inside of us, which I still call *parts,* will all have some preferred role, and each will be different from the others. But when the tribe has been hurt or is under attack, its members are forced into other roles, extreme roles they want to get out of."

Schwartz had learned that Gestalt therapists would often have patients talking to imaginary parts of themselves seated in empty chairs. "I started doing that, and I found that when a person was talking as the part in the chair, they would say things they weren't aware they thought or felt, and you could get a family-therapy-like interaction going that way. I had a lot of different chairs, and they'd jump around being different parts, and I was amazed at the very dramatic shifts they would make."

At that time Schwartz believed, in contemporary family therapy style, that he and the client were co-creating these different personalities, but the more he worked in his paradigm the more he çame to believe that the personalities (or parts) existed outside the consulting room. They were just *there*. People *had them*. And sometimes the parts in the chairs would fight with each other. "It occurred to me that when I'm working with a family and that happens, often it's because a third member is interfering—that's a basic family therapy concept. So I would say, 'Go in and see if you can find the part that's making you feel angry and ask that part to separate,' and I would find this immediate shift in the person's view from anger to fear, so I would find the part that was making it afraid and get *it* to separate."

The Self could take a position of "compassion or curiosity or perspective or acceptance" once those extreme parts had moved aside—thus everyone, even the most traumatized and symptomatic patients, seemed to have a symphony conductor, a "nondamaged part." Schwartz has now mapped out an internal society composed of three groups: the *"exile parts,"* which hold painful and often traumatic memories; the *"managers,* who try to run your life with an eye toward avoiding anything that might activate those exiles; who try to keep your life under control at all times and dissuade you from taking risks so you don't get rejected"—the "highly critical, evaluative parts"; and a third group, which comes into play when the managers fail and the exiles come out. This group is called the *fire-fighters*, "the parts that will take people into binge-eating or drugs or alcohol to pour something on the fire or dissociate the person from the painful feelings." This certainly resembles some Freudian theories of repression and defense, but it is organized differently.

"In the goals and stages of therapy, you first work with the managers, just as when you enter a family you work with the parents or whoever has control, because they're running things and you need their trust. I'll lay out exactly the steps that we're going to go through, like a dentist who says, 'Now I'm going to give you a shot.' If you open the door without being careful, you can set off the fire-fighters, so I then deal with those before I bring out the exiles."

I asked Schwartz how the model worked with children, and he said it worked well, with some adjustments. "Children can change more quickly—they're closer to the phenomena. They have less trouble seeing their parts and interacting with them. They have imaginary friends, but this all gets drilled out of them by the time they grow up."

While Schwartz and I discussed the theory at length, it was most useful to see it in action; he loaded the VCR with a four-year-old cassette of Rebecca, a fifteen-year-old bulimic anorectic, Bob, her father, a dentist, and Faye, her stepmother. "At this point they had been through two years of her struggling with anorexia: she'd been hospitalized four or five times in some of the best places, and now their insurance was totally depleted and she was in a state hospital. She originally went on a diet and lost down to a life-threatening point, sixty pounds, so she went into the hospital where she would gain up to a place where it felt safe to discharge her. Then when she was back home, she would immediately lose and be hospitalized again.

"Rebecca's mother, Sue, started having affairs when Rebecca was nine. She'd been a good woman all this time and now she went on a rampage, and so Bob got custody of Rebecca when the marriage broke up. Soon after that he married Faye, and they had their own child."

Rebecca, who has short black hair and weighs eighty pounds, is weeping. "I think a lot of her bulimic behavior is irritating to me," says Faye. "I find it sort of slovenly, and it really bothers me. I have a very short fuse when it comes to messiness."

"So you've been having to struggle with yourself," Schwartz says. Faye nods. "Would you like some help in that area? I mean that part of you that gets so activated by Rebecca's behavior? Do you think if that part of you wasn't so activated, it would be easier for you to help her?"

"Yes," Faye says. "If I could get help and not have to discombobulate my life."

Schwartz gave me a play-by-play, just as Chasin had. "You're hearing from this manager part of her, who can't stand slovenliness and time is such a big deal. But just using the word *part* frees her Self up to say *yes*. You can see the power of the language—it's so much easier for people to say yes about a part of them."

"Almost any parent gets irked by some particular thing the kid does

and will say, 'There's something about when he does that that sets off
something in me,' and that's a perfectly reasonable thing for a parent to
say," I proposed.

"Exactly," Schwartz said, "and he knows that something in him doesn't
really help the situation."

Schwartz turns to Rebecca. "And you would like to work on parts of you
that feel sad and hurt so they don't make you binge as much and hurt?"
Rebecca, sniffling, nods, and then Schwartz asks Bob what parts of him
get in the way. Bob says "I guess mostly in being passive, if anything," but
seems to resist the notion that he can change.

I remembered that one of the conventional family therapy formulations
for anorexia involves a passive father, but that eating disorder specialists
I'd spoken to in biological psychiatry reported that not all families of
anorectics necessarily conform to this pattern. Schwartz agreed that there
are many different types of families with anorectic children. "This one
happens to conform to the stereotype," he said.

In describing her irritation, Faye says, "You know if you spend money
on something it's going to get trashed. It's this sort of carelessness about
personal property." Schwartz says, "So the part of you that feels strongly
about those kinds of issues and then the part of you that gets outraged
about what you call the sneakiness . . . those two things, again, interfere
with the affection you have for her"—Faye is agreeing—"that you'd like
to show her."

"It's there someplace," Faye says.

Schwartz moves back to Rebecca, asking her gently about whether it's
hard for her to know that Faye doesn't approve of her or her behavior, and
whether feeling that makes her criticize herself. "Is there a part of you
that gets on your back and sort of agrees with her about yourself? Does
that part of you make you feel real sad? I want you to tell me if I'm saying
anything that doesn't fit." Rebecca can't do much but nod and weep.
There is an angry part of her too, which she's able to say she tries to push
away, "because if I get angry at Faye, she will get more angry at me, and it
will make me feel more sad." Rebecca, it appears, is capable of systemic
thinking.

Schwartz told me, "My goal here is mainly to define the sequence of
parts that happened between the two of them more clearly, so that Faye
will see the impact of this critical part on Rebecca. I'm trying to have
Faye see that Rebecca also has a part in this, that Faye's critical part

activates the critical part inside of Rebecca, which then activates the hurt part that Faye dislikes so much. And then she binges, and you enter this vicious cycle. I'm also trying to get Rebecca to talk a little more. I figured it would be easier for her to talk about the angry part than the sad part."

Faye tells Rebecca, "I love you, but I also feel a lot of disgust and resentment," and Schwartz reiterates the notion of parts. He is calm and firm—"leading with his Self" as he describes it—in stating his goals. He told me, "Just through this process you get a little more self-leadership in the various people. They're starting to come away from their parts, and Faye's voice is a little less hard-edged."

I asked Schwartz whether a whole session of parts-language might get tedious; once explained, it apparently didn't bother his patients. Faye described her ambivalence to Rebecca in powerful terms—"it's the garbage that has been tossed on top of the affection and love that is there." And Faye also had to listen to Schwartz telling Rebecca he would help her find "ways to not feel so vulnerable to those parts of her." For Rebecca's stepmother, that was a powerful message.

Schwartz says people's Selves have insight when the parts back off and stop interfering; it seemed to me, as I watched, that Faye was at last being questioned by someone who acted nonjudgmental, and this allowed her to stop and analyze her behavior. Schwartz described the cycle to Faye several times and told her she could break it at any number of points. During this session neither he nor the family could figure out where Bob fit into the cycle. Later he learned that Bob was a drug-abuser and that the marriage was far more troubled than it appeared in the beginning. This "family secret" took several sessions to come out.

Faye also models the early process of analyzing her parts before Schwartz moves on to work with Rebecca. He asks the girl what her own critical parts say when she senses Faye's anger, and Rebecca, in a little-girl voice, says, "I'm a bad person and worthless, and this is never going to get better." He tells her that is a standard reaction and asks, "What do you think would happen if you argued with them? If you said to them, 'No, I'm not bad, I'm not hopeless?' " Rebecca says that won't happen because she agrees with Faye's criticism. And Schwartz, leading with his Self, says, "One thing we need to change is for you to start to see yourself differently so that when those parts of you get activated, you don't just go along with them and agree with them.' "

To Faye and Rebecca together, Schwartz, once again leading with his own professional skills, says "there are some techniques that can make it a lot easier." But he also points out that "there's going to be a period where Rebecca's behavior is not going to change immediately, so you're going to have to work real hard to see what I call your Self."

Schwartz now demonstrates—on Faye—the technique of working with parts. This is an "intervention" in itself. He asks Faye for a summary of what happens inside her when she learns Rebecca has been purging or when Rebecca says something she knows is untrue, and Faye describes an inner voice that's "overburdened." Schwartz says, "Sometimes it helps people to close their eyes, but you don't have to. Try to focus exclusively on this part for a second, home in on that put-upon part. See if an image comes to you, something alive. What does it look like? Don't try to put images on, but see if something comes to you."

"It looks like a dragon," Faye says.

"That's a common image. Is that dragon in the room by itself?"

Faye nods.

"What's it doing there?"

"Doing dragon things," Faye says, laughing.

"How are you feeling toward him as you watch him?"

"It looks so *angry*."

"Are you afraid of it?"

"No."

Schwartz told me he was asking her these questions to see how differentiated her Self was: had she said she was afraid of the dragon or angry with it, he'd have known there were other parts he'd have to move in and separate. "She's amused," he said, "which indicates that her Self is fairly differentiated so that it's safe to have her go in and work with the dragon."

Faye says she wouldn't want to scare the dragon, and Schwartz says it looks upset, and she should go into the room and ask it why. The dragon won't talk; Faye leans back, stretches, and smiles, and when Schwartz suggests she find a way to calm him down without talking, she knits her brow and finally announces she has put her hand out to the monster to show she wouldn't hit it, "like with angry dogs." This interchange is all very playful, and Faye reports that the dragon likes her, gets upset because it's big and angry and doesn't know what else to do, is the biggest part of her life, and would like her to come in and calm it down.

Rebecca is transfixed by the scene of her stepmother mollifying her internal dragon. Bob is very fidgety and looks uncomfortable. When Faye "comes back" from the room with the dragon, she says it was fun and she feels eight or ten years old.

In a tentative tone I said to Schwartz, "She seems to be a woman with not a lot of softness and gentleness in her but who is on top of things and perhaps a bit defensive about herself."

"I would say that's an accurate description of the parts that generally run her life," he answered. "I wouldn't agree that she doesn't have it."

Faye was not an appealing character, but one could empathize with the part of her that felt trapped in a mess she didn't make: that is, she was Rebecca's *stepmother*. At least some of the child's problems had originated before Faye's arrival. As for Bob, Schwartz added that "he kind of abdicates, so she gets dumped with all the responsibility for straightening Rebecca up, and it's not the mess that she created."

That first session bore some fruit: Faye behaved a bit more calmly during the following week, and in the next session Rebecca, while she hadn't gained much weight, didn't look so wiped out. The problem, however, was that while the girl was vomiting less often than before, her parents didn't give credit for partial improvement so Rebecca thought there was no point making the effort. Rebecca asks to work with the sad part, which she envisions as a little rag doll. Schwartz told me he no longer allows this. While it worked with Rebecca, it is extremely risky to bring out the exiles too soon: some other patients developed iatrogenic symptoms (that is, symptoms inadvertently caused by the treatment) like psychosomatic pains or the desire to bolt.

We watched Rebecca talking about the rag doll and trying to comfort it, and Schwartz told me that, as he came to learn, she was going back to the sad and lonely time when she was six or seven years old and her parents—not Faye, but Sue, her mother, and Bob—were "totally out of control." I saw various sessions between Rebecca and Bob or Faye or both. In session with Bob, she asked for more time with him: he thought she was too demanding, she thought he was impossible to please. Faye became somewhat kinder.

It took about four months for Rebecca to stop bingeing regularly, but sporadic episodes occurred for a while afterward. But Faye and Bob continued to be critical of Rebecca, and ultimately they threw her out. So Rebecca went to live with her mother, Sue. Schwartz then worked with Rebecca and Sue, who felt apologetic and repentant about the past: what the rag doll was remembering was a dependent relationship between Sue and an abusive lover, as well as Bob's episodes of drug abuse. Now she and Sue, with Schwartz's help, arrived at "a pretty decent relationship": Rebecca got her weight up to 105 and got into a local college. After a long slog the crisis was over, and therapy diminished to biweekly sessions before terminating. "She called me not too long ago," Schwartz said, "to see if she could learn this model. She's majoring in psychology. I said no, she couldn't come down here and do it because it would be unethical for me to train a former patient, but she was interested in pursuing it. So it's a real happy ending."

Schwartz looks at his own four-year-old work-in-progress with a critical eye. "I can just tell from the tone of my voice and my face, I'm so eager. Every time she says something, I go, 'Good, terrific!' That is the part of me that is a little insecure about how things are going to go and wants to jump on things. Even there, when she had done this piece of work with the rag doll, she says she's doing fine, but now as I listen to it, there's something more I glossed over there because I was eager to make it go okay."

Schwartz has used the technique frequently with survivors of abuse; he has used it with dignified fathers and delinquents with attitude. "You can do it with most anybody, but you have to work with their managers first."

The sessions I saw, despite the complaints of Schwartz's picky, self-critical part, looked elegant and powerful: that is, the therapist knew where he was going, kept control of the proceedings, and drew a lot of information out of the people he was treating. I have often been asked, over the course of my research, what a professional can do that kind, compassionate Aunt Mary or a really good sixth-grade teacher or the local clergyman cannot. Even after a role-play where Schwartz and I talked to my impatient white horse, I was not sure I was wholeheartedly committed to the world of dragons, ogres, rag dolls, and indeed, white horses that make up the exiles, managers, and fire-fighters in our inner tribe—but I knew professional skills when I saw them.

I thought of Schwartz again after my research was finished and I sat down at the computer and began Chapter 1. There is, it seems, a part of me that writes nonfiction. What it writes uncannily resembles what it has written in the past. And it comes out only when there is a book or article to be written.

As for Schwartz's family systems colleagues, several of them have hotly debated Schwartz in *The Networker*. Like philosophers since nearly the dawn of time, they are arguing about whether there is really a Self.

PART V

THE RIGHT STUFF

Biological Psychiatry

CHAPTER 13

"WITH A MOTHER LIKE THAT . . ."

Starting with Bradley (1937), who introduced the use of amphetamine for behavior-disordered youngsters, innovative psychopharmacological treatment for childhood psychiatric disorders has offered both great promise and many disappointments. Today, demands from the public and the media for child practitioners to find easy, quick answers to complicated problems creates a temptation to use the psychopharmacological agent as a "magic pill." The unsophisticated clinician can be easily infected by the contagious passion of the public, the enthusiasm of those working on a new medication, and the general hope for a cure of chronic, painful disorders.

> —Harold S. Koplewicz and
> Daniel T. Williams,
> "Psychopharmacological
> Treatment" (1988)

BEFORE YOU CAN HELP PEOPLE with psychological problems, you have to get them into your office. In order to complete their therapy, you must induce them to return until you believe they have extracted the maximum from the treatment. That is why mental health practitioners of every orientation worry a lot about the social stigma associated with being a patient or having a mental illness. Indeed, for this reason "patients" are often called "clients," and their afflictions may be (or may not be, depending on the therapist's orientation) euphemized with an assortment of terms including "disorder," "problem," and even "issue"; instead of being "neurotic," "abnormal," or "defective," their behavior may be "dysfunctional," "maladaptive," or "inappropriate." Discussing psychotherapy

361

with professionals sometimes seems a lot like playing the childhood game of Coffee Pot.

Except among some psychoanalytically trained psychiatrists (who eschew what they perceive is sugarcoating the pill) and their biologically oriented colleagues, there is a widespread notion among mental health professionals that the "medical model" stigmatizes more than others. This point is made most often by nonmedical practitioners, for whom it is obviously convenient. While I, coming in as an outsider, found some complaints about lordly, authoritarian psychoanalysts quite legitimate and recognized a number of situations in which psychologists and social workers might be better equipped to solve a problem than psychiatrists, *this* idea appeared to me mysterious. It seemed far less stigmatizing to be told that nature has played us foul, that at times our bodies betray us, than to hear that our problems emanate from misperceptions of the world, distorted values, or an inability to face up to and control our impulses or form positive relationships; in theory, parents also should find it less demoralizing to hear that their child has a brain disorder, especially a mild one, than to be told he or she is, say, "insecurely attached." My reaction is apparently not universal, and mistrust of the medical model is fairly common in the general public as well as among psychologists and social workers, for reasons I can only guess have something to do with the old questions about predestination and free will.

Still, the more a theorist or clinician attributes our "coffee pot" to involuntary circumstances, the less likely it is that at least some of us are going to feel guilty and defensive. There is, of course, a downside to this: if our circumstances are *too* far beyond our control, there is not much point in working to change them.

Throughout my research I have encountered practitioners who came at child psychiatry through pediatrics. (The best-known ex-pediatrician in child psychiatry was D. W. Winnicott, described in Chapter 4, who followed the path available at the time, into psychoanalytic work.) They present the folksiness of the family doctor rather than the distant superiority of the specialist. They speak English. They often "join" with patients and families by freely admitting they have faced similar problems in their own lives.

One such clinician is Harold S. Koplewicz, chief of the Division of Child and Adolescent Psychiatry at Schneider Children's Hospital and Hillside Hospital, both part of Long Island Jewish Medical Center in New

Hyde Park, New York. Born in 1953, Koplewicz is the youngest of the lead therapists in this book. Charles Sarnoff is also on the staff of Schneider, but it would be hard to find two practitioners more different in viewpoint and style. Koplewicz respects Sarnoff's brilliance, but he has not chosen to emulate him; the younger man is a protégé of Donald Klein, M.D., and his wife, Rachel Gittelman Klein, Ph.D., two distinguished names in psychopharmacological research. The generational difference between Sarnoff's outlook and Koplewicz's is symbolic of the directions in which psychiatry is now moving.

Much of Koplewicz's clinical practice involves consultation, in which he evaluates patients, decides on the best plan for treatment, and refers them to the appropriate practitioner; he may consult for as many as a hundred patients a year. "When you see enough children who meet the criteria for a certain diagnosis," he says, "you get a clear understanding that this is not something their mother did or their family did, that this has a lot to do with either genetic or biological predisposition or a neuro-anatomical defect or biochemical defect. When the child is given this medication and not that or the other, and given it at the right dose, you can actually see him become symptom-free. Maybe not cured, but certainly treated so that his life becomes one that's functioning well, and there's a kid that's not distressed.

"When I take histories from the mothers of kids who meet the criteria for attention-deficit/hyperactivity disorder, the mothers will tell stories about their three- or four-year-old. They'll say, 'No one will baby-sit for my child. His own grandparents call him Sweet Destructo. We can't go to the movies. We can't take him to a show. He was thrown out of two nursery school programs.' And then you sit with this little boy in your office, and you think, 'I can take care of any little boy,' and the kid starts ripping the place apart.

"Rachel Klein and I decided to take a look at the mother-child interaction. We were going to give these kids Ritalin and placebo, triple-blind— the doctor wouldn't know, the patients wouldn't know, the mother wouldn't know—and after four weeks they would receive the other medicine. Before they got the medicine, we put them into a playroom and videotaped. First they were allowed to play with as many toys as they wanted. Next they'd have a cleanup period where the mother would be told it was time to clean up and she'd have to ask the child to clean up. Number three, the mother sat with the child and they were given forty things to do. They'd never get through all forty, but we'd say, 'Start at the top of the list and work your way down.' They were easy tasks, things we know three-, four-, and five-year-olds can do.

"The first child played with something like sixty-one different toys in a ten-minute period. The mother-child interaction was striking. We had this mother who was screaming, 'Joshua, Joshua, come on over here, play with this,' and Joshua is running to play with something else, and the mother says, 'Come on, let's have a catch,' and Joshua now's got another toy, and with the TV camera going, the mother takes the beach ball and tries to hit the kid with it while the kid's running around so fast she misses. You can see she's incredibly frustrated.

"When it comes time for cleanup, he throws a temper tantrum, and when it's time for the structured task, he's out of his seat moving around the room, and you see his mother getting even more frustrated.

"The kid was then put on what happened to be active medicine, and we did the video again. I showed these tapes to a group of Columbia medical students. I had around ten of these very bright students, and I said, 'This is what one of our kids looks like,' without saying 'hyperactive.' They looked at the tape, and they said to me, 'If I had a mother like that, I would be running around also. What's wrong with that mother? She's intrusive, she's not following the kid at all, she doesn't say anything nice to the kid.' They were a hundred percent right about those things, but they put the blame definitely on the mother.

"We then showed them the next tape when the kid was on Ritalin but they didn't know that. The child and the mother were sitting on the floor playing with something, and it was almost boring, because how many minutes can you watch a kid playing with a make-believe tool chest, banging with the hammer, whispering with his mother? So I said to the medical students, 'What's different about these two tapes?' and the majority of them said, 'What are you giving the mother?' The guesses ranged from Valium to Thorazine.

"It struck me so strongly. One of the reasons mothers are so upset when they come to see a psychiatrist is that society overall is blaming them. They come in with this incredible guilt on their head. If only they were a better parent, if only they were more attentive, if only they didn't work, if only they did work—whatever they were supposed to do that they didn't do, they wouldn't have this problem. They wouldn't think that way if the kid had a heart murmur or a brain tumor or diabetes. There's a certain amount of this that's really out of their control.

"It's true that having a child like this requires superparenting, absolutely positively superparenting, while some of us who have easy children get away with murder."

Koplewicz, who is on the tall-and-thin side and has abundant curly black hair, assumed he'd go into pediatrics but found, as an intern, "a certain cookbook quality to it." Seeking a more challenging pediatric specialty, he decided on psychiatry and applied to New York Hospital–Cornell Medical Center's Westchester Division, a unit known for its strong psychoanalytic orientation. "After spending a year in pediatrics, where I was able to help very sick kids with meningitis—I gave them a spinal tap and put an IV in and I could make them well—I was put on a unit with adults who were there on an indeterminate stay, which could be six or nine months.

"I learned a lot about psychiatry and about sitting with patients, but I can tell you that the most dramatic patient that year was a young girl who came in from another hospital. She was nineteen, diagnosed with schizophrenia. She had been treated for two months with Haldol, a major tranquilizer. She was very stiff, because Haldol has the side effect of causing you to have Parkinsonian types of symptoms. You can feel that stiffness when you hold someone's arm.

"She walked in with her parents and said, 'I have to be me. Who else can I be?' And she kept repeating this while she was stiff as a board.

"We took her off medication. It was standard procedure there, to see what the patients look like free of medicine. She lost the side effects but became incredibly manic, hypersexual with other patients on the unit, and very aggressive in her language with me, and she stopped sleeping.

"Once we got her on lithium and put her on the right dose there was a switch. There was the patient that the mother and father had been talking to me about—a delightful, funny, intelligent individual who a few months later was sent back to college and eventually graduated. She's one of the patients that drops me a Christmas card.

"That was an acute episode of a chronic illness—she was manic depressive. But for me the part that was so eye-opening was that there are certain diagnoses that have absolute definite treatments. For these kinds of patients, talking about their mother or their father or their dreams misses the point. They first have something biochemically wrong with them, and until that is resolved, there is no reason to discuss with them how they are going to cope with having a chronic illness or an intrusive mother or a neglectful father."

As a resident at Cornell, Koplewicz sought supervisors with various therapeutic orientations, from the most analytic to the most biological; he read whatever was available on psychopharmacology during those years from 1979 to 1981. One patient had obsessive-compulsive disorder, generally expressed in the compulsion to wash, check out, or count things over and over again: "He couldn't leave the room without counting, looking in the corner, and reciting a series of numbers, and then he would get stuck putting on his underwear because he would have to fold it over and over again. My analytic supervisors told me this patient was on the road to becoming much crazier, and if I took away his obsessions and compulsions—which held him together—I'd be left with a raving lunatic."

But Koplewicz, visiting Columbia for a job interview, stopped in to hear Judith Rapoport, a psychiatrist from the National Institute of Mental Health who is this country's leading authority on obsessive-compulsive disorder; Rapoport was presenting grand rounds that day. "Here was a woman standing up there and talking about my patient, saying these symptoms don't get worse, but if you give Anafranil the obsessional thought disappears, the behavior disappears, and these patients go on to have less stressful lives. There's an eighty percent remission in their symptoms."

Koplewicz granted the importance of learning to sit with patients and know their feelings, and "how certain patients would enrage you and certain patients would bore you, and it didn't always have to do with the patient's style, it was the content of the material and your emotional baggage." Early in his career he himself had gone through five years of analysis, hoping to become less irritable and competitive; having been analyzed, he says, he's more tolerant. But it was not a rebirth like Sarnoff's. And as a psychiatric resident, he wanted to learn more about the other half of the puzzle. Thus Koplewicz, believing psychopharmacology was the wave of the future, moved to Columbia, a center for psychopharmacological research.

Koplewicz's experiences proved to bear out my perception that of all the treatments available in the field of mental health, it is pharmacotherapy that most polarizes lay people. "I can't tell you how often,"

Koplewicz told me, "someone will come to see you when their child's three years old. Nice couple, father's a doctor, mother's a professional, and they tell you the nursery school the kid's going to is no good, it's mean, this nursery school.

"The kid is delightful, very bright, and you speak to the nursery school, and they say the parents are impossible. I grant you the parents are difficult people, but that's not the issue. When you ask what the kid's like in school, the school says he's disruptive, he's distracting, he's impulsive—the kid is all of three and a half.

"So you say, 'Let's talk to the parents about it.' You tell the parents, 'I've spoken to the school. There are some problems there, but there's one major problem in the way the two of you deal with things. You're very inconsistent, one says one thing, the other says another, and on top of that there's a lot of conflict, and you let your son see it.'

"The parents say, 'You're absolutely right. We're going to try to work on this ourselves and have less conflict.' Two years later they come back to you. Now the little boy's in kindergarten, and the father's saying, 'I don't *like* my kid. I love my kid, but I don't like him. He's a mean child. We can't take him places because he'll break other kids' toys. He gets into fights. It's often like he's a wild man. I can't tell where he's going.'

"You talk to the mother and the mother minimizes—it's not so bad, she says. You say to the parents, 'It really does sound like your child might have a shorter attention span than the average kid. He's certainly brighter than the average kid, but nonetheless he's not functioning in school as well as you'd expect, and he's not a happy kid.' You say, 'Your marriage is better now. Why don't you take these forms to the school and have them fill the forms out.' "

Koplewicz hands them the Conners Teacher Rating Scale, a standard form used in assessing children's problem behavior. "I tell them that when the forms come back, we'll talk about whether, based on these, your child is significantly, ninety-five percent more inattentive, more impulsive, more hyper, more disruptive than the average boy his age," he says. "And we'll discuss whether medication makes sense. The parents say okay, and you tell them to make an appointment once the forms come back.

"My secretary keeps a tick file, and she sees that more than three weeks have gone by and we never got the Conners forms back. So she calls the family and says, 'Hello, Mrs. Smith. We never received the

Conners forms back from the school.' The mother says, 'Tell the doctor we're not coming back to him. I don't want the school involved with this at all, and I certainly don't want a doctor who's going to drug my child.'

"Small world. I happen to have been at the child's school during those three weeks giving a speech, and the principal came over to me and said, 'I've heard that the John Smith boy has been to see you. I can't tell you what a relief it is, because we've been having problems for some time, and the mother's very difficult.' I said, 'You're right, she's difficult, but I don't necessarily think that's the problem, I think that's a little simplistic.' But the school is very aware of the kid's problem.

"The mother doesn't want the school to know about it, and more important, I've insulted her by saying we might possibly give medicine. She's not even ready to pick up the phone and say, 'Can we talk about other options, because medicine really disturbs me?' because it was so offensive, she doesn't even feel the need to talk to the doctor. She just tells the secretary, 'Leave us alone.'

"If you think about that, how frequently do you find a pediatrician who looks at your son's throat and sees some white patches on the tonsils and says, 'I think he's got strep throat. Start the penicillin. I'll take a culture, and I'll call you in forty-eight hours'? We don't hesitate to put our children on penicillin, even though there's a very good chance, statistically, that it's not strep throat. He calls you forty-eight hours later and says it's not strep, quit the penicillin. You wouldn't react like Mrs. Smith. Let's say someone said to you that your kid is peeing sugar, he's got sugar in his urine consistently, and it would be nice to control it with diet, but frankly his pancreas does not produce enough insulin, and we have to give him injections.

"I'm sure there are lots of patients and their parents who would say, 'No, no insulin, I can't do it,' but eventually they'll work it through. A kid who's hyperactive is not going to die, but he has a much more miserable existence than he'd have if he were properly medicated."

At the same time the perception that pills—pills unabetted—are the silver bullet for all mental health problems is increasingly widespread, and this development too inspires ambivalence. We want a quick fix, but we feel guilty about wanting one. We believe that both we and our children should face and sweat out the ups and downs of life, but we would love not to have to, and the prospect may even make us fearful. Since my visits with Koplewicz led me to conclude that both these conflicting emotions are irrelevant to the decision to seek pharmacotherapy (both for one's child and for oneself), it seems particularly important to understand what a pediatric psychopharmacologist actually does. What is the texture of the therapy? How does Harold Koplewicz interact with patients and their families, and how do parents affect the course of the disorder? What is it like when things go well, and what is it like when things go badly? I spent several days watching Koplewicz at work, and afterward we discussed what I had seen. The cases presented (for my purposes) a useful variety, and a good picture of the current state of the clinical art.

Psychopharmacologists, like behaviorists, are wedded to empirical research. There is, however, a less procrustean quality to this research than we saw in some of the behaviorists' studies, because much of what the psychopharmacologists are doing is traditional biochemistry. (In Chapters 14 and 15 I will discuss the work of researchers in psychopharmacology and how it is integrated into clinical practice.)

Koplewicz doesn't have a private office; the cubicle he inhabits at Schneider Children's Hospital is surprisingly free of the trappings of power and, indeed, without much character at all. I was ushered in shortly before the arrival of Amy Ratner for her fourth session, so he could tell me something about her case. Patients, parents, and teachers fill out detailed histories before a child or teenager sees Koplewicz, and he is impressively educated when they walk in the door.

Amy, a thirteen-year-old, had shown depressive symptoms ever since her father died two years ago, following a two-year siege of liver cancer. She began seeing a psychologist at that time, but a year ago her grandfather also died and things began to get even worse. She couldn't concentrate on schoolwork; her appetite and sleep patterns were disturbed; she was irritable and had trouble dealing with her friends and her feelings about her father. Her mother—whose own friends were worried about Amy—felt the psychologist, despite the fact that Amy liked him, wasn't helping much.

Koplewicz speedily rewound his account to Amy's prehistory: "She's the third child. She was an unplanned and uneventful pregnancy and delivery, her mother received good prenatal care. She was normal weight, natural delivery, and stayed in the hospital for five days with her mom. In kindergarten she had some reading problems and went to see a learning specialist. She's always been an average student, and her attention span has been a problem. Her father was an alcoholic, but it was well concealed from the kids. She had some separation anxiety when she was six and first went off to camp, but considering all the bad things going on in the family, it's unclear whether it was biological or environmental. Her mother has a history of depression, adequately medicated; one sib has minor learning disabilities, the other a small anxiety problem.

"Let's see, she says she's having difficulties sitting and focusing. She's daydreaming. Socially she feels she's in the second group in school. She worries about Mom, about being alone, bad things happening to her, what people will think about her. She says she's kind of rejection-sensitive—people can insult her easily by looking at her the wrong way. All this information came from the first visit. After that I called her guidance counselor, pediatrician, and therapist, who confirmed everything, giving us a diagnosis of major depressive disorder with atypical features." The language Koplewicz uses in describing a case tends to resemble that of the DSM.

"I took blood tests a month ago and started her on Prozac, twenty milligrams. Two weeks later she had all the bloods done. I explained the confirmation I got from the school, the pediatrician, and the therapist reporting the changes in her behavior and mood and explained the diagnosis. She came back for a third visit a couple of weeks after that and told me she felt somewhat more mellow. She was not as irritable, and her sleeping was okay but still not improving as much as she would like. She told me she went out for dinner with her sibs and really enjoyed that. What we did was continue the Prozac and start Desyrel at night. Desyrel's another antidepressant: it causes sedation, so we didn't use it as an antidepressant but as a way to help her sleep."

Now Amy—a heavyset girl with short curly red hair, wearing standard teenage jeans-and-flannel-shirt—and her mother, whom she resembled, came in. Koplewicz asked them various questions about Amy's diurnal rhythms: she was still having trouble sleeping and getting up. Moreover, one recent day she was late for school, and another she didn't go at all. "What time did you get up?" asked Koplewicz. "Ten thirty or eleven," Amy said. "What did you do then?" "Stay in bed." "You couldn't get yourself motivated to get the hell out," Koplewicz reflected. Mom said it wasn't coming together yet, but it was definitely better: her temperament had improved, but sometimes she forgot to take the Desyrel.

Koplewicz suggested Mom help Amy make a chart to check whenever she takes a pill—"It's hard for most people to take medicine"—and dispatched Mom to the waiting room while he talked with Amy.

The discussion suggested that Amy would jump at any good excuse to stay home and watch TV or hang out with her friends, and Koplewicz asked her, in a nonjudgmental tone, some pointed questions about schoolwork, tests, and attendance. For several years she had not been highly motivated in school, and it was difficult for me to pick up how much of this was depression and how much was just Amy's temperament. "I like to take tests," she said. "I think I do well, and then it turns out I did really badly. It's been happening since last year. I'm getting frustrated in math and in English too."

More discussion of appetite and exercise, and whether Amy was continuing to see Dr. Tom, as they called her psychologist, with whom Koplewicz was working. Koplewicz asked Amy how she felt about her upcoming birthday; Grandma would take her out. "Do you know why I'm asking? Because it was two years ago on your birthday that your Dad—"

"It's always gonna be like that," Amy said.

"How's Grandma doing?"

"She's tough."

"Are *you* tough?"

"No."

Amy no longer had the overwhelming feeling that something bad was going to happen, but she wasn't full of optimism either. Finally Koplewicz took her pulse and blood pressure, reviewed scheduling with Amy and Mom, and the Ratners left.

Before the next patient there was a bit of time to discuss Amy: I told Koplewicz she impressed me as an average kid of limited horizons, not, as they say, a rocket scientist. "It's not my job to judge her but to try to get her to reflect somewhat on her behavior," he said. "The fact that on Friday she couldn't get out of bed even though on Thursday she came home only at nine P.M., and then she watched television until at least eleven before studying for a math test the next day, certainly shows not only a lack of responsibility but a kind of lethargy. She can't get motivated. She cares about her grades, but at the same time her behavior is telling you, 'Hey, lady, what's going on? You're not getting into gear here.' She spends Friday lying in bed. She's really vegetating in bed, and that's a sign this is not a completely treated depression.

"There was a dramatic improvement from the first session. I find very commonly with kids who present with depression or with almost any other kind of psychiatric illness, that when you're able to tell them the name of the illness and that these symptoms fit together in a syndrome we can treat, you're validating what they thought was just crazy. Very often the secondary demoralization lifts right away." Koplewicz is not the only therapist who reports that phenomenon. Moreover, supplying a diagnosis is not unlike the "externalizing" treatment devised by the Australian family therapist Michael White in Chapters 10 and 11: once you have named the monster, you've gone a ways toward taming it. And like the poet's pen in the Shakespearean phrase Sarnoff cites, you "give to airy nothing a local habitation and a name."

"But she's only thirteen," he went on, "and she's somewhat immature, and it's a chaotic household right now. Even though Dad died two years ago, it's still a tough time for this family. She looks pretty good to me now. Remember when I talked about 'atypical' features? With me here she comes alive, she actually flirts a little bit, she's very engaging. It's when she's by herself that she feels her absolute worst, and even then she's not in hysterics. Is she going to be a top-notch student when I finish with her? I don't think so. However, I do believe she'll have more energy, and with that she'll be able to study better and then she has a chance of being a better math student.

"Overall I would say this is a patient who has had an incomplete response to medicine, her compliance is mediocre, and usually Prozac takes several weeks before it kicks in. But you see a change in cognition even after three sessions: she first came in and told me tearfully that everything was bad, the family didn't have enough money to go away for a vacation. Today she couldn't remember what was good and what was bad.

"We could switch to a more cognitive-behaviorally oriented therapist here whom I would work with closely, but she has a very warm relationship with Tom, so my treatment is going to be short-term. I'll see her maybe six times until we titrate the medicine to where it belongs, and then I'll see her monthly and monitor her blood pressure and pulse and symptoms, and she'll see Dr. Tom for regular treatment. This is crisis management, a young child who's had a tough time with the loss of her father. The psychologist agreed there was a biological component, and I told him I would be supportive of his treatment. There's no magic here. I don't care who makes her go to school, as long as she gets there.

"We don't believe that depression is like diabetes, where you need to take insulin all the time. It is more like an ulcer that flares up. You can treat it, it can disappear completely, and then you can recognize the warning signs. With a history of alcoholism in the family and a mother with depression, one can guess she's genetically predisposed to this, and she'll be taught to recognize when it's getting out of control. If all of a sudden three years from now she stops sleeping again, she can say, 'Hey, I'm gonna call Dr. Koplewicz fast, because I don't want to get into lying in bed and feeling like the world is crap and everything's dark.' "

"When she calls you in three years, will she also have to call Dr. Tom?"

Koplewicz took a deep breath. "I don't think anyone who really does psychopharmacology doesn't do psychotherapy. Even in this minimal interaction, I'm doing what you might call parent counseling with Mom. Mom's my ally here, and yet my real partner in this is the patient, and I can identify with her how difficult Mom can be if Mom does something outrageous. If psychotherapy is an alliance between two people to work on getting rid of something troubling the patient, that's what I do. Sometimes we use medication, and unfortunately there are lots of disorders that don't respond to biological treatment. Characterological problems and temperamental difficulties, sometimes interpersonal relationships. Self-esteem. Some of these things cannot be alleviated with pills, and they are much harder to treat. It's possible you could cognitively change your view of how you feel, but self-esteem could also be a function of the environment telling you you're pretty crummy on a regular basis—meeting frustration at school every day, or with a mother and father who are very nasty to you, so when you're twelve, you feel you're a crummy person. It's very hard to change that."

Next we were to see Zachary and Alexis Young, both adopted children with AD/HD, and their mother, a social worker, and once again Koplewicz clued me in beforehand. Zachary was a bright eight-year-old. Three years ago he had been referred by Judith Rapoport of NIMH, a family friend, for behavior problems in kindergarten: he couldn't switch activities without acting up, and the teacher saw him as defiant and undisciplined. "When he was three months old, Mom went back to work; at fourteen months he walked, then stopped walking for three months, then started up again. He talked early, was easily toilet-trained, had no separation difficulties, but he was a terrible eater because he doesn't like to sit still. Meals have to be *very quick.*"

Koplewicz launched into what I'd learned was his litmus test of peer relations: "He had lots of play dates at nursery school, was very popular, but groups were always problematic—trouble with birthday parties except his own. Bedtime was always 'I don't wanna go,' and he'd often be up at two in the morning. He had a good relationship with his sister, three years younger.

"There are several other problems with Zachary. He was diagnosed with asthma at four months of age and has had a few acute episodes. He's been wearing glasses since he was three. He had a hearing loss that required an operation, which was successful.

"He's a charming little boy. I diagnosed him as having mild to moderate attention deficit. This child had multiple reactions to every medicine we gave him. When we gave Ritalin, he developed tics and got separation-anxious. He started getting phobic about what would happen to his mother. When we took him off the Ritalin, he was so hyperactive he still needed help. His IQ recently tested at a hundred and twenty-five, with verbal higher than performance—which is often seen in hyperactive or ADD kids. He's currently receiving Ritalin, which he can now tolerate, along with Catapres, an antihypertensive patch used for tics and hyperactivity. The Catapres seems to improve his impulsivity, and the Ritalin improves his attention span. He occasionally sees a cognitive-behavior therapist at Schneider, and his parents sometimes see me for parent counseling. They were here last in December and weren't to come back till March"—this was January—"but they've come today essentially free of charge because I wanted you to see them in a session.

"Alexis, who's now six, has pure AD/HD. They lucked out with both kids. No ifs, ands, or buts, on twenty milligrams of Ritalin, this kid is a charm. She's looking much better now, she doesn't need behavior therapy, she just looks like a joy."

Alexis and Mom came in, and Alexis—who had long, straight black hair in a ponytail—twined herself around a chair. Briefly. Then she moved to another chair and twined herself around that.

She had made a book about herself and Zachary, which Koplewicz said was "very impressive," and then he asked her how things were going at school.

"Good," said Alexis.

"How good?"

"*So* good."

"What does the teacher say about you?"

"I forgot."

"Does she say, 'Alexis, sit down, don't get out of your seat, behave yourself'?"

"Yes," said Alexis, laughing.

"Does she say that a lot? More than she says it to everyone else?"

"She says it more to me."

Koplewicz asked her if she'd been to any good birthday parties lately and if she'd had any play dates. She had a sleepover date: "Did you miss your mommy and daddy when you were there?" Alexis missed them "a whole bunch to the wall," but not enough to call them to take her home. In response to another question, she'd been getting in trouble at home for hitting Zachary. She was giggling as she talked and gently slapping Koplewicz on the hand. She slid off the chair, moved some chairs around, and changed her seat to one that was "more constable." Next it was time to take Alexis's blood pressure and pulse and talk a bit with Mom alone, so Koplewicz ushered the patient out.

"Does she get any worse than this?" Koplewicz, returning, asked Mom, a pretty woman with a mop of curly blond hair. "She just looks very rambunctious now."

"She isn't," Mom said. "She's usually unmanageable after three. During mornings in school she's fine," although she had some alphabet problems that required tutoring and, especially in the afternoon, tended to blurt out answers impulsively, thus appearing "less capable than she is. So she looks like a dull child and she's being categorized. . . . And she is *absolutely* unmanageable. She gets fifteen milligrams in the morning, ten at lunch, sometimes five at three o'clock, but it interferes with her sleep. Not all the time but sometimes."

"When you say she's unmanageable . . . ?" Koplewicz asked. Mom said, "She's oppositional, and when you're going at a hundred miles an hour and you're oppositional, you're bound to find yourself in the most precarious situations. If she sees something across the street, she might run. When she's medicated, she's very easy, it's like night and day. The pediatrician saw it. The rebound is intense."

This is the "rebound" effect that Ritalin has with some patients when a dose is wearing off, and hyperactive symptoms become worse than they were before the child was medicated. "There's a possibility," Koplewicz said, "that the longer she stays on the medicine, the more the side effects will decrease. So if we can possibly give her a larger dose at noon, and then a five-milligram dose at three P.M., you're talking about a total dose of thirty-five milligrams versus thirty. It's not much more, but most of the time she's getting twenty-five milligrams now. So increase the lunchtime to fifteen milligrams, and give her five milligrams at three P.M., and watch what time she goes to sleep."

Mom said she'd try it, and she described how impossible Alexis had been in the afternoons during Christmas vacation, when the family visited Dad's parents in Santa Fe. "It's not good for her. My mother-in-law says she'll stay with her for a while, and all the time she tells Alexis, 'You're bad.' She gets such terrible feedback."

"She's told all the time she's a bad kid," said Koplewicz, furrowing his brow.

"Right," said Mom, "and behavior mod does not necessarily work with her when she's so out of it. What we usually use is time-out, but it can go on, in and out, for three hours easily, and taking away things means absolutely nothing. Once she gets going at that pace, she doesn't even hear you. She's so impulsive that from seven o'clock we take the puppy away from her, because she had said, 'Let me see the puppy do flips,' she was gonna flip the puppy over her head. She took the puppy to the bathroom, she was gonna hold her over the toilet. It's crazy. Yet at school they tell me she's an angel, so we're doing well."

"Okay," said Koplewicz. "Increase the Ritalin to fifteen milligrams, fifteen milligrams, and five milligrams. Let's have Zach come in."

Zach, living up to his notices, was an appealing little boy with huge glasses, wearing jeans, a Chicago Bulls sweatshirt, and black high-tops. He sat down.

"I want to talk to you a little bit," Koplewicz said. "I haven't seen you in a whole month, and I was supposed to see you even later, but we decided to see you sooner. One of the reasons why is that there is a lady here who's doing research on psychiatrists and how they help children, so it might be helpful for this lady to understand why you come to see a psychiatrist. Since you're a very *bright* kid and very *articulate*—you know what that means? You speak very well, and maybe you can explain."

Long silence. "I don't know," said Zach.

"When you first came to see me, you were five years old, and I told you I was the kind of doctor who takes care of kids when they have behavior problems, thinking problems, or feeling problems. If you had to pick any area where you could be more comfortable, what would it be?"

After a series of silences and I-don't-knows, Zach allowed that thinking was giving him trouble these days, particularly listening and paying attention. Mom said softly, "Can I interject? Zachary *asked* to come here. Zachary's having a problem following directions, doing math, remembering his books. In the last few weeks. I spoke with his teacher."

While Mom talked about Zach's problems, he looked crestfallen. His hand was on his mouth. He played with his hair. He rubbed his eyes. "You look so sad," Koplewicz said. "Why are you so sad? Are your problems so bad they can make you cry? Let's talk about problem number one and see if we can fix it. Listening? Following instructions? Give me a good example. Today in school."

"Reading," Zach said. He was slow to answer and answered in a tiny voice, eyes downcast. Koplewicz asked him small questions and gradually he got out that he doesn't pay attention when the teacher gives the assignment. Koplewicz asked about "leaving stuff behind," and Zach said yes.

With Mom's assistance it came out that Zach got 63 on a test and usually he gets 95, and that's why he was so sad. "It's not your fault," Mom said. "It relates to the medicine, honey. He can't stand it when the math isn't a hundred percent."

"I can help you with this," Koplewicz said. "Do the numbers really make a difference? Whether you get a ninety-five or a sixty-three bothers you a lot? Why is that so important to you? I think you think that if you get a higher number on a test, that means you're smarter."

Zach, in a small pained voice, said, "No."

"I think you're smart no matter what you get on a test," Koplewicz said. "You think I'm dumb because I think that? Why do you think I think you're smart? What would I be basing that on? Do you think it might be because I know you so well? The words you use, how you think? But it really bothers you when you don't do well in school. What are you worried about?" Koplewicz was leaning very far over toward Zach, looking into his eyes. He took Zach's hand away from Zach's face and held it. After asking—without success—what was troubling him and what could be fixed, he tried a new tack; "What's the thing we shouldn't change? You having any fun at school?"

This all moved like pulling teeth, and Koplewicz finally asked if it was "the lady behind the mirror"; Zach said firmly, "That doesn't bother me," and I was relieved. Through this difficult conversation Zach was not in any way sullen, just overcome with grief, and Koplewicz said, "You really *are* in a funk today." Gradually we learned that Zach ("Would you stop picking that nose, please? Thank you," interjected Koplewicz) is better on weekends and has three good guys at school he likes to have lunch with. Koplewicz and Zach were now affectionately tapping hands. The problem was the schoolwork, and they decided to fix the medicine.

Alone, Koplewicz and Mom reviewed the Conners forms and a list from the teacher that said things like, "Difficulties in writing. Rambling sentences." Mom said, "At night, if his Catapres patch falls off and we don't know it, it's like he's drunk. He's giggly, and he's unable to sleep and walks around. The tics are starting a little bit. They're not reporting them at school, but we see them a little watching TV."

The school problems, according to the teacher's report, were extensive. "My suggestion is we can increase some dose of medicine," Koplewicz said, "but I've got to tell you, it's hard to read Zach today. He's withdrawn, and I always worry if it's a sudden thing."

"No, it's not," Mom says. "I'm telling you straight out, he's very upset. If Zach doesn't do well academically, it's the most important thing in his life, and he really cannot stand it, and he cannot follow directions at school, which means he can't do the work, he doesn't know what math unit to study for the test. It's all related."

"Look," Koplewicz said, "we're on a tenuous balance here, because the more medicine we give him, the more chance of side effects. My suggestion is we just increase the morning dosage. I'm worried about the sleep with him, and if the morning is when he does most of his academics, five milligrams more for him could be a lot. Continue him on the Catapres, but I need to be called in a week."

While Koplewicz went out to check Zachary's pulse and blood pressure, I talked with Ms. Young. Both children were infant adoptions: the Youngs paid for Alexis's mother's prenatal care, while Zachary, the son of a teenager, came with very little history. "When Zach's upset, he usually tells Dr. Koplewicz," she said. "He loves him. They play checkers and do a lot of brain-teasers, and Dr. Koplewicz has become his advocate in the school. Theoretically, Zach should go into a gifted program, but he can't meet the criteria for test-taking in a group. So Dr. Koplewicz went to the district on his behalf. But they wouldn't give in."

"If an individual were testing him in a room alone?" I asked.

"He would do fine. We had an individual IQ done in the hospital. We sent him to a neurologist. The effect on the family until he gets in the right place is awful. With my second I didn't have to question. I knew exactly what was happening."

Koplewicz returned. "Classical AD/HD is what Alexis has," he told me. "If you saw her in school, she'd look much more compliant. Right now she's running back and forth. Her reality testing is good, but she's impulsive because her attention span is so small. Zach, on the other hand—and this is a no-fault brain disorder, it's probably the kind of thing that causes a kid to have to have eyeglasses at such an early age, and he's also hyperallergic, with the asthma at four months—unfortunately every side effect we can get, Zach has gotten, so we play games with the medicine, we keep changing and shifting, doing trials.

"As a psychopharmacologist, I have felt Zach should see other people, so he has seen Rachel Klein, he has seen Alan Zametkin at the NIMH, he has had reviews of this treatment. While he's a kid who's sensitive to tics, and Ritalin can induce tics, if you take him off all medicine, he's so disorganized, his attention span is so short that you don't tap into his hundred-twenty-five IQ. It's probably more than that.

"He also misses out on social cues, like when someone is saying, 'Hey, Zach, we're playing over here,' or, 'Zach, calm down,' or, 'Cool it.' So while it's very upsetting to see him so dysphoric, you have to know your mother, and if she tells me this is secondary to what's going on in school, it's very different from a mother I didn't know and didn't find a reliable reporter. I would say the sadness is a side effect of Ritalin or the Catapres. The therapy has to be done in partnership with Mom, so there are many phone calls. You can always make a whole formulation that it's the parents, that they're overanxious themselves, high-functioning, or neglectful." Pointedly, Koplewicz wasn't doing that.

Koplewicz observed that the two Youngs were very different cases of the most common disorder of children and adolescents, which afflicts between five and ten percent of American kids. Zachary's was much more one of attention-deficit than hyperactivity, although he also could do impulsive, dangerous things.

I asked Koplewicz how many years kids could stay on Ritalin. He mentioned Rachel Klein's controlled study of hyperactive children grown up (there has been some concern about whether the drug stunts growth): the matched controls reached full growth at age sixteen and a half, while the kids on Ritalin reached it at eighteen. "I also have kids who grow like weeds on it. The kids that did poorest on growth were the ones who stayed on the drug seven days a week without any drug holidays. Most kids you hope will outgrow some of their symptoms when they hit adolescence. A certain percentage lose at least one of the three symptoms, the attention deficit, the impulsivity, or the hyperactivity. A third lose all their symptoms, and a third keep all their symptoms.

"The symptoms won't kill you, but they'll make going through school difficult, relationships difficult. If you listened to what Ms. Young was saying before, the interaction between Alexis and Grandma is absolutely horrendous [when she is on the medication]. While a grandmother might say, 'Never give Ritalin,' she sees her granddaughter and she can sit with her granddaughter and really have fun with her. They can play checkers together, they can go to a museum, they can go to a show. All of a sudden the interaction and the building of self-esteem is wonderful."

At the end of the day, Koplewicz and I rode into Manhattan. He told me Ms. Young—an exceptionally sharp woman who probably has weeks where two teachers call her every single day—had paid for a psychologist from Schneider to come to school and teach behavior-modification techniques to the staff. "She felt it was cheaper to spend a thousand bucks that way than to move the kids to a private school," he said. "She's also been a terrific advocate. She doesn't see it as a stigma, she sees it as a no-fault disorder. I don't know if you noticed how all the mothers you've seen today look at their children in a positive light."

"Is that because you've trained them?" I asked. "Do you ever get a tense, awful scene?"

"I think this comes after time, with either training or exposure. I genuinely feel they're not bad parents. I formulate the cases the same way I would with a kid who has cancer. After a while, when they feel less guilty and they don't blame themselves, they can look at their kid and say, 'Hey, there are some wonderful qualities in this kid. The problem, biochemical or genetic or dynamic, or whatever is interfering with their functioning makes it difficult for me to be with this child, but I still love the child.' And then the parent's able to take direction when you say, 'Look, you can't do *that*, it will cause a problem.' That doesn't negate the fact that there are very toxic parents out there. There are parents who are inconsistent, who are inappropriate and say things—they don't know how to parent."

The next day I had reason to ponder how parents might affect the expression of a "no-fault brain disorder." We had no time for advance briefing before Koplewicz saw Andrea Moss, a fifth-grader with a perky blond ponytail, her mom (a nurse), and her dad (a successful lawyer). The Mosses were an entirely different kettle of fish from the Youngs, and Koplewicz's demeanor with them was different too. Andrea had brought in a scrapbook filled with various awards from school, Sunday school, gymnastics, swimming, and band practice, all carefully pasted in by Mom. Since Koplewicz had seen her last, she had written a prize-winning school essay on recycling cans, which Koplewicz read aloud in an admiring tone. He thumbed through the scrapbook, looking at the report that said "Andrea is working to her full potential! A delight!"

"Terrific, Andrea! Is there *anything* you don't get awards in? Your parents must be *very proud* of you!" A little more stroking, a review of the Ritalin dosage, and Andrea was shipped out while Koplewicz settled in with Mom and Dad.

"She has two or three hours of homework a night! It's impossible!" Mom said. "It doesn't come easy to Andrea, and as the medicine wears off, the attention drifts and it's very difficult.'

"She doesn't shirk from her work," Dad said. "Neither does my son. She plods along. He plods along, and *we* plod along. That's what you do. That's our style."

Sunday school was just terrible too. Koplewicz said his kids didn't like Sunday school either, and they commiserated. As he went over the usual questions with the Mosses, he said, "What about her mood? Does she seem happy to you?"

"No," said Dad. "No," said Mom.

"She's crabby with us, she's not pleasant," Dad elaborated. "She's not a sweetheart. You take her someplace, and maybe it's her problem, but you say, 'Let's go where you like for dinner,' and you get there, and she doesn't want it."

"Let's go through that specifically. Name a place," said Koplewicz. They ran over the scenario, how after band practice they asked her where and she didn't know, so Mom suggested some restaurants and they agreed on the Golden Palace, where they give you the little umbrellas. "Great. You're in the parking lot of the Golden Palace?" Koplewicz asked. "She says I don't want Chinese," Dad answered. "She wanted to go home. She was tired."

"Let's play it out," Koplewicz said. "What if she had gone home? What I'm looking for is, is she insatiable, you just can't please her, or is she so overworked from band practice that she's spent and needs to veg out at home?"

It turned out that she did this even on an easy day. And then there were the movies. "In the middle of a movie, she'll turn, like a younger kid, and say, 'I don't understand. What does he mean by that?' You say, 'Andrea, we don't have a lot of patience with that.' It's at the top of her lungs."

"Or it seems that way," said Koplewicz.

When Andrea keeps asking, Dad loses all patience and says, "You watch, it will make sense."

"Not necessarily for Andrea," Koplewicz said. "Just so you know, you're not telling the truth. Can you say, 'Andrea, remember that, we'll discuss it right after the movie'? Because that would be helpful to her. TV's also a great place to learn social cues because of the expressions and the canned laughter. It's a good time to say, 'Hey, did you really understand that subtlety there?' Her essay about recycling is good because it's starting to abstract. Andrea still has difficulty with abstraction, and that's a neurotransmitter again that's misfiring or not connected correctly."

Dad said these reactions were inconsistent, so it was hard to believe they weren't willful. Koplewicz questioned them in detail about Andrea's "annoying" and "unpleasant" behavior and their reaction to it, saying, "I know I'm nitpicking, but . . ." Mom and Dad described her moodiness, particularly with Dad. Koplewicz pointed out that this was a kid with average intelligence who was making the most of it. "While you may plug, there's no doubt that there's a lot more you're plugging *with*."

In this long counseling session on how to handle Andrea, the burden of Koplewicz's advice was twofold. First, the Mosses should "give her distance but at the same time maintain control. If we know that Andrea is always in a bad mood when she comes in, that's okay. We label it. We say, 'I don't know what the deal is, Andrea, but when you come home, you're very unpleasant. I'd like to do something pleasant with you, so maybe you should just mellow out for twenty minutes or so, and then we'll have a glass of milk and some cookies and play Monopoly.'

"The other thing we talked about, remember, is asking questions that are not performance-related. 'How's school?' is not a good question. So— 'Were there any special activities today? Is Mommy home yet? Were you given a lot of work tonight? Do you know what we're having for dinner?' Factual questions like that.

"This is very hard when I have to give people scripts for dinner with overanxious kids, who seduce you. You say, 'Hi, Josh, how ya doing?' 'I'm fine, Dad, played soccer today, I got six assists, two goals, the coach said wonderful things about me. That's sixty-two percent better than my last game.' Fathers get sucked right in. 'By the way, I'm thinking of running for president of the school.' 'When's the election?' 'In six months, but I want to start talking about my campaign.' The kid is eight years old. So when you say to the father, 'Look, we can't talk about performance,' the father says, 'What are you talking about? *He* only talks about performance!' "

Koplewicz—who seemed almost an educational consultant— suggested the Mosses tell Andrea's tutor to get her to tell stories: something exciting or funny that happened last week. "Most of the time, kids who have verbal skill problems can't do it. So on the weekend you take the Polaroid camera out. You take a few pictures, and she takes them to the tutor, and she has cues that help her. After six weeks in a row, what's supposed to have happened is she gets those photographs in her head, she says, 'I can now tell the story from beginning to end.' She gets better and better. 'What made you laugh about that story, Andrea? Can you now express that to me so I can laugh too?' "

"She's such an unpleasant soul," Dad said, and Koplewicz flinched. "What's the purpose of being unpleasant? I don't believe people are born unpleasant. If things are difficult for you, you get whiny." Dad said it reflected how disabled she is, and Koplewicz flinched again. "She's not that disabled. She experiences it that way. Don't say, 'You're being a bitch,' but say 'You're whining, and I'm having a tough time with it. Why don't we talk later?' That way she's not feeling a love-withdrawal."

They talked about sleep, appetite, and school in terms of dosage, and indeed, over the years the school had put the Mosses on a roller coaster, first insisting Andrea needed to be in special ed, then claiming her problems were their imagination, finally recommending a tutor. Now she was doing better, and Koplewicz, keeping up his barrage of reassurance, said, "She's adorable, and she's getting better looking too."

When I went out to Schneider two weeks later, Koplewicz filled me in on Andrea, whom he had seen only five times in the previous two years. She had a history not only of fidgetiness but of learning disabilities, irritability, moodiness and anxiety, and some difficulty making friends. Her relationship with her parents was tense. But she had done much better after the Ritalin and was now highly successful in school, with glowing reports from the teachers. "She's using every IQ point she has. The father and mother have made it clear that they are not candidates for psychotherapy. So the focus of most of the treatment now with this family I see so rarely is not Andrea. She just needs a pat on the back. It is not the Ritalin that's raising her self-esteem. It's that her life experiences are very positive, and she's feeling better about herself.

"Where we really need a little work is with Mom and Dad. I'm a little tougher with the father. I take the attitude of almost being a member of the family, and I want them to recognize that I'm a parent also. Notice how many times I tell them how lovely Andrea is and how wonderful and delicious she is. You have to remember who your patients are, and these people are very concerned about what other people think."

I had watched many therapists by the time I saw Koplewicz, and while his manner with children was engaging and supportive, I witnessed no particular feats of brilliance in drawing the kids out (although he did assess their problems astutely). His gifts—which were considerable— lay in talking to parents. When I asked him about this, he said, "I try to find that chord where we're talking as equals, not me as the child expert. The baby boomers—my age group—have expectations, they live through their children, and that can be problematic. The common ground is that most of the parents are from my generation."

Two years later I called Koplewicz for an update on the children I had seen. He had treated Amy Ratner for a total of eight months; for six of those months, she was on Prozac, which she no longer needs. She continued talk therapy with Dr. Tom for six months after terminating with Koplewicz. Her depression has lifted, and she's bouncy and much more focused on school—and has boyfriends. "What has remained is a kind of funny interaction with her mom, and Mom has dealt with that by actually going for help herself to be more firm and consistent with her kids. It's hard for her to be what she sees as punitive, and punitive is saying no."

Andrea is just fabulous. She gets straight A's and had a wonderful summer at sleepaway camp. She is embarrassed about the Ritalin, so her mother wraps it up with her sandwich instead of giving it to the school nurse. Whenever she has a chance to stop taking the medicine, she actively votes for that because "she's still on some level ashamed that she needs this medicine." Still, she sees the pill as helpful. Her relationships with her mother and father and friends have improved. Koplewicz says she could be a doctor, a lawyer, or a teacher: "Lots of colleges will want her eventually, and she's looked upon by other people as bright and capable.

"The nicest part about a good psychopharm case is that time becomes your friend instead of your enemy. With developmental milestones the kid becomes more mature, and the parents say, 'Look how well things are going.' To have an attention deficit disorder without Ritalin, time becomes your enemy because they start feeling angry at school, hanging out with kids who are also problems, and then we have maybe some delinquency, and time is not your friend. Andrea's father has told the family pediatrician it was like a miracle, but the miracle is not the medication. The miracle is that the parents now see their child differently."

The Youngs are more complicated. Zachary had a good summer at camp and is hanging in at school, where his intelligence is somewhat appreciated—but departmentalized middle school is tough for him, and Mom must keep constantly in touch to make the school more "user-friendly." He is disorganized without the medicine, and the medicine has side effects. Koplewicz can only hope he will luck out and lose the symptoms at puberty. Alexis is "a dream," responding to medicine during the school year and taking drug holidays during summer camp where rambunctiousness is acceptable. Alexis's calmer behavior in school enabled the teachers to pick up a learning disability they might have missed otherwise, and she's getting some helpful tutoring.

While Koplewicz himself would protest the size of the sample, my stint behind his one-way mirror offered compelling illustrative evidence of the role parents play. None of those I saw could be tarred with responsibility for their children's disorders. Mrs. Ratner seemed no different from parents I knew whose children weren't depressed; she'd had bad luck, and with help and education she was coping with her child's problems. The tensions between Amy and her mother looked more or less ordinary, and might be intrinsic to their relationship.

The Mosses, on the other hand, began as, at least, magnifiers of the problem—and ended up being part of the solution. Perhaps, in the end, they might prove to be a closer family than the Ratners.

Finally there were the Youngs, a miniature epidemiological adoption study on the role of biology and environment. These two utterly different children—with, incidentally, the same DSM diagnosis, thus also illustrating the limits of DSM—shared the largest part of their environment, most importantly Supermom. But there were limits to what even Supermom could do to ensure their happiness and the future course of their disorders, which were bound to be different. At the same time, however unscientific a hypothetical assertion might be, they'd surely be less competent without—well, a mother like that.

My final task with Koplewicz was to bring in Little Hans for treatment. Like Chasin, Koplewicz needed a refresher course on this case, so I summed it up for him, as I described it in Chapter 4. "Let's look at what specific fears he's presenting, not his parents' representations," Koplewicz said crisply. "At about the age of four and a half, he gets an illogical fear that horses will bite him in the street. He also starts developing bad dreams and worries about a threat to the integrity of his family, that he will lose his mom and dad. A sadness comes over him, his mood and affect seem quite depressed at times, but the symptoms wax and wane. He continues to have dreams about his mother, and some kind of phobia of giraffes develops also.

"If we just go with the behavior, take the history that at three and a half he had a sister, and he's had lots of interest in his anatomy, with normal sexual curiosity, and his parents didn't handle it well, but nevertheless the sexual curiosity is always within normal limits, we're left with a kid who has a lot of fears. From a diagnostic point of view, this child most probably meets the criteria for separation anxiety disorder. The key symptom of that disorder is the central preoccupation that something bad will happen to his parents or himself that threatens the integrity of his family.

"The other symptoms related to separation anxiety disorder include the stress upon separation, sometimes homesickness. Bedtime is problematic, and you'll find kids who feel very comfortable sleeping in the parents' bed or on the floor of the parents' room and feel discomfort when forced to sleep somewhere else. Otherwise—you don't report any reality-testing problems, you don't report any other major functioning problems except for the fear, but you can change his behavior and get him back in the park.

"So if you go with the assumption that that's the diagnosis, what is the etiology? Part of it comes from the child's having had parents who didn't teach him to sleep in his own bed and stay in his room at night when he was one or two years old. It was a very sudden and dramatic separation they gave him just at the time of his sister's birth.

"But there's also the possibility that this child is predisposed to having separation anxiety disorder in the same way that other kids are predisposed to other physical problems. This is considered a disorder after the age of four, but it's considered normal between the ages of eighteen months and three years. Kids become distressed when Mom and Dad leave them in a strange place or with a baby-sitter. By age four, they should be able to internalize their parents' image and know that even though their parents are out of sight, nothing terrible is going to happen to them.

"The treatment approach would be a very behavioral family approach, talking to the parents about some guidelines to help the child get over his symptoms. We might use a contract that will get the child motivated to strive for some prizes when he's able to separate from his parents. If he is able to change his behavior but the illogical fear and worry persist, then one would consider a pharmacological agent. That's if he can go to the park and separate from his parents but he's really uncomfortable doing it.

"The medications of choice at the moment, according to two studies, one in 1992, one in 1979 or 1980, are tricyclics like Tofranil. An anti-anxiety drug, Xanax, has been used in low doses in open clinical trials, and there's anecdotal evidence that the new drugs—Prozac, Zoloft and Paxil—would be effective as well."

I asked Koplewicz about Frau Graf's threats and the bloody scene Hans witnessed when his sister was born. He suggested that while this might have been a precipitant (and would surely be traumatic today), in those days middle-class Viennese families routinely had babies at home, and most children did not develop separation anxiety disorder. He also suspected the parents' discipline was the same as that practiced by most Viennese families in the early twentieth century. "It's amazing how many parents say foolish things, and clearly their children are able to be resilient and recognize that the parents didn't actually mean what they said. You would want to know more about what the culture held at that time, and about the family's history. Was it typical for Viennese families to put children in the parents' bed or in their room, or was this a very anxious, worried mother who had to keep an eye on her child? Does this family have a positive history for separation anxiety when they were kids, and are there any family members who had panic disorder or agoraphobia, both of which we know run in families and have a real correlation with childhood separation anxiety disorder?

"However, before we give medication, we'd want a family intervention and very directive and supportive behavior therapy. Most of these kids respond very quickly to the short-term symptom-oriented treatment." Koplewicz felt comfortable with Kendall's and Chasin's therapy, and only as a last resort, if these other treatments failed, would he put Little Hans on Prozac.

CHAPTER 14

BREAKING THE CODE

The personalities, attitudes and behavior of the parents . . . seem to throw considerable light on the dynamics of the children's psychopathologic condition. Most of the patients were exposed from the beginning to parental coldness, obsessiveness, and a mechanical type of attention to material needs only. They were the objects of observation and experiment conducted with an eye on fractional performance rather than genuine warmth and enjoyment. They were kept neatly in refrigerators which did not defrost. Their withdrawal seems to be an act of turning away from such a situation to seek comfort in solitude.

—Leo Kanner,
"Problems of Nosology and
Psychodynamics" (1951)

The high frequency with which the psychotic children developed fits during adolescence strongly suggests the importance of "organic" neurological factors. It should be noted that none of these children had any abnormality on a neurological examination when first seen at the Maudsley Hospital. The development of fits was particularly common among the children whose IQ was below 50 or 60. It is well known that many mentally subnormal children become epileptic, and indeed the control children (in whom overt brain damage was common) developed fits almost as frequently as did the psychotic children. Thus the development of fits does not differentiate the psychotic child from the child with severe subnormality or with brain "damage," but it clearly distinguishes him from the child with a psychogenic disorder.

—Michael Rutter and
Linda Lockyer,
"A Five to Fifteen Year Follow-up
Study of Infantile Psychosis"
(1967)

THE PATIENTS DESCRIBED IN CHAPTER 13, all regularly in Harold Koplewicz's care, exemplify the middle range of mental disorders. To varying degrees, the Ratners, the Youngs, and the Mosses, however painful their lives might be at present, could look forward to a better time, and Koplewicz himself to the satisfaction of helping bring that about. At other times in my research, I saw far more severely disturbed children, yet even those cases allowed room for therapists, having worked hard, to pray for some favorable conjunction of stars and planets that might reward their efforts (and the patients') just enough to paste together a decent life. One day, however, I sat in the observation room down the hall from Koplewicz's office and watched a scene of misery so intense that it remains with me now and will presumably forever. Most particularly in the months that followed, as I learned more of the history of biological psychiatry, I pictured the characters and heard again the dialogue of that January afternoon.

While the case was hopeless, there was still plenty for Koplewicz to do: the text for the day was Tolstoy's famous observation that every unhappy family is unhappy in its own way. If the therapist could not cure an illness that had perplexed researchers for decades, perhaps he might moderate that portion of the family's suffering that was self-inflicted.

As usual, I had arrived early to review the history, in this instance, of a new patient about to appear for consultation. He was a Connecticut teenager now under the care of Ivan Rothman (a pseudonym), an old professor of Koplewicz's. "The boy is named Baruch Avram Ostreicher, but I've been told not to mention the Avram," Koplewicz told me. "He's about to turn seventeen, and the complaint is neurological impairments, learning disabilities, and behavioral problems. His behavior's deteriorated, so the parents want a second opinion about medication. They have checked 'obsessive behavior that interferes with his everyday functioning,' 'relates inappropriately to others,' 'attention deficit disorder,' 'neurological impairment,' 'speech and language disorder,' 'bedwetting.' I would imagine also he's somewhat retarded.

"The symptoms first began with facial tics at six or seven, so he has a ten-year history." Koplewicz read from the questionnaire, " 'Obsessive tendencies have become progressively worse and are interfering more and more with behavior. Mostly problems occur due to extreme sensitivity toward what others say to him. Taboo areas include hospitals, calling him Avram, nightmares. Reactions of extreme anger, loud verbal objection, insistence on the culprit taking it back.' So they're right about the obsessive quality. He has seen some very famous people—one of New York's better-known pediatric neurologists treated him for quite a long time. Then another neurologist he's still seeing, a psychotherapist, and now Ivan, who's still seeing him.

"Here's a list of all the medicines taken." Koplewicz showed it to me, and I said, "Oh, boy!" Over the past ten years Baruch had taken—or flirted with—Haldol (a major tranquilizer), Ritalin, Tofranil (an antidepressant), Mellaril (another antipsychotic drug), Haldol again, Catapres, Cylert (a psychostimulant), Tofranil again, and Inderal (a beta blocker drug originally used for blood pressure and heart problems and later found to be effective for reducing aggressive outbursts in brain-damaged patients). Mostly these medicines were prescribed in low doses, then abandoned (often quickly) because the varied side effects were intolerable.

Continuing the list, Koplewicz said, "Okay, he took Prozac for almost a year. He was happier, with better attention, but he was also more hyperactive, and he had occasional suicidal episodes. I might question the suicidal episodes, but I can believe he got more hyperactive." In response to my question, Koplewicz discounted reports of patients on Prozac *becoming* suicidal: "A lot of the patients had characterological problems, and some had made suicide attempts before taking Prozac. Prozac is given to depressed individuals, who tend to make suicide attempts more than anyone else. David Kessler at the FDA is very fast to pull anything off the market, and he refused to pull Prozac.

"Then back to Mellaril. Anafranil maybe for the obsessive-compulsive disorder, but he became extremely hyperactive and violent; he took it only for a day or two, so you can't really tell. Then he took Tegretol, which is an antiseizure medicine, anti-aggression medicine, a nice-size dose, for a whole year. The mother says he got nauseous, lethargic, and suicidal. It's questionable. Then BuSpar, which he's taking at present. It's a new anti-anxiety drug, the mother's absolutely right, he's taken it for a month, it's too early to tell.

"Father is forty-three, a lawyer. Mom is forty-two, she's a computer programmer. There are two brothers, thirteen-year-old Mordecai, and eighteen-year-old Benjamin. He has difficulties with Mordecai. 'How do you punish? Take away TV.' 'Tension caused by the situation in the house, by having this child.'

"This is the form for the child to fill out. It's questionable whether he or his mother did this, but the ones checked off are: 'fairly easily annoyed or irritated, crying easily, temper outbursts that you cannot control, worrying too much, fearful, feelings being easily hurt, feel inferior to others, difficulty making decisions.' ... These are symptoms of anxiety and depression. 'Sometimes avoid certain activities' falls into anxiety. 'Trouble concentrating' can be anxiety or depression or hyperactivity. 'Tending to repeat the same actions such as touching, counting and washing' at least we're in that area, knowing where we're looking. 'Having the urge to break or smash things'—again the same kind of thing.

" 'Feelings of worthlessness.' Now this is the parent questionnaire. The kid picks his nails, has problems in making and keeping friends ... 'excitable, impulsive, cries easily or often, speaks differently from others the same age, baby talk, stuttering, hard to understand, denies mistakes, quarrelsome, fails to finish things, feelings easily hurt.' "

In sum, said Koplewicz dryly, "he's not an easy kid. You see disruptive behavior and also anxious behavior. Distractibility is very much a problem. He fights constantly, does not get along with brothers, disturbs other children. The parents have checked off that he's 'immensely more difficult than the average child.' "

The teacher forms mirrored the parent forms: the school had its hands full. "This kid had a lot of symptomatology. We can understand why he has been to so many doctors," Koplewicz said. "How his parents deal with this could either be stellar or terrible, it doesn't really make a difference in the symptoms. First we've got to take care of the kid, and then the parents are going to need some help in how to cope with him."

I settled myself behind the mirror, and the three Ostreichers walked in. Mr. Ostreicher was a tall, thin, dark-haired, fair-skinned man who wore glasses. Mrs. Ostreicher was a stocky red-haired woman in a black velvet hat. Baruch was slightly built and bespectacled; he and his father wore yarmulkes. In the standard reassuring medical tone, Koplewicz explained to Baruch how he works. Baruch was making faces and looking anxious. "No!" he shouted. "Dr. Rothman helps me with my problems! Dr. Weiss helps me with my problems!"

"You have enough doctors on your case, is that right?" Dad said pleasantly.

"Don't you wear a yarmulke?" Baruch asked Koplewicz.

"I am Jewish, but I don't wear a yarmulke, because I'm not that religious," Koplewicz answered.

"Are you one-step or two-step?" Baruch continued.

"One-step would be conservative and two-step reform? I'm reform. I'm all the way down there at the bottom, practically Unitarian," Koplewicz said cheerfully.

"How about Dr. Rothman?" Baruch asked, insistently and more angrily. It was extremely difficult to get him off this subject and to get cooperative, rational answers to basic questions. First Koplewicz asked, "If you had to pick one of your three areas—behavior, thinking, or feeling—which area would you say gives you the most trouble?"

Baruch whiningly demanded to know what these meant, and Koplewicz explained: "Behavior problems would be that you can't sit still, that you get in trouble in school, that you bother other people and other people bother you. Do you have some of those problems? Fighting a lot?"

"No, no. If I have a problem, I take the problem to Dr. Rothman and Dr. Weiss."

"We're just going to try to help Dr. Rothman help you better."

"Do people call you 'what's up doc?' "

"No, they don't. Let's go on. You don't have any problems with that?"

"Excuse me, do they have a thing in the hospital, saying, 'What's up, doc'?"

"No, people don't do that."

"They started that I'm Bugs Bunny, calling everybody 'what's up doc.' "

"Baruch, shift gears. You have to stay with me. What about feeling problems? Do you worry a lot? Everybody worries about something."

The interview went on in this style. It was an uphill fight for Koplewicz. Baruch sounded like a computer program gone awry, picking up key words and taking them on ever more bizarre paths. Putting his head in his hands and moaning, he said he was worried about hospitals, and he objected strenuously to the video and sound equipment and the one-way mirror, which Dr. Rothman didn't have. Koplewicz persevered too, explaining reasonably that people in the hospital need to watch him work, while Dr. Rothman works in a private office. Finally he suggested that Baruch have some food in the cafeteria while he had a private talk with Mom and Dad.

Koplewicz and Baruch left. The Ostreichers—who knew I was behind the mirror—were otherwise alone. "Would you say that he's getting an accurate picture?" said Dad to Mom, in a tone of irony that must be perpetual. Looking grim, Mom nodded.

Koplewicz returned; Baruch poked his head in; Koplewicz said, "Good-bye, Baruch"; finally the three were alone. "You want a review of his medication, or just a general review?" Koplewicz asked. "I'm not sure where we should go, and frankly Dr. Rothman doesn't know," Mom said.

"We're really at a loss," said Dad. "This morning we came from an appointment. He's been at private religious schools most of the time, but lately we're at the point of taking him out. We've met with the local board of education, and they too are at a loss. I can see it in their faces, and I can hear it in their voices." Mom and Dad also had stricken faces and stricken voices.

Koplewicz reviewed Baruch's history, analyzing the forms. "There are three areas with great difficulties. One is with disruptive classroom and group behavior. I don't think he has classical attention-deficit/ hyperactivity disorder, but certainly a lot of those symptoms come up. The next category is that there seem to be some tics that started when he was six." Mom thought the tics were minor; Dad thought they were major.

The third category was the anxiety symptoms, being unable to say "hospital" or use the name Avram or say certain things without compensating actions, and the fact that Baruch wouldn't shake hands. "If he shakes hands, he has to even out the other hand and people laugh at him. Mordecai laughed at him," Mom said.

"That's obsessive-compulsive behavior," Koplewicz said. "The obsession is that 'if I don't do this, something awful will happen.' The compulsion is to do it. But overriding that what we have just seen is that there is some kind of developmental delay, an immaturity. Whether it's intellectual or not, I'm not sure. We don't have intellectual or psychological functioning tests on him. The first three problems are very treatable. For his attention span, there's behavior therapy and also medication. You can get rid of tics with Haldol and with Catapres, you can get rid of OCD symptoms now with Prozac and Anafranil. However, when you have the other symptom, this kind of immaturity—that usually is related to some kind of brain dysfunction."

Koplewicz went on, "The damage that's done in this brain is so microscopic that an MRI, which is very sophisticated, can't pick it up. There are people that have a 150 IQ that have severe OCD. I can't tell you exactly which transmitter is misfiring, but that's where it's coming from. The part that makes it most difficult to manage with a child like this is, he's almost seventeen. You start to worry what's the future going to hold for him. How can we make him more functional, more mainstream?"

"He's rapidly become almost entirely dysfunctional," said Mom.

"Socially," Dad said—incredibly—"I've always had hopes. He has not quite made friends, but I felt that he was a likable enough kid, and he was not a bad-looking kid, and eventually I figured he would overcome that immaturity. If anything, he's taken a turn for the worse. Children greet him in school, and he curses them. They are working very hard to keep him even half a day.

"At ten thirty last night I brought home the newspaper. He needed to check the weather report. That's his thing. He doesn't just read the temperature in New York, he reads everything about how the weather patterns are changing—in Florida. He'll take a pen to trace the map carefully. I said, 'You're going to wake up exhausted. Save it for tomorrow'—no. I saw him *physically unable* to go up those stairs to bed until he had gone through that newspaper. He was crying, he was begging, he was insisting."

"But he still was able to do it?" Koplewicz asked.

"After fifteen minutes I brought the paper up. Then he shifted. I said, 'Okay, read the paper.' He said, 'But you just told me I couldn't. Why did you tell me I couldn't?' "

"I know exactly what you're talking about," said Koplewicz. "He gets stuck. You can't get out of it. That's the OCD symptoms. 'We Are Going To Tangle With Each Other, No Matter What You Do.' It's almost a dance. Once you say, 'Fine, I'll sit this one out,' he says, 'We're gonna dance anyway.' " Mom and Dad were grimly laughing about the dance: there was a lot of dark laughter among the three of them, as Koplewicz explained that kids do this from anxiety, which gets worse at night because of separation and things that go bump.

Almost apologetically, Koplewicz asked to review Baruch's history from birth, the pregnancy, the delivery. Had Baruch been a "floppier" baby than his siblings? Dad seemed to have a better memory for these details: the joy he felt that Mordecai was not like Baruch. It was Mom, it seemed, who tried to shut the memories out; it was Dad who was driven to pick every scab. This was helpful, of course, for Koplewicz.

Koplewicz—asking a question that seemed particularly bizarre because it was so ordinary—actually wanted to know if people invited Baruch to birthday parties. Dad said, "They were inviting our son." But "he didn't go when they said to go. He didn't stay when they said to stay." Yes, he had an IQ test, a while ago, it was 80, but it was hard to get him to sit still, so that might not be accurate. The school was pleased with the Prozac, but he was difficult at home, so they took him off it.

"What happens when he can't go to school?" Koplewicz asked.

"He stays home and watches television," Dad said.

"And what is he doing while he's staying home and watching TV?"

"He masturbates."

"He exposes himself or just rubbing? Does he really masturbate and ejaculate?"

"I haven't seen," Dad said. "It's not that often," Mom put in. Dad said, "He's gotten more sophisticated. He insists on watching television in private."

As the conversation went on, Dad described how Baruch didn't like to be touched and what happened when he took a shower. "He will first put on the water and let it run so it's not too cold, but he takes twenty minutes to go in. When we're in a hurry, I go up and try to supervise. I make sure it's not going to scald him or freeze him, then, 'Get in that shower.' I see him summon up his strength, his toes are curled, he is as tense as you can be—picture somebody walking on coals!"

"Or acid," Koplewicz joined in.

Dad's voice was loud and full of emotion, and he was curling himself up in imitation of Baruch. "As fast as this kid can move, that's how quickly he's out. He's out! I say, *'You didn't take a shower. You just got wet—that doesn't count!'* He goes back in there: 'Oh! Oh!' "

Koplewicz needed to move things forward. "The problem is that in the management of this child, you have *three* children. It contaminates life, it affects your relationship, it affects the time you can spend with your children, and naturally it starts to preoccupy your mind. 'What's going to happen? How do we plan? Are our other kids going to take care of him when we're not here?' There's a question he won't get a trade, a question he won't be able to live independently. I'm sure that's one of the major concerns you have."

This is not the immediate concern, Dad said. But the siblings— Benjamin, who has learned to deal with Baruch, is now away at college.

Mordecai—"he's very embarrassed, and he's very angry that he has this burden called Baruch."

Koplewicz wanted to talk a bit about medication before seeing Baruch alone. He recommended focusing exclusively on the obsessive-compulsive behavior, which was the most troublesome problem. There are other ways of controlling the hyperactivity induced by Prozac than with Mellaril, an antipsychotic drug: Baruch was not hearing voices or seeing things. Minor tranquilizers like Valium and Xanax are preferable for anxiety disorders. "Child psychiatrists used to give Mellaril like it was candy seventeen years ago. Today if you give that, we'd be very concerned why you didn't try other medicines first, because there's a possibility of tardive dyskinesia, a disfiguring lip-smacking motion that will not go away. Prozac really does work on the obsessive-compulsive symptoms. It's possible with a kid that's bouncing off the walls at night, we can augment the Prozac with Klonopin, an antiseizure medicine that also causes some sedation and seems to make Prozac work better."

As they went over the history, it was clear that medicating Baruch—or perhaps medicating the son of these parents—was a tricky business. Baruch was a good candidate for a thirty-day inpatient evaluation at Schneider or some other hospital where there is a school on the premises, a staff of therapists including psychiatrists, psychologists, and social workers, and a community of other child patients with normal IQs, more like the real world than a special ed class (this is the sort of evaluation we saw in Chapter 2 with Hector, the boy who liked to play dinosaur); it would be much easier to titrate the medication. Mom—sitting with her hands on her hips—saw a million problems. And, Koplewicz repeated, it was time to look toward the future—vocational training, a residential school or group home where he might begin to learn independent living.

Dad said they were planning to keep Baruch at home, in whatever day school would take him, until he was twenty-three or twenty-five. "He needs us more than he needs other kids his age." Mom said he would require a kosher, Orthodox environment: "This is a big part of his identity."

Koplewicz described the benefits of a residential school where kids are reinforced for good behavior, "the treatment of choice for this. His behavior can change with the right kind of reinforcers. The secondary gain is of course for your other children. Your younger son gets more attention, sees his brother as less of a burden. There's much more of a chance that later on in life he will be supportive of a handicapped brother who went to special school and came home on weekends, instead of a kid who contaminated his own childhood.

"Let me spend some time with him. I don't know how much we'll accomplish."

The Ostreichers left with Koplewicz, and I sat for what seemed eternity behind the one-way mirror. Finally someone found Baruch, and he and Koplewicz came back. When Baruch at last settled down, Koplewicz said, "Your parents told me you sometimes do a lot of silly things. Do you know they're silly? Like shake hands with me. I know you do a silly thing after you shake hands. If I shake your hand, your parents say you're going to go like this and like this." (Koplewicz shook each hand.)

"Because they're not *even* to me!"

"Okay, so explain that evenness. I have lots of patients who do that. If I touch you here, I have to touch you there, right?"

"This is not an even world. This is an uneven world," Baruch said in a whiny tone, putting his fingers in his mouth and playing with the wax his mother had put there so his braces wouldn't rub.

Koplewicz kept asking Baruch to explain, and Baruch agreed that if someone came and shook both his hands at once, it would not be necessary to even out the handshake. They talked at length, with Koplewicz trying to elicit the feelings that caused the boy to scrutinize the weather report and pick his fingers. They went around and around about Baruch's objection to his middle name, which apparently had started out as his first name. This sounded harsh, but it served a diagnostic purpose, which Koplewicz later explained to Mom and Dad. Meanwhile, running down the DSM list I had begun to recognize, he asked Baruch about his worries: Baruch reported, and then took back, that "I hear them fighting when I watch television."

Then Koplewicz said, "Do you ever have days you want to cry, you feel so bad?" There was a long silence, and Baruch said, "I think yes." Softly, Koplewicz asked him, "What kinds of things make you feel most sad?" Baruch was pulling pieces of wax out of his mouth and throwing them on the floor. "That's pretty disgusting. Stop doing that," Koplewicz said in the same gentle tone. "How could we make things at school better?"

"Fix my braces."

When Mom and Dad came back in, Koplewicz told them, "He wasn't terribly cooperative. He can perseverate on those braces. But there are times, I have to tell you, that he can be cajoled into moving on. Which will affect the treatment approach. He didn't freak out when I touched his hand, but he refused to accept that the habits were ego-dystonic, which was disturbing to me. *Ego-syntonic*, for example, means I hear voices and I'm really crazy, and God or the Devil talks to me—I believe it. *Ego-dystonic* is, I have to keep doing this, and I know it's peculiar and you're looking at me, but if I don't do it, I feel terribly anxious. I recognize that it makes me look silly, but I can't help it. OCD symptoms are usually ego-dystonic. He refused to fess up to that, and it's much harder to treat. It's easier when somebody wants to get rid of something, and if you really don't want to use medication, that would be the key."

But Koplewicz—almost as persevering as Baruch—reiterated the residential treatment theme, now describing what would happen in a behavior-mod environment if the boy insisted on publicly picking out his orthodontic wax. "There would be a consequence for that. 'You just lost five minutes of TV because it's socially unacceptable and disgusting.' The environment is controlled, not in a mean way. So with socially appropriate behavior—'Hey, Baruch, you happened to let me call you Avram without making such a fuss. That's really terrific—you get ten minutes of extra television time.' Families can't do that; your home has to become like a therapy lab. When you're in a restaurant and he has a temper tantrum, it's very hard to reinforce the consequences. For him the major deal is the social delay, not the eighty IQ. There are a lot of people who function in society with an eighty IQ, and I bet he probably has more, he doesn't allow you to test him. The only way to change the social problems is with a dramatic intensive treatment approach that will have to *bombard* him. So you have to shift gears. I can make him less OCD. I can make him have a longer attention span. The medication management is more challenging, but it can be done. We can make life more comfortable for him in school, but I don't really think that's going to address the long-term outcome for him. I can get you a good school counselor who places people. . . . I know I didn't give you good news. I'm sorry."

Dad was willing to talk turkey. Mom said, "I don't want to send him away to school." The conversation continued for a long time after that, retreading the same ground and covering his previous medication in great detail, until finally the next patient was due.

Two weeks later I went out to Schneider for a debriefing on Baruch, whose DSM diagnosis was "Pervasive Developmental Disorder Not Otherwise Specified"—PDD, in the everyday lingo of the field—a classification that is allied to but does not meet all the criteria for autism: one requirement for the full-fledged disorder, for example, is onset before the age of three, and the history supplied by the Ostreichers in this and other respects was highly ambiguous. And while three-quarters of autistic children are moderately retarded, Baruch's IQ was low-normal. Of all Baruch's symptoms, the crucial, overwhelming one was his inability to respond to people—what DSM-III-R called "a qualitative impairment in the development of reciprocal social interaction"—evident in all of Koplewicz's conversations with the young man. The obsessive-compulsive behavior and the depressive and hyperactive symptoms did not reflect separate disorders. They were by-products of his having a fragile, vulnerable brain; and they were the symptoms medicine could alleviate, thereby making both Baruch and those around him a bit more comfortable. But Koplewicz told me, "The parents, interestingly, have come to some kind of resolution by saying, 'We'll tolerate the PDD, and we'll deal with it as a delay. He's around eight years delayed, so when he's twenty-five, he'll leave the house, miraculously.' They were coming to me about a blemish on the child's arm, when I thought he was bleeding from the chest. The PDD wasn't being addressed at all." It is possible that a better history of Baruch might have resulted in a diagnosis of autism, Koplewicz told me, but the treatment would have been the same. Moreover, he felt the Ostreichers had not come for a diagnosis but for a pharmacological silver bullet—and this he could not give them.

The sudden deterioration in the boy's condition, Koplewicz said, was the result of some stressful precipitant, which might have been a maturation process in the brain, puberty, some change in school or family living; perhaps Benjamin, the older brother, was a stabilizing force and his going away to college threw Baruch off. This is a characteristic formulation for biological psychiatrists: that a disorder to which the patient is biologically predisposed flares up in response to stress. Of the parents, Koplewicz said, "They have chosen to live with their marriage under chronic friction."

In the past two weeks, Koplewicz had talked with Rothman, suggesting adjustments in Baruch's medicines. He would not risk putting Baruch on Prozac as an outpatient because his parents said he had become suicidal in the past, and "he has an abnormal brain."

He knew of a family who had successfully placed a child like Baruch in residential treatment and who might talk with the Ostreichers. "As I sat with them," Koplewicz said, "I thought that from a family therapist's point of view, you could have a field day. But they've had the worst catastrophe befall them that could come on a family because they have a child who is not going to grow up." He talked, movingly, about what we all want for our children—college, a profession, friends, a healthy sex life, independence, and to keep some of our values—what professionals of every orientation call "the developmental tasks of adolescence," which Baruch will never accomplish. "Did you notice my shift in the way of dealing with them?" he said. "My role as psychopharmacologist became minor."

Koplewicz had often made the comment that parents of children with a severe brain disorder could be either "stellar or terrible" and it wouldn't cure the actual disorder. Obviously Baruch's parents had been devastated by a tragedy for which they themselves were completely blameless. But it also seemed possible that repairing some of the devastation might make the experience of being Baruch—Baruch in the social world—less painful, and this was what Koplewicz was trying to do. One might surmise that he was also treating the parents of Mordecai and Benjamin and doing some couples therapy on the side.

At the same time his comments reflect an assumption that family systems therapists always blame the family for its problems, a premise that we saw in Part IV is no longer accurate. A family systems therapist—in this case it would have to be one of the world's best—might simply apply different techniques to breaking the Ostreichers' logjam. Despite Koplewicz's impressive skill in working with parents, the Ostreichers—with whom he hadn't the opportunity to build a relationship—were, as I learned two years later, not persuaded by him or anybody else to face up to Baruch's innate disorder. They did not try residential care. They continued to be resistant to his taking medicine. The drugs, each of which receives only a short trial, never seem to work right, and it is hard to tell how much of that comes from Baruch's abnormal brain and how much from a self-fulfilling prophecy: it is difficult to assess whether a medicine is effective without taking the time to watch it work at the optimal dose.

In Chapter 9 we saw some autistic children. While more appealing than Baruch, they were less functional, although small children, even atypical small children, are somehow still endearing. But the classification now called "Pervasive Developmental Disorders" in DSM-IV includes four related conditions marked by "severe and pervasive impairment in . . . reciprocal social interaction skills, communication skills, or the presence of stereotyped behavior, interests, and activities." ("Stereotyped" in the psychiatric world means "mechanical," not "hackneyed.") The most knowledgeable therapists now believe these children are best helped through behavior training that involves their families. Sometime in adolescence they are carefully weaned toward whatever degree of independent living is feasible—the long-range plan Koplewicz suggested for Baruch. But this regime would not make sense if one believed the parents had caused the disorder, and indeed if one hadn't classified the symptoms to see which might be helped by medicine, which by education, and which by psychotherapy.

It would be very difficult today to find a respectable mental health professional—of any orientation—who still believes that autism and its relatives are brought on by poor parenting, although I have encountered a surprising number of lay people who are not aware of current thinking and hold on almost truculently to their belief in "refrigerator mothers." It is difficult indeed to look at Baruch Ostreicher with a modern eye and not see a substantial organic disturbance. But how the profession as a whole came to alter its view of these most serious childhood disorders makes a good introduction to biological psychiatry (or psychopharmacology, because both terms are appropriate). It heralds the path researchers now take to explore other mental illnesses.

There are, indeed, two lines of inquiry now going on in biological psychiatry, and most investigators pursue both of them: one studies what medicines are most effective for children with particular disorders, and the other seeks to learn more about the origin and course of these disorders. While professionals in this school (which is dominated by psychiatrists but includes psychologists as well) complain mightily about inadequate funding, it is still an exciting and fertile period in neuropsychiatric research. Since recent biological study has made many fascinating and helpful discoveries and failed to make many others, these practitioners struck me as the most humble and flexible of all; at the same time they radiated the excitement of the chase. By teaching me to ask questions I hadn't thought of and to make fewer assumptions about the answers, they altered my way of thinking.

This story began in the thirties and forties, when researchers at various psychiatric hospitals began to study childhood psychoses. The heterogeneous group of children the clinicians called psychotic showed no common, specific, identifiable evidence of brain damage, but their functioning was severely disturbed. A summary written several decades later by Barbara Fish and Edward R. Ritvo, two specialists in the field, offers a detailed portrait of the children the various researchers observed, who exhibited pervasive functional disorders in speech, thought, affect, and social relations. Particularly when their symptoms had emerged before the age of two, they would present peculiar, irregular patterns of motor development and skills. Their demeanor—alternating rapidly between anxiety and indifference—made their whole personalities seem fragmented and chaotic. Disordered language and thought were critical to the diagnosis: the children ranged from being mute and never developing communicative language to losing their speech to mastering only simple nouns, adjectives, and present-tense verbs. In some patients, unintelligible and mature speech coexisted. Their comprehension was also limited. Intellectual levels varied: often they had low IQs, but even the more intelligent children suffered a dysfunction in logic and metaphor that made communication difficult. They spoke with strange juxtapositions, irrelevancies, fragments, and echolalia (see Chapter 9), and the content of their thoughts also seemed bizarre. Socially they were either inappropriately solitary or too clingy.

Since the disorders ranged in severity, it was tricky to diagnose the children: the lower-functioning might be taken for retarded, and the higher-functioning might be thought neurotic. Because each researcher tend to focus on a different segment of this still amorphous group, there was considerable controversy about the cause, the nature, and the developmental course of the children's illnesses, and indeed about whether there was one common psychosis or two.

In 1943, Leo Kanner of Johns Hopkins identified a syndrome he called "early infantile autism." Kanner's studies of autism continued throughout

the fifties and covered a group of children and their families that grew
from the original eleven to a hundred. His description of the symptoms
crucial to autism bears marked similarity to the current DSM list. But his
ideas about the parents' role in precipitating the disorder—articulated in
a compelling literary style that few current theorists can match—laid a
cloud of guilt over a generation of parents whose children showed the
symptoms. For lagniappe it struck no little fear in the hearts of intellectual parents whose families were untouched by the disorder. In truth, he
had been to some extent misinterpreted.

An overwhelming percentage of the parents of Kanner's autistic patients were, he said, "cold, humorless perfectionists" who were "more at
home in the realm of abstractions than in the world of people." As Kanner
observed in a 1951 paper, "They were anxious to do a good job, and this
meant mechanized service of the kind which is rendered by an overcon-
scientious gasoline station attendant." Some autistic toddlers memorized
names of the presidents, recited endless nursery rhymes, and reeled off
catechisms they couldn't understand. Kanner believed, "The emotional
refrigeration which the children experience cannot but be a highly pathogenic element in the patients' early personality development superim-
posed powerfully on whatever predisposition has come from inheritance."
With all this Kanner's formulation was moored in biology. He didn't
suggest that all professional or intellectual parents risked making their
children autistic—that's the misinterpretation. Rather he thought these
particular parents were themselves "successfully autistic adults," parlay-
ing a milder form of the disorder into optimum career achievement.

Kanner said early infantile autism was the first manifestation of what
Lauretta Bender, who headed the Children's Psychiatric Service at
Bellevue Hospital in New York, called "childhood schizophrenia," with
some characteristics all its own. The children Bender was studying, more
heterogeneous than Kanner's, ranged in age from two to ten; she ultimately followed them into young adulthood.

Bender concluded that her patients had a disorder in the central
nervous system that prevented them from developing "biologically patterned behavior," thus producing the symptoms described above. Some
predisposition to this biological defect was inherited, and clinical variations were due both to the age at which development went awry and to
"varied defenses to the biological disorganization": Bender believed
there was one basic disorder called "childhood schizophrenia" that ap-

peared sometime before the age of eleven. Many of the children's distorted perceptions of the world—apparent, for example, in their artwork—stemmed from skewed or stunted motor skills. The syndrome of social withdrawal, stereotyped behavior, and speech difficulties so important to Kanner was in Bender's formulation often the characteristic defense of a child placed in a situation with which he can't cope.

In the forties and fifties, many other theorists believed childhood psychoses were wholly psychogenic. But while both Kanner and Bender disagreed with this proposition, Bender offered a different explanation for the way a psychotic child's mother behaved:

> The mother . . . shows a specific mechanistic patterning due to her efforts to help the child in his distorted identification processes, to understand what is happening and to identify herself with the child. The mother bears an intolerable burden of anxiety and guilt, and is more bewildered than the child himself. She will try every mechanism for denying, evading, displacing, or absolving the child's psychosis. The motor and physical dependance of the child, his intriguing charm, his distressing anxiety all bind the child to the mother while she cannot identify with his problems or follow his disturbed thought process and development.

To some degree that description might apply to Mrs. Ostreicher, although no one could accuse Baruch of displaying "intriguing charm." Bender was observing, most profoundly, that the mother's apparently dysfunctional behavior was the *result,* not the cause, of her having a disturbed child; this, as we remember, is what Harold Koplewicz and Rachel Klein, many years later, recognized in the mothers of hyperactive children.

Until the seventies there was wide disagreement about whether "infantile autism" grew into "childhood schizophrenia." And was the latter continuous with adult schizophrenia (a diagnosis that, then and now, requires the existence of delusions or hallucinations)? Some children had family histories of schizophrenia but no known brain damage; others had brain damage and no family history. Resolving this question was, of course, crucial to the patients' prognosis and treatment. But the resolution carried a more cosmic significance: it encouraged the shift from psychoanalytic to biological dominance in the field of child psychiatry. (Another piece of the continuity puzzle, as described in Chapter 2, was

oppositely resolved, with the agreement that depression exists in childhood, and children's depression is continuous with adult depression.)

In 1967 the British psychiatrist Michael Rutter (see Chapter 1), and
Linda Lockyer, a Ph.D. candidate in psychology, reported on "A Five to
Fifteen Year Follow-up Study of Infantile Psychosis." Rutter and his team
compared the behavior of unequivocally psychotic children at the
Maudsley Hospital Children's Department with controls matched for age,
sex, and measured intelligence, who had been treated at the Maudsley for
a gamut of nonpsychotic disorders.

The psychotic children's histories and symptoms were quite similar to
those of Kanner's group. Most them had shown signs of disorder from
infancy, while the rest had appeared to be developing normally until the
age of two or three. While both the psychotic children and the controls
exhibited delayed and retarded speech development, the psychotic children's abnormal communication was more persistent and pervasive. They
also displayed the other autistic symptoms that should now be familiar
and that existed despite varying intelligence. None of the children's
parents were psychotic, and psychotic symptoms were rare among the
siblings.

Several factors stood out at follow-up. Most notably, even though none
of the psychotic children had presented with brain damage, a good
number of them developed fits in adolescence, most particularly those
with IQs below 60. While the fits did not particularly distinguish autistic
from retarded children, it clearly set them apart from children with
psychogenic disorders.

The psychotic children who were able to go to school made some
progress, both educationally and socially, but even those who became a
little less "autistic" continued to be handicapped in speech and intellect,
making it unlikely that these problems were the result of social withdrawal. About half the children remained "incapable of any kind of
independent existence," and very few could hold a job.

The next significant diagnostic advance was made by another British
psychiatrist, I. Kolvin, of the University of Newcastle upon Tyne, with a
team of colleagues. Kolvin's study distinguished two different psychoses,
dependent on the age of onset: infantile psychosis (known here as IP),
which appeared before age three and conformed to Kanner's and Rutter's
descriptions of autism, and late-onset psychosis (LOP), which showed up

between the ages of five and fifteen and included hallucinations and the other symptoms of adult schizophrenia.

Were there only one disorder, Kolvin reasoned, the children with IP would develop LOP symptoms when they reached the appropriate age: they didn't. Moreover, there were other ways to distinguish the two groups, including family and social class, differences in maternal personality, and evidence of cerebral dysfunction. (The higher prevalence of autism among educated upper-class families, which appeared in early studies, is now attributed to a sampling error: such families would read about the disorder and seek out famous experts, while parents with little schooling might simply assume a child was retarded and not send him for sophisticated and expensive care.)

Most interestingly, in refutation of Kanner's formulation it was the mothers of the LOP children—the schizophrenics—who tended to be more socially isolated than the mothers of the autistic children, and usually a deep-seated withdrawal had been part of the mothers' personalities before their children became ill. By contrast, the mothers of autistic children who were socially isolated had withdrawn only after their children showed symptoms, and simple counseling served to draw them out. On psychological testing the mothers of schizophrenics proved sensitive and suspicious (an innate characteristic), while the mothers of autistic children were overprotective (a situational reaction to a fragile child).

More autistic children than schizophrenic children were retarded. Evidence of brain damage in both groups was fairly substantial but not universal, and it varied: thus autism and schizophrenia seemed to be heterogeneous in their etiology and best defined by behavior. But the evidence for nature over nurture in both disorders was compelling.

Meanwhile, genetic studies of adult schizophrenics were going on. The most significant was that done by Seymour Kety, then of Massachusetts General Hospital, David Rosenthal and Paul Wender of the National Institute of Mental Health, and Fini Schulsinger of the Kommunehospitalet in Copenhagen. (Denmark has continued to be a treasure-trove for epidemiologists because of its exhaustive record-keeping.) Kety and his colleagues combed the lists of unrelated adoptions that had occurred in Copenhagen between 1924 and 1928, searched Copenhagen's psychiatric records, chose a group of adoptees who met American diagnostic criteria for schizophrenia, and then found normal controls matched for age, sex, the socioeconomic status of their adoptive parents, the amount of time they had spent with their biological family, and other aspects of their preadoption history.

Finally the researchers traced adoptive and biological relatives of their subjects and searched psychiatric, police, and military records for mental aberrations. They found a "highly significant concentration of disorders in the schizophrenia spectrum in the biological relatives of the index cases as compared with the similar relatives of the controls." This concordance became even more significant when the authors compared subjects and controls who had been adopted before they were a month old: among 13 of the schizophrenics' biological relatives who had schizophrenic disorders, 7 were paternally related half-siblings who hadn't even shared an *in utero* environment, just some genes. Meanwhile, the adoptive relatives, like the controls' relatives, were hardly inclined toward schizophrenia at all.

The concordance was not, of course, complete, so environmental features were still important. The biological relatives shared only a vulnerability or predisposition that required interaction with other factors in order to flower.

By 1968, even Kanner was willing to recognize that "autism is not primarily an acquired, or 'man-made' disease." (He claimed he had been misquoted, but he didn't utterly deny that parents played some role.) But Fish and Ritvo's comprehensive fifteen-year-old account of "childhood schizophrenia"—important to us because it shows nonprofessionals, some of whom still haven't caught up, how long ago clinicians scuttled the notion of autism and schizophrenia as psychogenic disorders—takes note of this and other genetic studies of adults and children. It points out, significantly, that biological children of normal parents, who are reared by schizophrenics (an odd occurrence, one would think, suggesting sloppy work on the part of some adoption agencies), don't have an elevated risk for the disease. They acerbically comment that unlike biological theories, psychodynamic explanations of pathological parenting "have not led to objectively definable hypotheses which could be tested by generally accepted scientific methods. Neither have they led to therapeutic techniques which have been demonstrated to affect the course of the disease in patients treated by psychoanalysis or psychodynamically based psychotherapy."

Indeed, they observe, the work of John Bowlby and others on maternal deprivation shows that parents can make their children very sick. Without a biological predisposition, however, they can't make them autistic or schizophrenic. And conditions stemming from maternal deprivation can be helped by the restoration of nurturing.

The next task diagnosticians undertook was to separate autism from ordinary mental retardation. While autistic and retarded children had some symptoms in common, retarded children did not display social withdrawal, and their social and language skills matched their IQs; children with autistic symptoms were not all retarded.

Where are we today on what used to be called "childhood psychoses"? DSM-IV has refined the classification of "Pervasive Developmental Disorders" even further. The highest-functioning patients with PDD, for example, have something called Asperger's Disorder; one of them, a college professor of some distinction, was vividly described by the neurologist Oliver Sacks in a 1994 article in *The New Yorker*. As for schizophrenia proper, it is something else completely, experienced rarely in childhood but continuous with the adult, hallucinating kind. And while schizophrenia runs in families, autism generally doesn't.

Professionals now agree that absent the biological predisposition, parents can't give their kids a PDD, and clinicians cannot cure the disorder. Life circumstances can affect the course of the illness, and patients can be helped to live with it. As we have seen, it's difficult to imagine that some of Baruch Ostreicher's difficulties don't come from the social experience of being Baruch, but it's also hard to tease out which problems are which.

The second line of research in the biological psychiatric world, pediatric psychopharmacology itself, has a surprisingly long history. In 1937, Charles Bradley gave the stimulant Benzedrine to thirty behavior-disordered children during the middle week of a three-week period. The effects were dramatic, including school improvement, a "subdued" emotional response that enhanced their social relationships. (The degree of success varied among the children, as did less widespread side effects including sleep and digestive problems, malaise, and anxiety.) In Bradley's report each child was his own control: the effects appeared immediately when he gave the Benzedrine and disappeared the minute he stopped.

There were other studies of Benzedrine for hyperactive and enuretic children during the thirties and forties by Bradley, Lauretta Bender, and others. Bender said that in order to use the drug effectively, clinicians needed to choose the right children through careful diagnosis and to supplement the pharmacotherapy with psychotherapy and tutoring. By 1950, three hundred and fifty children under thirteen had received Benzedrine—which helped hyperactivity for more than half, relieved shyness for a fifth, improved school performance without behavior change in five percent, and had no effect on the rest. Some 15 percent suffered unfavorable responses, becoming either overstimulated or oversubdued. In other studies during the fifties, some children did better with Dexedrine—another stimulant that is still used for AD/HD—at half the dose. Ritalin, now the stimulant of choice, was first synthesized in 1954 and helped children and adults with a variety of problems: it improved the attention span and the ability to follow instructions and complete tasks and decreased hyperactivity and impulsiveness.

The explosion in psychopharmacology had begun in 1950 with the synthesis of Thorazine, the first major antipsychotic drug. (Thorazine is the brand name for chlorpromazine. While professional literature uses generic names for drugs, I will for simplicity's sake refer to medicines by the names nonprofessionals recognize; this is not, however, meant to be an advertisement.) Thorazine is a "major tranquilizer" or "neuroleptic," prescribed for schizophrenia, mania, and very severe depression; neuroleptics are also sometimes used for Tourette's disorder, conduct disorder, and autism. They calm agitation and reduce hallucinations, aggression, and tics; at the same time, as Koplewicz pointed out in talking with the Ostreichers, they can produce numerous major and minor side effects.

Judith L. Rapoport, chief of the Child Psychiatry Branch at the National Institute of Mental Health, graduated from Harvard Medical School in 1959. "My medical school and residency training years," she told me, "were spent watching the hot packs, the cold packs, and the seclusion rooms disappear in psychiatry with the use of Thorazine, and watching people stay a much shorter time in hospitals because of tricyclic antidepressants. People forget because now they've been around for forty years, but these drugs were a real revolution in psychiatry. What's more, they gave an impetus to research because in order to get a new drug on the market, for the FDA you have to have things like placebo control and blind raters and rating scales. To an experimental psychologist that is a trivial concept, but in psychiatry, which had been outside a scientific and medical model for so long, it was an enormous impetus to bringing it back to where it was before the 1930s—more closely tied to medicine, biology, and research science."

Rapoport paused. "I had been an experimental psychology major at college," she said. "I was much more comfortable with the medical and scientific model than the following-a-charismatic-leader model. What people in the other areas of therapy tended to talk about was which guru was particularly wonderful—which to me was intellectually sterile, though very good for the flavor of intimate gossip. In my social life I enjoyed it enormously."

By the mid-fifties, studies began to appear on the use of Thorazine for severely disturbed inpatient children who didn't respond to psychotherapy, but pediatric psychopharmacology didn't begin to take off until the late sixties, with further studies of stimulants for hyperactivity. Research and diagnosis had been fairly unsophisticated; now professionals needed reliable criteria. The Conners Teacher Rating Scale was developed in 1969, and the Conners Parent Symptom Questionnaire in 1970; like most practitioners, Koplewicz still uses the teacher form. His own parent form reflects the Conners. Researchers also began studying tranquilizers and antidepressants for children from the sixties on, and the more varied the medicines, the greater the need became for careful diagnostic studies. Thus the two kinds of biological research proceeded in tandem.

Before going further, it makes sense to sketch out some of what researchers now know about the biological basis of mental disorders: this knowledge comes from a range of sources, including epidemiology, animal behavioral research, studies of stroke victims and other brain-damaged patients, new brain-imaging techniques, and developments in molecular biology. Activity in the brain occurs when electrical impulses, carried over the length of one nerve cell (or neuron) cause the cell to fire packets of chemicals called *neurotransmitters* across a minute space, the synaptic cleft, to the next neuron. This transmission is, in effect, a message, telling the recipient, in its turn, to fire or hold back its own neurotransmitters; each neuron is part of an extensive network from which it receives many such messages simultaneously and totals them up to respond positively or negatively. Moreover, once the first cell has discharged its neurotransmitters, it may reabsorb them for future use (a chemical process called *reuptake,* which metaphorically resembles recycling the paper a note is written on). Thus the brain's response to stimuli is affected by each cell's ability to manufacture, release, respond to, and on occasion recapture the neurotransmitters. The networks of neurons send and receive messages to and from various parts of the body.

The operation of this highly complex process—for example, the speed with which brain enzymes synthesize the neurotransmitters; the type of stimuli to which the enzymes respond; and the structure of the neurons—is to some extent under genetic control: that is, it is hard-wired. To what extent, and how this control is exerted, is the subject of much research in biological psychiatry. What medicines do is intervene at some point in the process to alter it.

There is, however, a role for "nurture" in the biological explanation of brain activity. First the prenatal environment affects the development of the neurons; much of the hooking up of neural networks occurs after birth, particularly in infancy and early childhood; and early in life and again in adolescence, the brain actually sloughs off unnecessary neurons according to the environmental requirements of the individual organism. Activity in the brain often occurs in answer to some outside stimulus, and each neurotransmitter governs many different types of responses. Which ones are fired and the path they follow may be affected by the way the whole person assesses the stimulus: for example, if he sees it as a challenge to his control, the neurohormonal "fight or flight" response may be activated, part of which is then involuntary; if he sees himself as powerless to resist the stimulus, a similar withdrawal-and-depression response is set off. His perception depends on a mix of temperamental hard-wiring and attitudes learned from prior experience, which brings us right back to where we started and gives an opportunity for followers and descendants of Freud, Skinner, and Minuchin to do their stuff. "Nurture" or "environment" helps get the whole process going in the first place; "nature," including heredity, determines how well the equipment operates once this complicated chain of hormonal events is set in motion. Finally, since the hormonal activity, in turn, affects the intensity of an individual's response to a particular stimulus, the whole process is circular. It works both from the outside in and from the inside out. And, of course, future research may change the way professionals balance the nature-nurture equation.

The aforementioned flexibility and humility of biological psychiatrists come from understanding the many points at which clinicians might intervene in the sequence, and from knowledge of innumerable research efforts, successful and unsuccessful, to tease out how this whole cocktail is mixed.

I spoke to several of Koplewicz's colleagues who were applying the biological, interactive view to a variety of mental disorders more tractable than PDD. Their investigations followed a trajectory similar to that pursued by earlier researchers in solving the riddles of autism and schizophrenia (and indeed, depression and attention deficit disorder, as we saw in Chapter 2). Since the illnesses they studied held at least a modicum of promise for researchers (and thus clinicians), their work offers not only illumination of the clinical present but a tantalizing glimpse of the future.

One line of research is exmplified by the experiments of Markus J. P. Kruesi, who is primarily a researcher and administrator and sees only a few patients. He now heads the Institute for Juvenile Research in Chicago; the IJR, readers may remember, is the home of two of the family systems therapists discussed in Chapter 12, and Kruesi's predecessor there was a family systems—oriented psychiatrist. Before coming to Chicago, Kruesi worked in the Child Psychiatry Branch of the National Institute of Mental Health in Bethesda, one of the centers of psychopharmacological research. His main interest is the role of neurochemistry in various childhood disorders, and his work illuminates how this is studied and what biological psychiatrists are learning.

While he was at the NIMH, Kruesi and six colleagues, including Judith Rapoport, did a two-year study of the levels of serotonin, a neurotransmitter important in regulating moods, in children with disruptive behavior disorders. (In the DSM that was current when the study began, these disorders included attention deficit disorder, oppositional defiant disorder, and conduct disorder, all of which we defined in Chapter 2.) The results appeared in two articles in the *Archives of General Psychiatry*.

When serotonin is metabolized in the brain, it produces a substance called 5-hydroxyindoleacetic acid. (Readers don't need to pronounce or even remember the full name of this substance, which is usually shortened to 5-HIAA. But they should recognize it.) Thus a measurement of 5-HIAA in the cerebrospinal fluid, obtained in a procedure called a "spinal tap" or "lumbar puncture," is one way to gauge the level of serotonin in the central nervous system. A low concentration of 5-HIAA has been linked in various adult studies to impulsivity and aggression toward self, others, animals, and property. Aggression is a characteristic of those disorders Kruesi's group was studying, which form an often-overlapping spectrum: while many children have plain ADD, it is rare to see pure ODD or CD without coexisting ADD. (These papers use a slightly older terminology.)

Previous studies of adults with low 5-HIAA levels in their cerebrospinal fluid have revealed, by the adults' own report, a history of behavior problems in childhood. But studies of hyperactive attention-deficit children, by contrast, have not found particularly low levels of the chemical. That research, however, as the authors note, has excluded antisocial, aggressive children.

So Kruesi and his colleagues wanted to study the connection further. But they ran into one of the fundamental problems of research on children. Not surprisingly, it is almost impossible to get permission to do spinal taps on normal children, who according to the rules of rigorous research would provide the optimal control group. Instead, for contrast the authors used a group of children and teenagers with obsessive-compulsive disorder who were already part of another ongoing study. In both groups they measured not only 5-HIAA but metabolites of dopamine and norepinephrine, two other neurotransmitters.

Kruesi and his collaborators sought to learn whether a low level of the serotonin metabolite characterized the most aggressive and impulsive children among a group with disruptive behavior disorders that ran the gamut in type and severity. In addition, they asked, did the measure of this chemical differ significantly between the children with the behavior disorders and the contrast group of obsessive-compulsive children? They also tested the children for social competence, psychosocial stress during the past year, and something called "parent and child expressed emotionality" (shortened to EE), which is a presumed indicator of family functioning. All of the psychological tests were matched against the level of serotonin metabolite in the children's cerebrospinal fluid.

The researchers took spinal taps on 29 children and adolescents aged six to seventeen with IQs above 80 and at least one disruptive behavior disorder diagnosis (most had two); the kids had no medical or neurological disorders and weren't psychotic. The contrast group (what would be called "controls" if they were absolutely normal) was made up of young obsessive-compulsive patients, many of them matched for age, sex, and race with the main group. The researchers found a relationship between low levels of lumbar cerebrospinal fluid 5-HIAA (as compared with the contrast group) and disruptive behavior, especially aggression. Moreover, aggressive children also had low concentrations of the dopamine metabolite—unlike aggressive adults, who had been shown in other studies to have high concentrations of it: the researchers didn't know if this discovery was a matter of chance or a real developmental difference.

At the same time impulsivity and the psychosocial problems did not significantly correlate with the serotonin metabolite. But the authors still believed, on the basis of primate studies, that there is some linkage between serotonergic systems (those that involve serotonin in the transmission of nerve impulses) and social competence that might show up in a less socially disabled population. (In other words, these kids were so impaired that they didn't find themselves in many ordinary social situations.)

What does this mean clinically? It suggests that drugs that alter the serotonergic system are likely to alter pathologic aggressiveness, but they won't do much for attention deficit per se or for ordinary hyperactivity. It also suggests that a low concentration of 5-HIAA in the cerebrospinal fluid may be a risk factor for subsequent aggressive behavior.

The researchers' next step was to follow their subjects for another two years. They found that low serotonin metabolite concentration significantly predicted the severity of physical aggressiveness. Follow-up studies of hyperactive children usually show antisocial behavior in about a quarter of them, and about a third of the children with conduct disorder, the most serious of the childhood behavior disorders, end up as criminals and substance abusers. In general, the most significant behavioral predictor of adult antisocial behavior is aggression in childhood, with the probability of this increasing according to the age of onset (the earlier the child becomes aggressive, the worse the prognosis) and the number and variety of aggressive behaviors the child shows. Most studies of factors that predict delinquency have dealt with psychosocial measures, but some researchers have argued that biological factors may be more important.

In their second paper, Kruesi and his co-authors point out that low levels of CSF (cerebrospinal fluid) 5-HIAA in depressed adults have been predictive of violent suicide attempts; another study linked the serotonin metabolite to military discharge for unfitness. Here the authors traced and re-interviewed the children to see whether this measure similarly predicted physical aggression and suicide attempts and also whether levels of the dopamine metabolite and various other biological measures predicted suicide attempts. Finally, they wondered whether any of these neurohormonal factors might herald lower overall functioning, institutionalization, and substance abuse.

As a whole, the group continued to experience significant problems. Nearly half had been hospitalized or incarcerated. Four of the 29 had attempted suicide. The group's mean score on the global functioning test was low. All but one of the 29 subjects had had some kind of therapy—be it medicine, inpatient or outpatient psychotherapy, or family therapy, not to mention such other interventions as tutoring and out-of-home placements. It is interesting to learn that aggression was linked to serotonin deficiency, while it was low levels of the dopamine metabolite that predicted suicide attempts. Small studies like this are limited by the population, method, and variables chosen, and it is the gradual accumulation and reconciliation of narrowly defined results that lead professionals to broader formulations.

By the time I met Kruesi, I was filled with excitement about new discoveries in neurochemistry. I started by asking him what the implications of his work were on disruptive disorders for the IJR's inner-city population. Kruesi said, "There's been a great to-do about biological research, particularly research pertaining to conduct disorder or antisocial behavior, which has been misinterpreted as being negatively related to race. The evidence suggests that this couldn't be further from the truth. When epidemiological catchment area studies were done, despite the fact that African-American males are incarcerated at a much higher rate, when one looks at Antisocial Personality Disorder [defined in DSM-IV as 'a pervasive pattern of disregard for, and violation of, the rights of others that begins in childhood or early adolescence and continues into adulthood'], which is one of the negative sequelae for conduct disorder, there's no racial predilection for it whatsoever. But there's another very interesting part of this story that hasn't been teased apart yet, and I hope if I get another forty years of life I will tease apart some of it." (Kruesi was born in 1949.)

"There are good suggestions of a clear environmental influence on violence, and at the same time some circumstantial evidence that between environmental events and their ultimate expression, there is biological mediation. That's where part of the future and part of the real excitement are, but it's a very difficult thicket to get through.

"You asked me, for example, if conduct disorder is biological. If you look at the studies comparing identical and fraternal twins for juvenile delinquency, there's no appreciable evidence there for a genetic cause. If you look at the twin studies of adult criminality, you then do see differences in the concordance rates between identical and fraternal twins."

While there are, Kruesi told me, a range of possible explanations for that information, all waiting to be tested, "there's one general phenomenon, which is that genetic expression appears to increase with age. Children appear more environmentally sensitive, so you may well see greater environmental influences early on. But we don't yet know to what degree those environmental experiences go on and permanently, as opposed to transiently, alter biological expression."

We have seen that environmental stimuli influence the developing brain; this was an even more radical turn of the nature-nurture screw.

"With all my caveats about extrapolating from animal studies," Kruesi went on, "there was one study that fascinated me when I was studying nutritional variables that affect children's behavior. It turned out that rats who had undergone severe malnutrition and then been refed did not perform any differently from the control animals, but when both groups were exposed to a subsequent insult of some sort, you saw the earlier damage revealed."

I asked Kruesi whether he meant more than the familiar principle that a body part becomes weaker with each trauma it suffers—that every time you throw your back out, it becomes more vulnerable. He cited Cathy Spatz Widom's study of whether abused children go on to commit violent crimes more often than nonabused children (see Chapter 1): they did, although not invariably. "We've got an increasing number of children exposed to a whole number of traumatic events. I can offer you no proof as yet, but it's not implausible to consider the idea that we may really be altering the biology of subsequent generations. How would we be going about that?"

Taking me for a stroll on the research trail, Kruesi first described a genetic study that crossed beagle and coyote hybrids. He told me there are certain social behaviors that appear in beagles and are mutually exclusive with others that appear in coyotes. The researchers had crossed enough generations to feel sure that some of these behaviors had now disappeared permanently. "But it was discovered, quite by accident," Kruesi said, "that under stress this behavior that they thought was no longer there reappeared: there must be parts of the genome that were silently being carried along but became expressed only under very stressful conditions. So—my colleagues and I have been looking at a biological marker that appears to be related to aggression. We don't know where that marker comes from.

"But adoption studies of violent crime in Scandinavia show clearly that it's not crimes of personal violence that have evident genetic loading, it's property crime. That's one clue, and another is Widom's report that exposure to violence does increase the risk of committing subsequent violence. Now, the only study I can point to in humans that looks at the relative contribution of genetics and what the researchers call 'cultural heritability' of the concentration of cerebrospinal fluid 5-HIAA suggests that the cultural heritability was greater than the genetic heritability.

"I am giving you part of a very interesting trail. I am giving you further clues that suggest—just circumstantially—that there's a biological marker that does appear, at least with some consistency, to be related to aggression, whether it be suicide or aggression against the self or aggression directed at others."

"Or property violence," I said.

Kruesi nodded. "A number of clues point to the idea that there may be environmental events that are affecting this biology. One possibility— purely speculative—is that exposure to certain adverse events in susceptible individuals turns on part of a genetic expression that otherwise would remain silent. Let's say you carry some genetic material that predisposes you to aggression. The expression of that part of the gene may be brought out only by some environmental insult, but now the question becomes very interesting: once it's been expressed, does that change the way it gets passed on? Have you passed on an even greater propensity to violence? The suggestion is there. There's no proof yet, but it makes you suspicious. And if we know how, then we can try to do something about it. I would love to know the answers to these questions. There may be a chance of intervening."

Kruesi pointed me toward the story of phenylketonuria (PKU), in which a researcher at the National Institutes of Health linked a metabolic defect, revealed in measures of the amino acid phenylalanine in the urine of some retarded children, to the retardation itself; now it is possible, by adjusting the diet, to alter the metabolic defect when such children are infants and thus improve their mental functioning. "With the cerebrospinal fluid 5-HIAA we're at a much earlier point on this trail," he told me, "and it's a very good reason to get excited. But on the other hand, Mother Nature reveals her secrets slowly and puts all of us in our place frequently. So I may be chasing after this one for a long time."

What, finally, was the role of talk therapy in Kruesi's world of biological psychiatry? "I will freely confess I am a biologist and I plan to continue doing biological research, but a great number of the problems people face are chronic conditions for which we do not have absolute cures. I can think of no medication in child psychiatry that's absolutely curative—you take it and the problem's gone and it never comes back again in any way, shape, or form. So if you haven't got an absolute cure, the questions are much like all the others medicine has to deal with: How does one accommodate, live with, and diminish symptoms as much as possible, and how does one manage and go on and enjoy life? These are human conditions."

CHAPTER 15

LIVING WITH THE PUZZLE

I think we can effect a presentation of the probably very complicated etiological conditions which exist in the pathology of the neuroses, if we establish the following etiological concepts:

(a) Predisposition, (b) Specific Cause, (c) Contributory Cause and, as a term not equivalent to the former, (d) Exciting or Releasing Cause . . .

The factors which are to be described as predisposition *are those in whose absence the effect would never come about; but which, however, are incapable of alone bringing about the effect, no matter to what degree they may be present. For the specific cause is lacking.*

The specific cause *is one which is never absent when the effect actually takes place, and which also suffices, in the required quantity or intensity, to bring about the effect, provided that the predisposition is present as well.*

As contributory causes *we may comprehend such factors as are not necessarily present every time nor able . . . to produce the effect alone, but which co-operate with the predisposition and the specific etiological cause to make up the etiological formula.*

—Sigmund Freud,
*A Reply to Criticisms of the
Anxiety-Neurosis* (1895)

THE PSYCHODYNAMIC AND FAMILY SYSTEMS THERAPISTS I met, however distinguished they might be, were in private practice or at clinics; the behaviorists were mostly academics whose clinical practice fed their research. Several of the biological psychiatrists, however, tended to be chiefs of hospital units. They saw a lot of patients for a few sessions and

420

only a few patients, if any, for a long time and frequently; their patients were either sick enough to be institutionalized or sufficiently puzzling and desperate to need a consult with an eminent practitioner.

It was these conditions as well as the biological approach that shaped their attitudes. The flexibility and humility I noted earlier, acquired by dealing with so many complex, hard cases, were paradoxically accompanied by absolute confidence in their basic method and impatience with those who differed with it, a not unreasonable position considering that every child who came into their purview was clearly having great difficulty functioning and had been unreachable by traditional talk therapies alone. They didn't suffer fools gladly and might have small tolerance for more trivial problems. But their kindness and skill in dealing with the families they saw were impressive and a pleasant surprise: parents seeking a biological psychiatrist, I concluded, ought to set high standards in the realm of art as well as science.

At Koplewicz's suggestion I made a foray north of the border to see Stanley Kutcher, who heads the Division of Adolescent Psychiatry at Sunnybrook Medical Centre, the hospital arm of the University of Toronto; both clinically and philosophically Kutcher proved as strong-minded and distinctive as his advance notices had predicted. As usual, I read some of his papers to pave the way for our meeting.

A review of adolescent depression, which he wrote with a Sunnybrook colleague, jibes with (and extends) what we learned from Gabrielle Carlson in Chapter 2; it bears reviewing to set the scene. The authors start with the contemporary understanding that depression in adolescence doesn't just come with the territory. Still, the old view dies hard, and clinicians sometimes fail to diagnose it: they are especially prone to this oversight when they don't use a structured interview that makes sure all the right questions are asked.

Depressed teens have some symptoms in common with adult depressives and others that are unique. Both adults and adolescents reproach and think poorly of themselves and lose interest in their usual activities; both may have suicidal feelings and difficulties eating and sleeping. But if depressed adults sleep too much, depressed teenagers sleep too little, and indeed, those at Sunnybrook have fewer vegetative and more cognitive symptoms like discouragement, helplessness, or what they perceive to be emptiness, irritability, or boredom. Other studies bear this out.

Perhaps the most graphic argument I have encountered for the structured DSM-diagnostic point of view is the statement that reports on how many adolescents are depressed vary from 2 to 50 percent of this population. Epidemiologists are apparently not always consistent in whom they talk to, and teenagers claim to be depressed more often than their parents say they are. Moreover, there is a difference between having symptoms of depression—which, in fact, a fifth to half of all adolescents experience at some point (perhaps giving support to the old comes-with-the-territory view)—and having the full-blown DSM disorder.

More systematic studies collecting information from a wide sample of teenagers, their parents, and their teachers via structured interviews suggest that 2.6 percent of boys and 10.2 percent of girls experience a depressive disorder during early to middle adolescence. Gender differences are dramatic: before puberty, more boys than girls show depressive symptoms, and while all the symptoms shoot up for both sexes in adolescence, girls leave boys symptomatically far behind.

Studies report neuroendocrine and electrophysiological abnormalities in depressed adults, but the biology of adolescent depression, less widely researched, may be different. Kutcher's own group has found differences in the secretion pattern of growth hormone between depressed adolescents and normal controls; most particularly, the pattern of growth hormone secretion after taking desipramine, a tricyclic antidepressant, was different for suicidal teenagers (just a portion of the depressed population) compared with normal controls. The group found variations in the sleep electroencephalograms of depressed teenagers at different ages, suggesting that developmental and medical history affects the individual's biology.

Adolescents don't respond as well as adults do to tricyclic antidepressants. And there are particular risks in the psychopharmacology of adolescent depressives: according to one of Gabrielle Carlson's studies, about a fifth of depressed teens develop mania—and thus a full-fledged bipolar disorder—three or four years after being hospitalized for severe depression. That mania can be precipitated by antidepressants, which may also be lethal in overdose. Finally some adolescents meet the criteria for an enduring personality disorder even after the depression has abated. Thus talk therapy by psychopharmacologists who treat teenagers is copious: contrary to the notion that many lay people hold, the very last thing you want to do is just hand the kid a pill.

Another paper Kutcher sent me—"The Pharmacotherapy of Anxiety

Disorders in Children and Adolescents," a collaboration between Kutcher, two colleagues at Sunnybrook, and Rachel Klein of the New York State Psychiatric Institute at Columbia University—is a blueprint for his clinical approach. The authors begin by pointing out that while there have been studies of medication for anxiety disorders, there haven't been studies of the talk therapies. (Philip Kendall's study of cognitive-behavioral therapy for anxiety disorders, described in Chapter 7, had not yet appeared.) Clinicians can't draw any real conclusions about pharmacotherapy until nonmedical approaches have been evaluated.

The clinical problem in treating anxiety is that it presents three sets of symptoms: the primary anxiety, whether it is about separation from mother or speaking in class or going to parties; the anticipatory anxiety kids feel when they know they are about to face the frightening situation; and behavioral signs like staying home or crying. The general treatment strategy is to prescribe medicine, when necessary, to relieve the child's anxious feelings and work with the child and the parent to modify the behavior. As Koplewicz observed in his hypothetical treatment of Little Hans, the therapist uses medicine only when other approaches, after about six weeks of trying, don't work. (That, of course, is what "when necessary" means: the biological psychiatrist is relatively impatient with talk therapy unaided by medicine.)

The clinician's diagnostic workup includes the standard structured interviews and a two-week tracking of symptoms with a rating by an "independent third party"—usually the mother. Next the therapist gathers the patient and family around and has a long educative talk with them, at a level appropriate to the child's age, about the nature of the disorder, explaining theories about it, how it affects functioning, what treatments are available, and why the therapist prefers one over others. They discuss therapeutic goals, and the therapist fills them in on what medicines can and can't do. They review possible side effects and the risks of not taking the medicine, drug interactions, and any family problems that might sabotage compliance. Finally they embark on the sort of treatment course we saw with Koplewicz and his patients, where dosage is monitored, stabilized, maintained, and reassessed.

Before visiting Sunnybrook, I had a hearty lunch with Kutcher in a nearby fern-wood-and-brick restaurant. His background is somewhat unusual for a biological psychiatrist. The eldest son of a Presbyterian minister from the Ukraine who worked in inner-city churches, Kutcher, born in Toronto in 1947, grew up in a family that prized debates and discussions in which all participants found their views subject to constant challenge. Logically enough, he majored in history and political theory at McMaster University in Hamilton, then set out to get a graduate degree in the history of science.

Somewhere after his master's degree, Kutcher switched to an experimental medical program that took students with nonscience backgrounds. "I went to medical school not knowing the difference between a cell and a molecule," he told me. One mentor was an analytically trained psychiatrist who said, " 'The only two books you really need to read about psychopathology are Shakespeare's collected works and the Bible.' On the question of adolescent depression, you read *Hamlet*. On the sociopathic personality, it's *Richard III*. If you want to look at psychotic depression in older age, you read the Book of Job. They go beyond illness, they go into the human condition." Other mentors, of course, were neuropsychiatrists and endocrinologists. Meanwhile, Kutcher had long worked in recreational programs with teenagers, and ultimately he went into child psychiatry because it was the only route to treating adolescents.

I asked Kutcher if adolescence got a worse press than it deserves: he cited Granville Stanley Hall, the first "scientific" student of adolescence, from whose 1904 book modern theories stemmed. Hall had been the first president of Clark University and the host of Freud during the master's famous visit to the United States. "He was also a tremendous fan of Wagner, and his view of adolescence bears more resemblance to the *Götterdämmerung* than reality," Kutcher said. What Kutcher calls "the mythology of adolescence—that to be normal is abnormal" comes, he says, from the psychoanalytic theoretical tradition. "What do you use for the validity of your theoretical framework? In this mythology you use case studies, which are very interesting and raise hypotheses, but they offer no validation, so it's a perversion of scientific method. When people start doing empirical research on adolescence, they don't find anything like that. They find that about twenty percent of teenagers fit the profile the analysts dealt with. Right now there's a tremendous reworking of the concept of adolescence."

My interest, I told Kutcher, was when a child needs therapy. "What is a really terrible adolescence, and what is a clinical problem? If you as a parent had a fairly mild adolescence and you have a kid who's having a somewhat stormy one, you might say, 'I assume that everybody isn't like me. This child is stormier than I am, so let's sit back and wait it out.' Or you might say, 'I had a mild adolescence and this kid is much more emotional. There's something wrong—I'm going to get the kid shrunk.' The parent is trying to figure that out."

Kutcher talked about different conceptual models of disease—the analytic, that "everybody is ill, which is bullshit," the model that "disease is what the sufferer says he has, which opens the door to everything and is also nonsense," and the empirical argument that disease is two standard deviations from a relevant norm, which alone is insufficient. What it comes down to is "some impairment of functioning, and symptoms that are not usually there when a person is well."

He said, "You think of treatment as a bunch of concentric circles. The middle circle is the symptoms the person is having—pain, depression, panic attacks—and that's a focus in treatment, obviously. And then there's a wider focus, the social interaction, and a still wider focus, vocational and academic functioning, and the next is family and interpersonal relations. You can go on and on, so you have to look at what you are trying to restore or improve. It's important that you have a way of evaluating your outcome that is more than healer and sufferer simply agreeing that the outcome is positive or negative, that you are a priori determining how much improvement will be enough, and when will outcome not be sufficient and how long you want to take to reach that. You can set up a way of evaluating everything you do in a systematic, objective way, and that has to be the basis of therapeutic practice."

Kutcher cited his own willingness to question the hypotheses of his tribe. He had done a study on the effectiveness of desipramine for depressed adolescents. "If one were to accept the current neurobiological theory of depression, this medicine would improve eighty percent of all patients with the disorder. And for our adolescent group there was no difference from placebo. This study not only challenges the theory of depression but makes a treatment that has been applied for a long time useless."

"But desipramine has been effective with adults, or nobody would use it," I said. "So doesn't that suggest there are differences in effectiveness between adults and adolescents?"

"Very much so. I think the brain undergoes particular maturational phenomena between the teenage and adult years. The other thing it suggests, which is more exciting from a neurobiology point of view, is that the brain actually, after repeated episodes of illness, develops an ability to heal itself, using a different neurotransmitter system. It tries to regain its equilibrium using the noradrenergic system in order to change mood." (The noradrenergic system secretes norepinephrine, a neurotransmitter related to adrenaline and involved in the fight-or-flight response. Desipramine acts to make more norepinephrine available, thus relieving symptoms of depression with a feeling of competence.)

"Does this mean everyone is just going to get better?"

"No, it means that if you're an adult and have had two or three episodes of illness, you have a very different brain than a teenager who's just had the first episode. Maybe the first insult to the brain has nothing to do with the noradrenergic system whatsoever, and maybe what happens over time, after the initial insult, is that the brain's built-in way of healing itself is to increase activity in another system, the noradrenergic system—and what these medicines do is simply accelerate the brain's ability to heal itself. You don't find this in the first-onset adolescent depressives because they have only recently gotten sick, and it takes time for the brain to rework itself."

I was confused, having been taught to manage a chronic bad back, and I used this simile with Kutcher as I had with Kruesi: without strengthening exercises, I had been told, the back would be cumulatively weakened, and a lesser stress would produce the same, then a worse effect. If these brains have had five episodes, wouldn't they be worn out, more vulnerable, less resilient?

"The two ideas are not mutually exclusive. To be more susceptible to stress doesn't mean that you don't have another process in place that tries to heal when stress occurs. I am suggesting simply a hypothesis, with no idea whether it has any validity. But when you apply empirical methods to measure outcome, it raises interesting questions, and that's one area where child and adolescent psychiatry has been sorely lacking. Therapeutics have been prescribed on the basis of theoretical etiology or empirical observation, which is okay to a point. But we have to go beyond that and evaluate what is actually occurring, in those concentric circles I mentioned. Because it could be, when you give a medicine to a kid, that you get rid of the symptoms, but the medicine also has something that impedes their ability to integrate socially."

Kutcher was pointedly *not* embracing the psychoanalytic notion that the patient needs the symptom, "a totalitarian construct that you're sick because you want to be sick, and if you don't want to get well, it's *your fault*. No blame or responsibility is ever put on the person treating."

Now it was time to get down to cases and how Kutcher manages them.

"If you have a kid with panic disorder," he said, "the likelihood of their having a family member with panic disorder or another anxiety disorder is sixty percent. Not only is it important to understand how the family interacts, but we have to identify others in the family with a psychiatric disorder and make sure they're being treated, because behavioral interactions develop out of the pathology. If you have a panic disorder, you feel much more comfortable when you're with somebody else. You go out accompanied, you drive a car accompanied, you go to a shop accompanied. You can't go to school accompanied, so you stay home. If the mother or father has an anxiety disorder and the kid has one, very often they will use each other as a crutch, and you get enmeshment. The most amazing thing is that when you treat the kids and they get better, all this goes away.

"The panic attacks respond beautifully to pharmacology. The phobic avoidance—not going on the subway, not going to school or parties—*that* doesn't respond to medicine. It's the psychological add-on to the initial insult. So what they need is some behavior therapy, and they benefit beautifully once the anxiety disorder is under control. You show them that no longer are they going to get these panic attacks, so they don't have to avoid situations. 'What are you going to do if you get a panic attack? What kind of strategies can you take? What are your chances of getting an attack now, when you haven't had any for two months?' "

What he was doing was what Kendall does, plus a pill. And, in fact, as Koplewicz had suggested, a biological psychiatrist finds plenty of situations when the pill is not appropriate.

En route to the hospital Kutcher told me about another tricky case: "We have a sixteen-year-old girl who comes in with a major depression with psychotic features. She gets delusionally guilty, she stops eating, she thinks the food is poisoned, and her parents bring her in. We take her family history and find a bipolar disorder that runs in the family: the dad's mother had it, his grandfather had it, the father himself has mood disturbances. Alcoholism also runs in the father's side.

"So right now we have a kid where we know the natural history of the disorder. We know that very often bipolar disorder in teenagers will manifest itself as a psychotic depression, and the chances of any teenager who presents with a psychotic depression—regardless of family bipolar history—having a first manic episode within five years is forty percent. We know that if they have a family history of bipolar disorder, the chance is eighty percent. We find out that the kid in six months prior to illness has broken up with her boyfriend. How many kids that age have broken up with their boyfriends?"

"Seven million and forty-three," I said.

"Exactly. And what's more, now she has a new boyfriend she's quite happy with, and the boy is a very nice kid. She has been out drinking and partying and doing teenage kinds of stuff, a bit more than her parents would like, and there is some conflict at home, and before onset she went on a school trip to Quebec City. She was there for about a whole week with the kids, carousing, skiing all day, and partying all night."

"And she's worn out," I said.

"This is a very common pattern for the onset because the illness is associated with the sleep-wake cycle. Tremendous stress that throws the sleep-wake cycle out of whack, associated with alcohol use, often brings it on. So this is not a response to the loss of a boyfriend, this is a major medical illness with a clear-cut family history. This kid is an A student, she has lots of friends, she comes from a great background. We looked at her academic history, and we found that about a year before she got sick, her math started to go down. All other subjects stayed fine, which is very interesting because we've noticed this pattern in almost every other bipolar patient. We're actually setting up a study to check this out, because we wonder whether the part of the brain that controls mathematical reasoning is different from what controls verbal reasoning and is associated with the part that controls mood in bipolar illness.

"Now—how do we treat this kid? There's very little literature about psychosis and depression in teenagers. We know the best treatment is ECT [electroshock or electroconvulsive therapy], but you don't go to it first. So do we go with a combination of medicines, a major tranquilizer and an antidepressant? When we begin with antidepressants, we know the chances of flipping them into mania are very high, about forty percent. You give them lithium instead? The response rate of a person who's depressed and given only lithium is very poor. So now you're left with some very difficult decisions, and you bring them to the family and the kid. 'Maybe what we should do is have the tranquilizer and an antidepressant that we know from the adult literature is least likely to be associated with flipping you, and as soon as your psychosis starts to go away, we'll start decreasing the tranquilizer and give you lithium instead. You don't have to have the lithium if you don't want—we'll follow you.' This particular girl didn't want to have anything to do with lithium, because we told her about the side effects—acne and weight gain. So she stayed on the antidepressant.

"And she flipped."

By now, we had arrived in Kutcher's office. My eye lit immediately on a poster on the wall: it was a patient's cartoon of two heads, one with the "mania bug" and the other with the "depression bug." Each had a large bubble of dialogue attached to it. The mania bug said, "Thoughts race so fast in your mind, you can hardly complete a single idea. You lose your ability to rationalize. In your mind you are fine and everyone else is worrying about nothing. You feel great. What's wrong? Feeling as though you can do anything, you will probably do things you normally wouldn't. You think you are far superior and much more intelligent than anyone and will strongly verbalize your viewpoints to anyone who will listen. Good friends will hopefully stick by you, but with your new personality you will leave most friends behind you or they will just get fed up with you. . . . Spending sprees will happen a lot until you run out of money. . . . Europhia [sic] is more like it. You might think you are God, Jesus, the Second Coming, an angel, or several other religious figures. You are here to help and save the world. By this time I hope you are hospitalized."

The depression bug said, "You need a good cry, but your feelings are so deep, they can't get out or you are constantly in tears. You feel you are useless and capable of nothing. Sometimes you think you can't even speak, so you don't. People ask you, 'What's wrong?' but you don't know and say nothing. When you do speak, your voice is very low-pitched and depressed. You probably feel that no one likes you. . . . You can't explain what's bothering you, and this frustrates you, thus more tears. Everything scares you. . . . Your thought process has nearly slowed to a halt. Then come the suicidal thoughts. I mean, who would care, do you think? When this happens, be sure to tell someone. You don't really want to kill yourself. It may take some time, but things will get better." This patient's bipolar illness, Kutcher said, was secondary to a head injury received in a car accident.

I sat down, and as I set up my tape recorder, he filled me in on Robyn, the eighteen-year-old patient I was about to meet. She, too, was bipolar, and a "slow learner." She had been having psychotic breaks for several years; her father was unemployed; her mother was a waitress; her parents had split up a while back. There was a history of mood disturbance, psychosis, and alcohol and drug abuse throughout the family. After her first break a couple of years ago, she had been hospitalized, put in restraints and isolation, pumped full of medicines, and discharged, then taken off the medicines by her father, who later pulled her out of two other hospitals against medical advice. She came to Sunnybrook, Kutcher said, "utterly, totally off the wall."

I was not going to watch Robyn behind a one-way mirror: the three of us were going to talk. "We try to work with the kids to teach them what the illness is, that it's chronic, like diabetes or arthritis, but it happens to be in their brain. We try to teach them illness management techniques."

"I have a manic-depressive illness that goes up and high, I mean up and low, I mean up and down," said Robyn, a pretty young woman with short, curly black hair. "I could be like, very high and blowing my money and be calling up some friends at certain times at night that were unnecessary. I lose control. I don't recognize the things I'm doing. It first started happening this year. I never had manic before." It showed itself, Robyn said, "by me talking so fast, interrupting people, and not letting other people say their speech. It's very scary because I don't recognize it as a problem."

Robyn told me she had been suicidal three years earlier. Her answers to my questions were informed but slightly circular, and Kutcher, reframing for me in a matter-of-fact tone, said, "Can you tell Ms. Fishman what happened when you were depressed, how you felt, and what you did at that time?"

"I had suicidal thoughts. I wanted to hang myself. I tried to take pills, I tried to stab myself, and that's how I got into the psychiatric hospital. I was fifteen, under age, so Children's Aid Society took me away from my family, and my dad had to go to court, and everything was a mess. After that they were treating me with medication, and I was paranoid. It was like an angel and a devil inside. It's like there was a demon controlling me, but then somewhere in my head I said, 'Do you want to live, Robyn? You have so much going for you. Stop, don't do it."

Robyn was taking Eprivel—the Canadian name for Depakote, a drug used in the past to treat epilepsy and recently discovered to be effective for mania as well—three times a day. She was also being weaned from Thorazine, the major tranquilizer necessary when the disease was at its peak. Her speech was slurry, like a patient with a mouthful of Novocain, and she seemed to radiate an aura of tension, as if she were a time bomb waiting to go off. She was not particularly insightful. With all this, however, what struck me as most dramatic was her complete lack of embarrassment in discussing her case; Robyn talked of the most extreme psychiatric symptoms as I would talk about the flu. "I don't feel any different after I take the pill," she said. "I just feel the pill's controlling the parts where I'm manic."

When I asked Robyn what life was like in the hospital, she stated a theme that recurred in her conversation throughout the time we spent together: "I don't like it here at all. The doctors are nice—I'm talking about the atmosphere. I don't like it here. I'm a young teenager, I should be having fun and enjoying myself. Here I'm stuck in the hospital, trapped, trapped! I have nothing against the staff, it's just this brick wall I stare at all day long—a brick wall! It feels like I'm not free. When my dad comes and gets me, I feel free, and I smell that fresh air!"

Robyn was due to go home in a couple of weeks and was being taught to manage her illness as she made a life outside the hospital. Kutcher's unit worked with a youth agency in Toronto. "They help with schooling and social integration and family work. We'll do the medical management and crisis work and intervention, and they'll do all the psychosocial and rehab work," he told me. In addition, Robyn had a primary therapist in the hospital, a ward nurse, and participated in group activities and school at the hospital.

Another theme of Robyn's conversation was "I won't get sick again," which Kutcher always countered with, "We hope you won't get sick again, and taking your medicine will help."

Today Kutcher was examining Robyn for side effects of the drugs. The Thorazine, she told him, "gives me a burned feeling and it stings, and it gives me a pain when I get up in the morning, pains in my legs."

"It's a terrible medicine," Kutcher agreed.

"It gives me blurry eyes, itchy skull, red face."

"I totally agree with that," Kutcher said. "And what have we been doing with that medication for the past three weeks?"

"We've been decreasing it."

"And what's the idea with that medicine? It calms you down. It gets the crazy thoughts out of your head. We will try to get you off the medicine completely, that's our goal. By the time you leave the hospital, you should be on just the Eprivel. The first thing we are going to go over is the subjective side effects. I'm going to ask you a bunch of questions, and you tell me if you have any of these."

Kutcher went through a standard form devised by the hospital pharmacy for monitoring side effects every three or four days; it served to jog the practitioner's memory. "You and I both know that sometimes these things can change. They can be worse one day and better another. Have you had any shakes in the last few days?"

"Yeah, when I pick up a mug, I have a tremor."

"And how bad are these tremors? Are they there all the time?"

"No, sometimes."

"If you had to rate those tremors from zero to four, zero never being there at all and four being there all the time and really bugging you, what would you give it? One is only when you pick up a mug, two would be you're sitting down and shaking a little bit, three would be a shaking all the time but it doesn't bug you. So what would it be?"

"Two," said Robyn.

"That's what I would have thought, so we're on the same track," Kutcher said, and turned to me. "Part of the discussion is to teach them how to evaluate. So what Robyn is going through is perfectly normal. We help kids understand the severity of their symptoms and whether the symptoms are present. Robyn will show you her mood charts, and how she's learned to identify when her mood is normal and when it's abnormal."

In this manner Robyn rated sleepiness, headaches, double vision, balance, numbness, tingling, muscle weakness, appetite, stomach pains, diarrhea, weight gain, hair loss. She and Kutcher reviewed the original purpose of the Thorazine. "It was helping you control your thinking so you wouldn't get these crazy thoughts, and the other things when you were really high—you couldn't sit still, you were running around and jumping up and down."

"And throwing food," Robyn put in.

"Throwing food and jumping on the furniture. You were pretty hostile. Now you're controlling that by yourself."

"I didn't know what was real and what was not. I was seeing movie stars."

"I was disappointed," Kutcher said, "because I was the only person you didn't think was a movie star."

Next Kutcher gave her the weekly physical examination for side effects: she had, for example, something called annular chilitis, little red rings on the sides of her mouth, which she treated with ointment. The rings would go away a few weeks after she finished the Thorazine. She stood with her feet together, closed her eyes, opened them, stood at ease, put her hands straight out with her fingers spread: Kutcher was checking the tremor, which he called "one plus." There were various exercises to check her movements and vision. "Now say this for me: 'No ifs, ands, or buts.' "

"No ifs, ands, no buts."

"No ifs, ands, or buts."

"No ifs, ands, or no buts."

She had to swing her arms and walk around. She opened wide and showed her reddish tongue, another mild symptom of Thorazine.

After the physical examination Kutcher, using a checklist, asked Robyn about her worries: these questions were similar to those I had heard Koplewicz asking. She worried about the future and the past—"I dwell on it," she said, worrying herself sick, worrying every day about her previous and possible future hospitalizations. This, Kutcher told me, would be a focus of the talk therapy Robyn was getting on the ward.

When the examination was over, Kutcher asked me if I would like Robyn to show me the ward while he made phone calls. Feeling a one-plus tremor, I went off with her, suspecting I was now a participant-observer, enlisted in some self-esteem-building part of Robyn's therapy. During the tour she repeated her themes, both the psychoeducation ("I couldn't help the fact I reached fifteen and got a mental illness") and the sadness at what the illness had done to her life; from time to time she wept a bit.

After leaving Robyn, I talked briefly with Kutcher alone. "She still has one of the hallmarks of the disorder, mood-lability," he said. "She can talk with you perfectly normally and all of a sudden she'll start to cry.

That's classic in manic-depression for teenagers. Before, her mood-lability was so intense that all of a sudden she'd throw things at you for no reason. She'd be sitting here just like you are, and then, boom, out it would go, or she would become totally grandiose, dance and sing and you couldn't even touch her, or she would become profoundly, abjectly, totally depressed to the point where she would just curl up and weep."

I asked Kutcher how the illness affected what professionals call "life-cycle tasks" of adolescence. "It gets in the way of completing the tasks," he said, logically enough. "The medicine is given to control the illness. It won't help them deal with their developmental tasks except for stopping the illness from interfering further. So adolescents learn to take care of themselves, to cook, to sew, to go to the bank, to take the bus—the normal social competencies. A lot of times the illness will hit the kid at fifteen or sixteen and when they turn eighteen or nineteen, they don't know how to do any of that. Other kids pick it up normally on their own; these kids have to be taught. Another thing is interpersonal relationships. These kids will hit the period of early dating not when they're fourteen or fifteen but when they're eighteen, nineteen, or twenty, and they need a lot of help because kids their age are way beyond." This is done by social workers after the kids leave the hospital.

Bipolar kids, Kutcher told me, develop normally until they get sick. Then, when "their cognitive functioning goes, it takes them months and months to get back to concentrating in school. It really rots your brain. We try to get them back up as much as we can." Robyn, of course, had started out as a slow learner before her first attack. Kutcher drew me a diagram of the bipolar patient, who declines in small steps with each attack. "The more times they get sick, the worse their outcome. So if they get sick once, and we can control it—I have patients who have one big illness. They've stayed on their medicine and done well. They've gone back to finish their master's degrees, and they're on their way."

Kutcher is now doing research on predicting the outcome of the illness; the stepwise effect of multiple attacks is one negative factor, and the kids' getting into drugs is another. Attention to self-esteem, he said, is of secondary importance relative to the real substantive help the kids need in doing their schoolwork and living their lives. In contrast he drew me another diagram of a schizophrenic teenager, who develops in a long, almost flat line before the first episode: "The illness manifests itself in subclinical form many years earlier. The kid starts out behind, and then they break."

As my own psychoeducation was finishing, Kutcher summed up, "We look at the whole patient, and that includes their biology as well as their psychology, their sociology, their institutions and networks. We are totally committed to people knowing what their illness is, and the treatment, and being very open about the pros and cons of everything, so Robyn knows exactly—and she's a 'slow learner,' so she doesn't quite have the grasp some other kids have."

Research in biological psychiatry has improved and altered the understanding of another elusive, mysterious adolescent problem, eating disorders. In view of the publicity they have received, these disorders are surprisingly rare: only 0.5 to 1.0 percent of girls and young women meet DSM-IV criteria for anorexia nervosa, and 1 to 3 percent meet criteria for bulimia nervosa; what the DSM calls "Eating Disorder Not Otherwise Specified" (in which the patient doesn't quite satisfy all the criteria for one or the other full-blown disorder) is more common. But since 90 percent of the patients are female and tend to be in the upper and upper-middle classes (including some celebrities), they have fascinated and frustrated practitioners of every therapeutic orientation, offering theorists the chance to have a field day expressing their views about gender issues.

Contemporary formulations add a surprising new dimension to the old clichés and thus another reason to give these disorders careful attention: once one starts questioning the conventional wisdom about some mental illnesses, it opens the mind to more pervasive revelations. My guide was Katherine Halmi, a former supervisor of Koplewicz's who heads the Eating Disorder Program at the Westchester Division of New York Hospital–Cornell Medical Center in White Plains. Halmi has devoted herself to the study of anorexia nervosa, bulimia nervosa, and their variations for the past twenty-five years; these days she is a researcher and administrator and no longer treats individual patients.

A book chapter Halmi sent me sums up what researchers now know—and don't know—about these disorders, which were first documented in the behavior of Saint Catherine of Siena. One reason eating disorders lend themselves to such varied interpretations is that, as Halmi observes, they are "entities or syndromes and not specific diseases with a common cause, common course, and common pathology." They provide a most dramatic illustration of the complex interaction between psychology and physiology.

The mechanisms for hunger and satiety are regulated by hormones in the hypothalamus and the gastrointestinal tract. Eating behavior varies according to the balance of certain neuropeptides and neurotransmitters, the individual's metabolic state and rate, the condition of her gastrointestinal tract, the amount of storage tissue she has, and the sensory receptors for taste and smell; quite obviously, it matters whether the food is or isn't appealing and the ambiance is or isn't stressful. As we learned earlier about psychiatric disorders in general, there are many points along the way where the system can be derailed.

In efforts to understand the biological side of eating, researchers have studied feeding patterns in animals and humans. With human subjects they have used drugs to probe and alter the onset and duration of eating—that is, one can induce anorectic behavior pharmacologically. Animal studies have probed the effects of stress on eating: researchers can bring on overeating by opening and closing tubes inserted in the esophagus and the stomach to determine whether satiety signals arise from oral, gastric, or intestinal sites.

The major criteria for anorexia nervosa as laid out in DSM-IV are refusal to maintain body weight over the minimal norm for age and height (at least 15 percent below normal is the figure cited); intense fear of gaining weight or becoming fat, even when underweight; disturbance in the way one's body weight or shape is experienced (in lay English, the individual thinks she's fat when she clearly isn't); and three months of amenorrhea—the cessation of menstruation—which, most important, can appear before noticeable weight loss has occurred.

There is, however, some characteristic behavior that does not occur invariably but should suggest to parents, pediatricians, and gynecologists that a teenager with amenorrhea should be checked out by a specialist in eating disorders. Anorectic patients may handle food peculiarly, hoarding cookies and candies in their pockets and purses; they "spend a good deal of time cutting food into small pieces and rearranging the food on their plates"; they may be preoccupied with collecting recipes and baking for friends and family (future chefs and people who just like to cook enjoy eating what they've made; anorectics only feed others); they may set up extremely rigorous exercise regimes and be constantly checking the mirrors to see if they're thin enough; and they may also follow an obsessive pattern of cleaning house and studying.

Anorectic patients come in two varieties: the restricting type, who simply starve themselves, and the bulimic type, who binge and purge. (Bulimia nervosa is a somewhat different disorder and is discussed hereafter.) Restricting anorectics tend to have delayed psychosexual development; bulimic anorectics, on the other hand, are often impulsive and may lean more toward suicide attempts, self-mutilation, stealing, substance abuse, and promiscuity. There are serious physiological and metabolic changes that result from starving or purging, although most go away once the patient is restored to normal weight. But because severely anorectic patients can starve themselves to death, they are often hospitalized.

The seriousness of the disease varies widely, ranging from one episode with complete recovery, through off-and-on rehabilitation and relapse, through a relentless lethal course. Less than a quarter of the patients in several long-term term studies were free of the psychological attitudes of the illness in middle age, although many were in better nutritional shape. Patients who got sick when they were older, remained ill for a long time, were hospitalized, had social and personality difficulties earlier in their lives, and had disturbed family relationships had a poor prognosis.

It is most important to understand that beyond the fact that anorexia nervosa always begins with a period of dieting or starvation, researchers and clinicians do not know of any specific etiology for the disorder: that is, everybody who diets is at risk, but only some individuals become anorectic. Which ones do is the source of controversy. Psychodynamic theorists have suggested that anorexia is a phobic avoidance of stress brought on by the physical changes of puberty; or fantasies of oral impregnation and dependent seductive relationships with warm, passive fathers, and guilt over aggressive and ambivalent feelings toward mothers; or untoward learning experiences that lead to cognitive misperceptions of body image and physical sensations.

The reasons anorectic patients began to diet, however, vary widely. Thus biological researchers suggest simply that some stressor disturbs hypothalamic function, which triggers amenorrhea. Malnutrition perpetuates this but doesn't cause it. Support for this hypothesis comes from the fact that when patients regain their body weight, they still don't return to normal menstruation for some time, and that marked psychological improvement is tied to the restoration of the menses. Neurotransmitter studies also support the hypothalamic theory, and twin studies show a better than 50 percent concordance for anorexia among identical twins, with only a one-in-fourteen concordance for fraternals: once again, we have, according to biologists' theory, a genetic vulnerability that is catalyzed by inappropriate dieting or emotional stress.

The vulnerability factor might be a personality type, a tendency to affective disorder, or a direct hypothalamic dysfunction. Family studies show, however, that while mood disorders are particularly prevalent among parents, children, and siblings of anorectics, the vulnerability doesn't work in the other direction: people with mood disorders don't have an unusual number of anorectic parents, children, and siblings. So being vulnerable to depression is not enough: one needs some particular vulnerability to anorexia. Halmi herself found a high prevalence of obsessive-compulsive disorder in the mothers of anorectic subjects.

Bulimia nervosa—the separate disorder—is marked by recurrent (meaning at least twice a week for three months) episodes of bingeing and what DSM-IV calls "inappropriate compensatory behavior." A binge episode means eating, in a two-hour period, a definitely larger amount of food than most people would eat in a similar period of time (this doesn't mean overdoing it at weddings and Thanksgiving dinner), and a sense that one can't stop eating or control the amount one is eating. The purging type of bulimics either vomit or abuse laxatives; the nonpurging type may compensate by dieting or exercising. Bulimics' self-esteem also hinges on body image. There is a milder form called binge eating disorder now listed in DSM-IV, which doesn't involve the purging but does include embarrassment, self-disgust, or guilt that may cause the patient to eat alone; the bingeing goes on twice a week for six months, and when the patient isn't hungry.

Bulimia nervosa usually follows a diet of several weeks to a year or longer. Some bulimics have scars called "Russell's sign" on the backs of their hands from sticking their fingers down their throats to induce vomiting, although many soon learn to vomit without the finger. Most bulimics don't eat regular meals and have trouble feeling full at the end of a meal; they prefer to eat alone at home. A significant minority will choose a reasonable weight as their ideal, resorting to inappropriate behavior only to maintain it. Most bulimics show symptoms of depression, with interpersonal problems, low self-esteem, anxiety, compulsiveness, impulsivity, and substance abuse (like the bulimic anorectics: indeed, up to a third of bulimics have a prior history of anorexia). Bulimics also steal—most often food, clothing, and jewelry.

Although bulimia is less often lethal than anorexia, purging leads to electrolyte imbalance and kidney dysfunction: thus bulimia can result in sudden cardiac arrest. Bulimics who abuse ipecac, an emetic syrup generally used to treat accidental poisoning, can also incur heart failure and death. Vomiting can lead to dental problems, esophageal tears, and shock. Except for the most severe cases, bulimia can more often be treated on an outpatient basis provided there is careful medical monitoring.

Studies—including Halmi's own—have shown disturbed perceptions of hunger and satiety in patients who binge and purge; moreover, patients with various eating disorders differ from each other in their tastes for sweetness and fattiness. Bulimics also often have affective disorders, substance abuse, and personality disorders and have scored significantly lower on social adjustment ratings than normal controls. Antidepressants have been moderately helpful in improving bulimic patients' mood, but the current treatment of choice is cognitive-behavioral therapy.

I talked with Halmi one winter Saturday at her home, a roomy and comfortable townhouse in Brooklyn. She drew me a diagram of the "Multimodal-Dimensional Model" of eating disorders, which essentially has three etiological aspects—the biological, the personality-and-family, and the sociocultural—all pointing to one circle, dieting, which then leads to varying degrees of malnutrition and bulimia. When dieting starts, the three etiological aspects are all in place. "A personality develops from birth on, affected by the influences in the environment, and the early environment, of course, is the family."

I asked her if this was the interaction between temperament and environment that Stella Chess and Alexander Thomas had described, and she said, "Exactly. This is an accumulative effect as the child grows up, and it expands into peers and the rest of the environment. What we have found in personality studies is that anorexia nervosa patients tend to have more of what we call a 'Cluster C' personality: they are more inhibited, more rigid, inflexible. That is a characteristic personality type that produces a vulnerability. This kind of person exists in a family milieu. The families are very complex, and they can vary a great deal. The family systems people like to promote a profile of all the eating-disorder families that simply is not true. If you have a theoretical bias about the illness and how the families are dysfunctional, you cannot accurately interpret the problems in front of you."

The families of patients at Halmi's eating disorder unit vary widely, she said. "Some are really very normal. They work with us beautifully, and we have few problems with them. Other families are extremely chaotic, with interfering problems of alcohol, drug abuse, or severe depression in the parents."

I asked Halmi about the old family systems view that the child is the symptom-bearer of conflict between the parents, and she said, "It's not universal at all. It's important when an eating-disordered child comes to a therapist that a family analysis be done, including an assessment for psychiatric illlness in the family, for the family's strengths, and not just focusing on their interactions with this child. The child also brings what I call biological vulnerability."

Halmi didn't want to talk much about the sociocultural aspect of eating disorders "because everybody talks about that. Dieting often starts because of pressures of society and culture, that's where I stand on it. We know there's a much higher prevalence of eating disorders in professions that demand eating and weight control. That again is your 'society and culture,' so it's highly prevalent in ballet dancers, actresses, models, male jockeys, gymnasts, and wrestlers. There's a high percentage of bulimia in wrestlers, all of whom binge and vomit, but not all have a psychiatric diagnosis of bulimia. Bulimia is bingeing and vomiting that is out of control."

I found it amazing that anyone could binge and vomit without being "out of control," and Halmi told me that the wrestlers do this during their competitive seasons and then resume a normal diet when not competing, all in the interests of fame and glory.

Halmi cautioned me that women between the ages of twenty and forty have actually significantly increased their weight since 1959. "The population is heavier, so there probably is some realistic need to diet and lose weight. I think that more women are working, they don't have time to prepare a lot of healthy foods, the quick foods are mainly high-fat foods, and people graze. All of that affects this realistic need to diet, and therefore more people are dieting and so putting themselves at risk for developing anorexia and bulimia. That's why I think bulimia has increased. I've gone to several conferences of pediatricians, and they are constantly emphasizing exercise, mobility—the amount of hours spent watching TV is enormous, and kids are no longer in good shape. This is an area of controversy, but there is some realism." In answer to my question, Halmi said she believes that people who obsess about weight and healthy eating are in a restricted socioeconomic class and are found especially in New York City, L.A., and San Francisco. "The minute you get out to the rest of America, the serious problem is obesity and inactivity.

"People diet for a whole variety of reasons, and to oversimplify that is inaccurate. A child can diet out of response to family stresses because Mommy and Daddy are threatening a divorce, and the child learns that if she becomes ill, that might hold them together. A child can diet because she's slightly pudgy and the boys make fun of her in junior high school and she gets very humiliated so she tries to get as thin as possible. A child can diet because she's a gymnast and needs to lose a little weight because she thinks she can perform better."

Whatever the teenager's reason for dieting, once she begins, big changes can occur. "For those who we think have a biological vulnerability," Halmi said, "this becomes an addictive cycle. Physiological changes reinforce the psychological motivations, and they cannot break out of this cycle."

I asked Halmi what constituted a biological vulnerability, and she told me that three neurotransmitter systems deal with food control. We have encountered them before: serotonin, norepinephrine, and dopamine. "We know from animal studies that they all influence appetite, satiety, the feeling of fullness, hunger, and eating behavior itself. These neurohormones are very interesting because changes in them are also present in depression, in obsessive-compulsive disorder, and in a lot of the associated problems we see in eating disorder patients.

Halmi explained further the neurochemical research process I had heard something about from Kruesi and Kutcher. "To go in and accurately measure the functioning of these neurohormones is next to impossible. There are only certain ways we can do it. We can measure the neurohormones and their metabolites in the blood, in the urine, in the cerebrospinal fluid, or we can use what we call neuropharmacological challenge tests—that is, we give a person one pill, a drug that we know will attach to a certain neurohormone receptor site, and that will produce a reaction, a release of another hormone into the blood that we can measure. A neuropharmacological challenge test is the closest way we can get some idea of what's going on in the brain.

"So one thing we're doing now is using a pill called fenfluramine. This facilitates the action of serotonin. Now serotonin causes humans and animals to feel satiated and end a meal. So it makes sense to see if the serotonin neurotransmitter system is functioning normally by testing it with a drug like fenfluramine. We give these patients a pill in the morning, they've fasted overnight, we put a needle in their arm, and the fenfluramine brings about the release of serotonin in the serotonin-containing cells of the brain."

Researchers cannot, of course, go right into the brain and measure the serotonin. They pick up the trail after an ensuing chain reaction in which the serotonin acts on the pituitary gland, which releases another hormone called prolactin. "We can measure prolactin in the blood, so after we've given the fenfluramine we draw blood every hour for five hours and measure the amount of prolactin released. What we're finding is that the bulimics are significantly deficient in this response compared with normal age-matched controls, so that indicates to us that there's something dysfunctional in the serotonergic system of bulimics."

The crucial issue is whether this kink in the serotonergic system of bulimics is there before they get sick or only after the illness has come on. And *that*—the inability to do prospective studies—is the bête noire of biological research in psychiatry.

"You would have to take a huge population in some school district and test them yearly. It's just prohibitive—the costs, and you couldn't get enough cooperation. So the prospective studies are virtually impossible to do. We study these people when they're ill, and we restudy them after they have returned to normal behavior. Our studies are showing that after they have stopped bingeing and vomiting for a month, they still have this abnormality in serotonin function. What we need to do now is test them after they have abstained from bingeing and vomiting for a year to see if the system is still abnormal.

"Some investigators have also measured serotonin metabolite products in the cerebral-spinal fluid. This neurotransmitter serotonin is metabolized in the brain. It's metabolized to something called 5-hydroxyindoleacetic acid, 5-HIAA." That is the substance Markus Kruesi measured in the cerebrospinal fluid of children with behavior disorders.

"This has been done in anorectic patients with and without bulimia,"

Halmi said, "and the study that did this showed that anorectics with bulimia had less of an accumulation of 5-HIAA compared with those who just restricted, again indicating that people who binge and vomit have something amiss with their serotonergic system. This is the way we approach this kind of research. The other thing I should mention is that many of the medications being used to help bulimics also affect the serotonergic system."

I asked Halmi about those wrestlers she'd mentioned who binge and vomit but are not abnormal. "Have they got a funny serotonergic system also?"

"Nobody has studied them," Halmi said. "It's extremely difficult to go in and study populations like that. There's enormous resistance from the coaches. It was virtually impossible to study anybody in the New York City Ballet. They have their own psychologists, and they are closed to the world in terms of any kind of study of eating behavior and disorders. That's not true with the Canadian Ballet Theatre, and so there have been some good studies done there that show they definitely have a higher prevalence. To do biological studies on those ballet dancers that restrain without getting sick and those that are sick is almost impossible. Maybe in ten or fifteen years, they'll be willing to allow people in—it's only to their benefit to learn how they can induce proper eating behavior and control it without the development of these illnesses."

Halmi is also interested in dopamine, "because animal studies show that neurotransmitter hormone to be implicated in self-stimulating behaviors—that is, addictions." Opiates are interactive with dopaminergic neurotransmitter systems. "The body's natural opiates, the endorphins, interact with dopamine in a self-stimulating type of addictive behavior," Halmi said. "So once it starts—with an anorectic dieting—the patient cannot stop, she's obsessive about it. She really cannot stop dieting. It has an addictive quality to it, and one becomes concerned about dopamines. I must say that in research there is a trendiness of getting funded for things, and the big trendy thing is serotonin, that's the neurotransmitter hormone of the decade. I have a certain amount of cynicism about all this.

"Dopamine is no longer as fashionable, but we did the same kind of challenge studies assessing dopamine, and we found abnormal responses. So there is something amiss with the dopaminergic system as well in both anorexia and bulimia. It was also abnormal after the anorectics gained their normal weight and maintained it for a month. I cannot answer whether these neurotransmitter systems are functioning normally a year or two later, because people will not come in for this kind of study. Once they get over it, they want to put it behind them. They don't want to be identified as having had this, and often their spouses do not know.

"Again, some studies with anorectics have shown dysfunction of the norepinephrine system. It has a lot of influence on the autonomic nervous system—heart rate, blood pressure, and so on. It does have definite effects on appetite and satiety, but they're not quite as marked as with serotonin and dopamine."

It isn't widely known, at least by nonspecialists, that as Halmi's papers point out, amenorrhea is often the first anorexic symptom and, surprisingly enough, not the result of starvation.

"Amenorrhea," Halmi said, "occurs first only in about one-third to a half of the population, but it is another indication that there is something primary going on, that starvation is not the sole cause of many of the hormonal abnormalities we see in anorexia. The whole complex hypothalamic pituitary ovarian cycle is not solely dependent on or manipulated by weight status. It's more complex than that."

"So people who have become anorectic have got a bunch of hormonal abnormalities?"

"Yes," Halmi said. "They're very subtle. Something is not functioning quite as robustly as it should, which makes them vulnerable to developing anorexia. When we weight-restore anorexia patients, many of them do not start menstruating right away. In fact, the average time of recurrence of menses is about a year after weight restoration. So those women who are maintaining a normal weight but not menstruating are more psychologically disturbed than those who have started again. The psychological well-being is very strongly related to the return of normal menstruation."

"Then there are aspects of depression or cognitive disorders that are secondary psychological effects of the patient not menstruating?" I asked.

"That's correct," Halmi said, "and that kind of psychological stress can influence the secretion of neurotransmitter hormones in the brain and other hormones that are necessary for normal menstruation to occur."

In other words, as I reviewed it with Halmi, this process *feeds* on itself, so to speak—and Halmi agreed. "Some of my readers are going to be parents," I continued. "What do they do when they see the beginnings, whether it's amenorrhea or some other early stages?"

"In very early stages," she told me, "they need to express their concern to their child and also give some thought to what's going on in the child's life, in the family life, and to the sources of stress that are encouraging dieting behavior or the fact that she's not menstruating. They need to try to talk to the child about it and get her onto a pattern now of facing whatever problems there are, including eating normally."

"But if the child is that way, it's going to be a constant fight with the parents."

If so, Halmi said, they should get some counseling. I asked whether pediatricians and gynecologists can "grab people before it gets too bad." She told me there is still no biological test for anorexia and bulimia. "It's not like phenylketonuria [the metabolic deficiency that produces retardation], where you have one enzyme that's abnormal, you can draw blood and measure that enzyme, and everything is cut and dried. These illnesses are disorders: they don't have a common etiology or even a common physiological path. They have multiple influences, including the biological influences. I'm not talking about one neurotransmitter hormone, I'm talking about *three*, and I haven't even told you yet about the neuropeptides that affect appetite and satiety. There are about ten peptides produced in the body that affect hunger, and all of these also interact with the neurotransmitters. So the whole system regulating food intake, eating behavior, and weight is extraordinarily complex, and there's no one thing that is wrong. There are different things that are not functioning well together as a system.

"This is not something the public or the drug companies or anybody else likes, because they like to find one simple thing you can give a pill for and cure. You're *never* going to be able to do that with eating disorders. There is no single cause. We're never going to find a single etiological basis for this—there is a confluence of a lot of different things that produce and sustain these abnormal eating behavior disorders."

I asked Halmi whether the biological aspects of anorexia and bulimia necessitate treatment by an M.D., and she told me, to my surprise, that since cognitive-behavioral therapy can be quite effective with mild cases, licensed clinical psychologists and M.S.W.s are acceptable; ministers, chaplains, and counselors are problematic because they have not been vetted. "I think it's necessary that a physician examine the child and get some baseline data—height, weight, certain blood studies—and that the therapist who is not a physician have a physician back up, so that if the bulimic has a whole streak of vomiting and goes into a severe electrolyte imbalance or cardiac arrhythmia, she can be hospitalized. An anorectic who is more than fifteen percent below normal weight or has not gotten back to normal weight within six months absolutely has to be referred to a qualified M.D. for further care, because the longer she stays underweight, the less chance she has of being cured. It's important to aggressively treat anorectics and get them up to normal weight and into an intensive psychotherapy program right away."

The million-dollar question in eating disorders is why, of the many people who diet, only a few develop anorexia or bulimia; the million-dollar subquestion is why most of these people are women—and this is most often answered in cultural terms. But after our talk Halmi sent me two studies done at the University of Oxford that showed that dieting— three weeks of ordinary calorie-cutting by male and female subjects with no personal or family history of psychiatric disorder—altered the sero- tonergic functioning of women but not men. And as the studies pointed out and as Halmi had told me, reduced serotonin function has been linked to impaired satiety, binge eating, poor impulse control, amenor- rhea, and depressive symptoms: that is, women more than men, and some women in particular, may be biologically vulnerable to developing eating disorders when they diet.

At the end of my conversation with Halmi, I remarked on the high burnout rate among therapists with her interest. A number of clinicians I'd met described this as a *former* specialty, and indeed, Halmi herself had just changed assistant directors. "The people who stay with the disorders," she said, "enjoy the challenge of it. The patients are extraordinarily difficult to treat, especially the psychotherapy of an anorectic. Once this gets going, there's a reinforcement of this maladaptive behavior that is so strong that she can't give it up. She gets an enormous amount of control and power. She's controlling literally the entire family, her entire environment, with her illness. That control issue really frustrates the family because you can't beat up on an emaciated kid. The child has made everybody in her environment completely impotent. I find it a fascinating problem and an extremely clever adaptation. Who would ever want to give up this power and control? It's meeting all the needs of this kid."

"I suppose you respect your opposition in a way," I said. "Now and then I have encountered therapists who will laugh in fascination at what a patient will do—at how clever the patient is in maintaining pathology."

"Those are better therapists in the long run," Halmi said. "If the patient starts controlling you or you can't see the humor or you can't stand back and be fascinated, then you burn out."

Our visits with Koplewicz focused on individual cases; those with Kruesi, Kutcher, and Halmi, as well as Gabrielle Carlson, the biologically oriented psychiatrist in Chapter 2, showed us some zealous bloodhounds on the research trail. After all this specificity I felt the need for a wrap, and so, I assume, does the reader. Toward this end I talked with Charles Popper about how he weaves the biological viewpoint into observing the clinical course of illness and therapy. Popper, born in 1946, is a clinician, writer, and editor who doesn't do formal research. He is the former director of child and adolescent psychopharmacology at the Hall-Mercer Center for Children and Adolescents at McLean Hospital and Harvard Medical School; to land at McLean—recently in the news as the setting for Susanna Kaysen's best-seller, *Girl, Interrupted*—a patient needs a serious disorder. Popper, now in private practice, is one of two editors of the *Journal of Child and Adolescent Psychopharmacology,* writes a quarterly column on the subject for the *Newsletter of the American Academy of Child and Adolescent Psychiatry,* and has edited or co-authored two books.

"Almost all of the disorders of children that are currently labeled in the DSM have at least some evidence of a genetic basis," Popper told me. "For attention deficit disorder there is perhaps stronger evidence than there is for others, but certainly for depression, bipolar disorder, anxiety disorders, certain phobic disorders, to a degree for autism, definitely for Tourette's disorder, for obsessive-compulsive disorders, and anorexia, there is quite good evidence that these can be conceptualized as medical disorders with metabolic abnormalities that are inherited, transmitted, or at least modified by gene function. What we can't say is that the genes are the cause or even the predominant factor. A person may be, at least in theory, quite loaded genetically for a particular disorder and still wind up not having it.

"Parenting experiences," he said, "certainly are one of many environmental influences that govern the way life works: like genes, they may be stronger in some cases, weaker in others. A person may have genetic loading for depression and lead a relatively ordinary life and still end up with a tremendously severe depression, either very brief or very lengthy. They may have a very severe genetic loading and not wind up with any depression at all, or they may have minimal genetic loading but because of life circumstances look as though they have the medical disorder and may perhaps even have it.

"There's no absolute determinism about this. But although this really hasn't been shown, my clinical sense is that some people have a sufficiently strong genetic load that despite a very supportive family, very reasonable ordinary life circumstances, and all the cards stacked in the right direction, they may still wind up with a depression. What's different in these 'high-ego' kids coming from 'high-ego' families is that they may get a depression that presents in a different manner from other kinds. Let's say they're manic-depressive. They may come into the hospital psychotic or nearly psychotic or severely depressed. They may get drug-treated, get some supportive help from staff and their parents, be given some education about the nature of the problem, and basically with medication and relatively minimal support, they will be able to be back at school three months later, and for all the world, you can stand on your head, there's no psychotherapy to be done. The family is supportive, the kid has a solid self and is able to understand that by staying on medication they can significantly decrease their risk of having a recurrence.

"The same kid, though, perhaps coming from a less supportive family, with parents who may be totally well-meaning but quite depressed and overwhelmed and they don't know how to handle it— the father may be alcoholic or absent or violent and not able to stand the symptoms the kid brings into the family—that kid may be drug-treated, and although the biological component of the disorder is in relatively good shape, the kid may, even with simple kinds of support and education, have a very complicated course of illness that would look as though they've made relatively little progress. They may still tantrum because they're scared of what their father might do, or they may feel enormously guilty and avoidant of people because they had a fantasy that it was their own depression that caused their mother's depression."

"So some psychodynamic therapy may be needed for such kids?" I asked.

"Intensive psychotherapy for a long term can be used often, typically in combination, for complicated situations. Drug treatment may make a difference to the biology and stabilize some of the impulses and too-strong feelings but still leave the child looking quite symptomatic."

I asked Popper whether any child would walk into McLean Hospital with those symptoms and without *any* biological factor at all—a child, perhaps, from a truly chaotic family. Popper said that without biological loading "the odds of the environment getting so horrendous that they wind up being hospitalized is very, very small. I maybe have seen it once or twice out of the probably fifteen hundred kids who have been hospitalized here."

I pressed Popper—"Megasexual abuse and violence and beating around?"—and he said, "One person in the environment can make a huge difference. Many kids have a grandmother or a next-door neighbor or one parent who doesn't beat and will be supportive, and those islands can go a long way. In terms of hospitalization, usually if there's some support, most psychiatric hospitals do everything they can to keep kids from being hospitalized unless they really need it, which generally means there's no one who can pick up the slack.

"Usually in cases of abuse several factors operate that blur the boundary between biology and the social environment. Much child abuse comes from families that are already rife with medical disorders of a psychiatric nature, so there's this whole genetic line running through this family. Secondly, a child who's abused sexually or physically in many cases winds up with posttraumatic stress disorder, which can be conceptualized in a variety of ways. You can think of it as a purely psychological trauma that's created a disorder of feelings, thoughts, and behaviors, and that corresponds to older kinds of thinking about what early trauma might do. These days it's becoming increasingly clear that there's a very large biological effect.

"The old way of thinking medically would lead one to think, 'There is a problem. Here's a symptom.' In psychiatry genes don't operate that way, trauma doesn't operate that way, no single environmental factor operates that way. Each factor may be more important in one particular case. A child who is quite sturdy with environmental stress at one point may become vulnerable to a lesser environmental stress later on. We don't know why. It could be psychological factors, it could be developmental factors, it could be biological factors, it could be the next-door neighbor who wasn't available. I don't mean somebody becomes chronically depressed if the grandmother isn't there, but there are a variety of factors."

"Perhaps," I suggested, "the biggest advance we've made in a couple of decades is knowing what we don't know."

"That's fair. Even if you sum up all the biology, all the environment, all the medical factors of different sorts, the sociological factors you might put together, you can never say, 'Now I know why this child has this problem.' "

There is some art involved in understanding individual cases, Popper said, but translating impressions into treatment plans requires a move into a sort of quasi-science: that is, the practitioner must make some choice from a range of possible treatments. "It's very rare—and pretty weak thinking—to say 'Here is the symptom, there is the treatment.' Actual treatment incorporates continual modifications."

As we've seen, modern clinicians, particularly those who are biologically oriented, are less likely than their predecessors to lay blame on parents for a child's disorder. But the responsibility of parents, once the disorder has appeared, is very clear. As Popper says, "A kid with very severe biological and psychological depression who comes from a family that knows to *get* the help, knows *how* to get the help, knows how to help the kid *receive* the help, that kid may be able to have a very ordinary life course, even if the biological illness is long-term and severe. They may go through school—they may even become a senator, and if they know how to get treatment, no one except their intimates may ever know anything about it. But someone with a very mild depression who avoids treatment, who's scared of treatment and doesn't like being put in the position of being a patient or receiving help, even with a mild depression, may end up with chronic underachievement, a lower level of employability, a lower income, lower satisfaction. It's really not the diagnosis or even the severity that necessarily indicates the course. The ability to get help can in some cases be a stronger factor."

Popper, like the other psychopharmacologists I met, often works with children and their families together. He points out that parent and child have different information, that both are inclined to distort some data, and the therapist has to figure out how best to judge, from not totally reliable sources, what's going on. He prefers to get them together so he can hear—and they can hear—their reactions to each other. Often one person will have very good evidence that something is getting better when others haven't seen it yet, or the child may be denying problems that parents can help clarify.

This isn't, however, actual family systems work as, say, Richard Chasin would understand it. But dynamic issues, Popper says, do come up. "They have to do with recognition of the problems, the choice to get help for them. The pill gives a concrete focus to this: one can see it, one takes it at a particular time of day, and the resistances, the fears about the therapy, the exaggerations about what the drug might be able to do are much more discussable. These real factors are loaded with individual and family transferences, so I end up dealing with some of the deeper issues that would eventually go on in the child's or the parents' psychotherapy. It's not just writing a prescription: there's real work that needs to be done."

Popper's training, at Harvard Medical School and Massachusetts General Hospital in the early seventies, was, according to the attitudes of that time, psychodynamic in emphasis. "What I kept running into," he said, "was supervisors who would be very skilled in dynamics and in being able to demonstrate how empathy can be a tool in therapy. But I kept being frustrated that there was a failure to empathize with the child's body, to experience the depression that a child would have as a physical thing, or they wouldn't readily *feel* how the attention was continually being disrupted by invisible but powerful forces like ADD.

"The dynamic people say every child has a conflict, or every child has a developmental stickiness. I know that the very occasional psychiatrist who thinks purely in biological terms is surely missing all the other stuff that needs to be done. What I do with a child is move back and forth very quickly between psychological and biological, family and cognitive-behavioral. If I find myself really getting into one particular area for a lengthy period of a session, it may be valid, but it's a red flag for me to see if I've let go of something theoretically that may be relevant. I will typically do the medication piece first and then go on to what other things there are. I want to know what happens once the medical disorder is getting clearer.

"The whole field is very young. There is a lot we don't know. We don't know about the efficacy and safety of many of the drugs. They're not as well studied in children as they are in adults, we don't have that long a track record in using them, and parents should be aware of that. It's easy to view different schools of treatment as opposing each other, and certainly there has been some historical sense of territory or property or rivalry or competition. But I think that to a large extent that has passed, and the average psychiatrist embraces a complementary role for different types of treatment."

PART VI

PUTTING IT ALL TOGETHER

CHAPTER 16

"ALIVE WITH PATHOLOGY"

Since what bothers us most about normal children is the problem of behavioral control and the question of just how to help them in their ability to cope with their emotions and impulses from within in a "well-adjusted" way, we have set about to study this same problem with the severely disturbed, hyperaggressive child. The extremeness of his behavior makes some of the details look different, but the basic machinery involved in the task of self-control and the problems of influence techniques remains the same. . . .

There is still a wide gap between the hatred which a well taken care of middle class child develops as a side line to his anxiety or compulsion neurosis and that of the slum area delinquent who has had to survive by aggression in a world of struggle. And there is still a great difference between the child who occasionally kicks back at frustrations or expresses the negative side of an ambivalent feeling toward brother or sister and the child who has been reeling under the impact of cruelty and neglect to such a degree that the acid of counter-aggression has eaten itself by now into the very stomach linings of his adaptational system.

—Fritz Redl and David Wineman,
Children Who Hate (1951)

THE READER SHOULD BY NOW HAVE PICKED UP my own view that each therapeutic orientation has something compelling to offer but none has the whole truth, that it is very likely that a child with a psychological disorder will need exposure to more than one type of therapy, and that this need increases with the seriousness of the child's problem; moreover, to the extent that clinicians assess children's disorders through only one diagnostic prism, they resemble the blind men and the elephant.

455

This judgment is not novel; it reflects the direction of most good practitioners' pious hopes. It is only early training, clinical habit, and the pressures of daily life—plus human defensiveness about all one's sins of omission—that interfere with their movement toward some greater degree of what is known in the field as eclecticism. Still, the term *eclecticism* is unfortunate: it implies a sort of undirected grabbing at any old thing. *Synthesis,* on the other hand, suggests not only a more meaningful selection but a second step, that of combining what one has selected in the most useful and powerful way.

Is anyone doing this optimally? Can we see how it works?

Early in my research for this book, two therapists—one psychodynamic, one cognitive-behavioral—suggested I take a look at Wediko Children's Services, an organization that provides short-term residential treatment for seriously disturbed children in a pastoral setting in Windsor, New Hampshire, as well as outpatient therapy for these and similar children and their families through the Boston public schools.

Wediko was founded in 1934 on the principle that camping itself could be therapeutic for troubled children; originally under the aegis of Harvard's Judge Baker Guidance Center, it was, in fact, the country's first treatment camp. Over the past twenty-four years it has become increasingly clinical (having individuated in the Mahlerian sense, it is no longer affiliated with the Baker), adding programs, staff, and ever more purposeful and sophisticated individual treatment plans, education, and research. During a recent summer when I spent considerable time at Wediko, half of its funding (by way of fees for the children referred) came from the Boston Public School System, 17 percent came from New Hampshire cities and towns, 7.5 percent came from the Casey Family Institute (a Connecticut-based adoption and foster-care agency), and smaller amounts came from the Massachusetts Department of Social Services, the federal government, the New Hampshire Division of Child and Youth Services, and private foundations. Up to 170 children participate in its forty-five-day summer program, and two winter programs—three and four months long—accommodate nearly thirty boys. (Girls are less often referred for residential care, and there haven't been enough to constitute a winter group.) The word *camp*—which suggests a frill beyond the current budgets of government agencies—is now X-rated at Wediko, and at least while the directors are listening, counselors are called "staff."

I first visited Wediko for three days in the middle of the summer. The following summer I spent five days at the beginning, three days in the middle, and three days at the end of the program, following two groups of children to watch their progress. A couple of years later, I returned during the winter season to update myself, and over the course of my research I also visited Wediko's Boston offices from time to time. I had many long conversations with Hugh M. Leichtman, the administrative director, Harry W. Parad, the clinical director; and various members of their senior staff. I came to know the organization and its people quite well, and as my own general knowledge increased, so did my fascination with their intricate blending of therapeutic approaches. Wediko is something of a family business: Leichtman's and Parad's wives work year-round in the Boston office, and Leichtman's sister-in-law and brother-in-law are on the staff in New Hampshire. It is not an overstatement to say these two families have been eating, sleeping, and breathing Wediko 365 days a year for two and a half decades, a commitment of particularly daunting intensity to anyone who has spent time in that environment. Leichtman and Parad don't write papers for journals: there are, after all, only thirty hours in a day.

Moreover, the place doesn't stand still: each time I returned, the two directors were absorbed in some new clinical phenomenon. Like all the lead therapists in this book, they gave me, at my request, a basic reading list. Unlike the other therapists' lists, theirs drew from every orientation. It ranged from Bettelheim to Minuchin to Chess and Thomas to Garmezy and Rutter. In a conversation with Leichtman or Parad, I might hear Margaret Mahler one minute, B. F. Skinner the next, and Abraham Maslow, the humanistic psychologist, the next. The spirit of Donald Winnicott hovered over the explanations of staff members; people even occasionally cited Freud.

What was the reason for this? First of all, there were the children themselves. "Outside of autism, frank psychotic presentations, and the mild clinical symptoms you see in most outpatients, we've got everything," Leichtman told me the first time we drove from Boston to New Hampshire. "If you eliminate those two ends of the spectrum, there's nothing in childhood pathology you can't see here: eating disorders, moderate-to-moving-toward-severe depression, every symptom of trauma you can possibly think of, borderline and narcissistic personality disorders, conduct disorders, antisocial, bipolar, various neurological disorders, learning disabilities, the range of ADD subgroups, schizotypal, pervasive atypical developmental delays, mild atypical developmental delays. All moving from that moderate-to-serious to severe end of the spectrum. Not in the profound range, but most of the children show indicators that if we can't turn their development around, they'll keep sliding."

In the season I spent time there, about 70 percent of Wediko's summer children were boys; just over half were white, and most of the rest were African-American, with a sprinkling of Latinos. More than four-fifths qualified for food assistance, and at least one in four lived with caretakers other than their biological parents. A number of these children had middle-class foster parents: as Parad told me, "The family may drive up in a Volvo but the child didn't grow up with a Volvo: the child grew up being switched from home to home every few months." Several years later Parad, discussing differences in race and socioeconomic status among Wediko's population, pointed out that "the New Hampshire children— who are virtually all white and who come from communities where gangs don't exist in the conventional sense—don't look one whit healthier than the Boston children. They're just as aggressive, just as likely to have tantrums, just as likely to affiliate in aggressive delinquent ways, just as likely to do *everything,* and they're arguably more likely just because they've received fewer services. I can't say that the cultural surround has made one group easier to work with than another group."

Leichtman and Parad, who both have Ph.D.s in clinical psychology, are opposites both in temperament and in familial and educational backgrounds. Leichtman, born in 1943, is an intense man with sharp eyes, boyish features, and receding silver hair; while his route into child psychology was circuitous, the fact that he was what family systems people call a "parental child," in the custody of a father who frequently left him to care for siblings and cousins, can hardly be irrelevant. His early training was cognitive-behavioral; postdoctoral studies leaned toward the psychodynamic. Parad, on the other hand, born in 1949, is the son of two therapists with D.S.W. degrees who actually worked at Wediko during his childhood: his father, Howard Parad, was later dean of the School of Social Work at Smith College and is a well-known theorist in crisis intervention. The younger Parad—who looks a whole lot like Groucho Marx and whose manner is as dryly humorous and understated as Leichtman's is frenetic—did graduate study in social work and special education and then received training with a strong classical psychodynamic emphasis; in essence, he is doing what he was born to do. But these days Leichtman tends to focus on individual "pivotal" children whose cases he finds illuminating, and he often (though not always) sounds psychodynamic, while Parad thinks more about the overall program and often (though not always) sounds behavioral.

When we first drove from Boston to Wediko, Leichtman told me, "These are children who are showing at least two-year lags in social adaptive skills. They have many problems that disrupt growth in at least two of four basic spheres: the development of the 'self-system,' the capacity to function in school, the capacity to function in a family, and social functioning. About four-fifths of the girls and one-fifth of the boys have been sexually abused, and four-fifths of the boys have been physically abused. More than half the population show ADD characteristics, and another significant percentage show what Chess and Thomas call 'difficult temperament': they're out of sync with their parents. With these children you never think in terms of a cure—you're always thinking in terms of *process*: How do we realign this child's development so it begins to approach age-appropriate levels of functioning?

"Do one thing: hang with the complexity. If you talk globally, I'm going to jump all over you. Think in subgroups of children, never in unified ways. You will see a child in one context functioning quite well and another where his functioning falls apart. Things we thought in the past were entirely psychogenic have a neurological component, particularly when there's ADD. But very often, under stress, the residue of early trauma overwhelms children, and they cannot process information. They are not hallucinating, but they are having a transient breakdown in reality testing. They just lose it: they have severe tantrums. Kids get here because the school system says, 'You're not making it in this school.' Parents are telling adopted kids, 'You're destroying this family,' and ADD kids, 'We can't contend with your impulses anymore.' For younger children, the Department of Social Services is saying they're at such high risk for abuse that they need protection. For adolescents, the law is breathing down their necks.

"At some point we always develop a historical perspective of where things went wrong. But we're not interested in history at first. It's irrelevant until they're on track; that's why many of these kids fail in therapy. When your life is chaotic, what good does it do if you understand it's because your parents beat you? It takes the first three to four hundred hours of back-breaking work with these kids to define limits, label behavior, make sure consequences are absolutely consistent, and teach them to listen so that information is processed and sequenced and the children own their behavior and recognize its impact. We never ask children how they feel: they just say, 'I dunno.' They don't identify gradients of emotion, like 'Now I'm getting pissed; I'm pissed; I'm *really* pissed; now you've really got me going; now I'm furious; I've lost it.' Our guys have nothing between 'I'm mad' and 'I've lost it.' "

This was as clear an explanation of the psychobabble cliché "getting in touch with your feelings" as I'd heard.

So the children themselves need more than one kind of therapy; what's more, the milieu dictates it, as Parad explained when I met him. After three weeks as an outpatient, a child has had about six hours of therapy. After three weeks at Wediko, a child has had 336 hours of therapy—or more precisely, therapeutic interventions.

"We live with severely disturbed children twenty-four hours a day," he said. "All the staff works all the shifts, with only five days off while the children are here. We don't leave at five o'clock or go home on weekends. What that does is, we care about what behavior means, which would be a psychodynamic perspective—the way each of us chooses to behave today reflects unconscious parts of ourselves and experiences that go all the way back to our childhood. But when you've lived with these children, somewhere between day seven and day ten, virtually everybody here is going to have moments when they feel incredibly frustrated with the way these children behave. In those moments they won't care why the children are doing things. They won't care what the symbolism is. They won't care that they've had horrible experiences early in life. The empathy will be out the window. All they'll want at that point is for the behavior to change, and that's the feedback we give the children. We need the behavior to change, and that forces us to say, 'How am I going to change the behavior?' A host of techniques have come about from that need."

The staffing pattern at Wediko reflects the way therapy is done: each group of eight to ten kids has a staff of six, four living with the group and the other two spending part of the day on other duties. The staffers are college juniors and seniors and recent graduates deciding whether to enter the field; the supervisors are graduate students and professionals, including an upper level with ten or more years of clinical experience. "We decided to put our resources into the people that spend hour after hour with the kids," Parad told me. "That's making a conceptual decision that what's more important for children than one hour a week of talking and reflecting and symbolic play is helping the children see the pattern of their own behavior as it unfolds across carefully structured situations hour after hour, situation after situation, day after day. We like one-liners at Wediko, so we say we believe in psychodynamic formulations—and the best techniques to use with them are cognitive-behavioral. If Freud were around today, we're sure he would agree with us."

Thus the senior staff is expected to be conversant, at minimum, with Freud, Erikson, Mahler, and Sullivan. At the same time each kid during the summer works with a staff member to develop a cognitive-behavioral contract that, in psychodynamic terms, expresses the child's basic developmental conflict (a teenager is replaying late-two-year-old struggles around autonomy, for example) and the behavioral choices that flow from it. This is all framed in snappy kid-language: Shawn must decrease his "my way or no way behavior" (which is the way Parad remembers his own children as toddlers) and act like "Mr. Elastic," who is able to compromise.

A psychopharmacologist consults to Wediko, visiting once a week. While medication is not the cutting edge of therapy here, the children come up with the full gamut of medicines. "This is a very safe place to try them out," Parad said, "because we can observe the child around the clock. Medication often has quite a dramatic effect: it doesn't change how the children think or what they think about, but it makes the difference between 'The impulse is in my head, and I do it' and 'The impulse is in my head—I feel like sluggin' you. I'm gonna walk over here. Now I can talk about it.' It buys the child a few split seconds to think."

While Bruno Bettelheim is credited with originating the term *milieu therapy* in the United States, the therapeutic milieu is a mode that goes back to August Aichhorn's work with delinquents in Vienna, described in his 1925 book called *Wayward Youth*—with a foreword by Freud himself. The first to apply Freud's theories to this population, Aichhorn believed, with Freud, that "emotion blocked in its direct outlet seeks discharge over a devious pathway"—an idea now considered old-fashioned but abundantly visible at Wediko—and while much has been learned since Aichhorn's day, some of his formulations, particularly that "a predisposition to delinquency" is "the factor without which an unfavourable environment can have no power over the child," might have been written yesterday by Markus Kruesi, the biological psychiatrist we met in Chapter 14. (Indeed, Aichhorn observed that "thousands of children grow up under the same unfavourable circumstances and still are not delinquent. There must be something in the child itself which the environment brings out.")

Aichhorn differentiated between what he called "border-line neurotic cases with dissocial symptoms," dissocial children in open conflict with the environment, and normal or neurotic children; each requires a different treatment approach. In Leichtman's phrase, he was beginning to hang with the complexity. From his Freudian base he proceeded intuitively and creatively. But what is most dramatic is the accuracy of his observations and the effectiveness of his interventions, measured against what I saw at Wediko. Aichhorn was in the trenches, and he observed, up close, the same skewed development, short attention span, and poor judgment. Among his worst cases, "aggression which had proved effective in the old environment did not bring forth the expected and desired response," so the child kept escalating his behavior to provoke the worker; absent the severe punitive response, the child "would no longer have any justification for his whole attitude toward life." The aggression would reach a climax, finally bringing forth "violent emotion which spent itself in weeping with rage," a period of emotional instability, a series of less intense outbreaks, and finally an emotional bond between the boys and the workers; after this the boys would follow the rules. I watched this happen sixty-five years later; the Rudolfs and Ottos were reincarnated as Tony and Lance and Jeff and Earl.

Bruno Bettelheim, the articulate and theoretically fecund founder of the Sonia Shankman Orthogenic School at the University of Chicago, is now a controversial figure, both because of his despotic behavior (actually irrelevant to his theories) and because many of his formulations have been disproven; while he also contributed a number of still-useful ideas, the highly speculative nature of his writing seems dated to the modern reader. His friends and peers, Fritz Redl and David Wineman, who briefly ran a school called Pioneer House in Detroit and wrote a powerful book called *Children Who Hate,* seem more relevant. Leichtman and Parad mentioned Redl and Wineman often to me, and I frequently felt Wediko was Pioneer House reborn.

Essentially Redl and Wineman—who were wonderfully perceptive analysts of children's behavior but didn't concern themselves with biological factors—said that delinquents face the same developmental challenges that confront normal children, but their brutal histories have altered them: there is "a great difference between the child who breaks out in some minor aggressive rebellion from time to time in the classroom, or who betrays deep-seated death wishes against us through the medium of finger paint, and the child whose aggression seems to flow uninhibited, skipping even the in-between stage of fantasy, into direct action of reckless destruction or into flare-ups of blind and murderous rage." It is important that nonprofessionals enamored of simplistic solutions keep this in mind. Redl and Wineman also noticed the behavior of foster children, "under the impact of trauma or fright . . . [who] become unmanageable or run away as soon as the foster parent begins to be really loving and accepting . . . they can take anything but affection, even though they seem to need it so much." For such children, conventional methods don't work: in mainstream groups they menace the other kids, but cold and restrictive institutions only feed their "persecutory interpretation of life," so that neither friendliness nor punishment is successful. And the atmosphere of a private psychiatrist's office, not to mention the expectations of talk or play, is utterly foreign to them.

Like Aichhorn and Bettelheim, Redl and Wineman began with unconditional love and affection, programmed activities the kids could handle, and worked via "the clinical exploitation of life events." Once again, I saw interventions used at Pioneer House carried out at Wediko. I also met the children Redl and Wineman wrote about: almost every descriptive phrase in *Children Who Hate* echoed down the years with eerie resonance. Wediko, however, has been able to refine its techniques over four more decades of knowledge and experience. (Redl and Wineman, interestingly, were terrific therapists but hopeless fund-raisers, which is why Pioneer House didn't survive.) There are other such milieus around the country, some more famous than Wediko. But the personal commitment of its staff—enforced and exploited by the design of the place—and its synthesis of approaches are distinctive.

My first sight of Wediko took me back to the camps of my childhood, the piney paths with bunks on stilts, the buggy playing fields, the lakefront, the complex of New England clapboard houses that form the nucleus of activity. It was pouring rain, and the hooded ponchos looked familiar too. It required a few minutes to zero in on what was not quite right: small groups on the muddy lawn, always triads, two young adults and a child. The child was struggling to bite, kick, and punch and sometimes succeeding. The adults were using all their strength to hold the child and were talking softly to him or her. From a distance it looked like cockroaches mating.

I was walking with Tod Rossi, a (then) forty-one-year-old Ph.D. who was (and still is) the *primus inter pares* supervisor. Rossi darted over to two women holding a ten-year-old boy in a turquoise sweatshirt. The boy had straw-colored hair and the face of a cherub, which was then red and swollen with rage and tears. In a matter-of-fact tone Rossi said to me, "Billy has had a hard life, and he sometimes has trouble listening."

"Don't tell her about my fuckin' life," said Billy.

"Okay," Rossi said pleasantly. "I'm respecting your privacy. I'm not doing what you tell me. You've got to separate those two things."

"I don't give a shit," Billy said.

Rossi, a dark, wiry man, continued talking softly to the staffers and me. He said all this rain was hard for everybody and asked if that was Mary's car over there. Suddenly Billy, who had been quieting down, began to kick and struggle again.

"I just want you to know that I'm not taking my attention away from you, Billy," Rossi said gently. "I'm giving you my attention back." Gradually Billy got calmer, and Rossi and I resumed our walk.

"This kid has been hospitalized," Rossi said as we sloshed up the trail. "He has been in residential institutions for much of his life. He is used to impersonal restraints and being loaded with Thorazine. We don't go in those directions here. We don't have time-out rooms, we don't have padded cells—we have people. What we do is hold a kid with as many people as are necessary to keep that kid safe for as long as he needs to work out of where he is. The reason a kid would get to this state almost invariably is because of the absence of what we call self-soothing mechanisms.

"The most primitive self-soothing mechanism is eating. Often the mother is cooing into the baby's ears, babbling while breast-feeding or bottle-feeding is going on, so the next phase of self-soothing is babbling.

If you have kids, you know at around seven months they stop waking up with a cry: suddenly there's this blissful period when they're babbling to themselves, representing you as the mother. That's the next self-soothing mechanism that happens. After food comes the human voice. When you have a kid in a restraint like this, you hear us babbling like a mother soothing a baby.

"It's very important," Rossi went on, "especially in this state of increasing agitation, to make it clear that we retain the ability to control them, because what is very consistent with the earliest stages of psychological development is periods of omnipotence, feeling that one is in fact the whole world and able to control everything. For somebody with the almost adult-size body this boy has, the perception of omnipotence can make one very dangerous.

"So I made it very clear that I was still in charge of my decisions and my body—and at that point his body too—by saying that I was not talking about his life because I respected his privacy, not because he was bossing me around. We must be very careful about those distinctions. Had he continued to have the sense that he could boss me around, that could escalate out of hand within moments—you can see it.

"Likewise, these poor kids live in a dilemma: although he said he didn't want me talking about his fucking life, he was really engaging me so that when I started to talk about other things, his body became very tense and he began to kick and struggle. Then I had to reassure him. With an infant-size body one would hardly notice. An infant might experience the precursors of rage and stiffen up momentarily, and if you were holding him, you would barely notice it. It would be a fidget. The infant might even swing out a fist, and that might be cute.

"So we need a very careful process of reintegrating the *affects* into the size body and size intellect and size world that the children now have."

Rossi's discussion was pure Winnicott. But therapists in hospitals and other residential facilities disagree about what kind of restraint is optimal. Some believe that holding can evoke sexual memories in a child who's been abused. Parad, on the other hand, points out that since some mode of restraint is inevitable for very troubled children, holding the child offers the potential for doing something therapeutic: "We don't have a room where we just lock the door on them and watch through the window while the child goes bananas."

The next time I looked down on the lawn, there seemed to be even more triads. "Good God, it's alive down there," I said. "Alive with pathology," said Rossi.

Shortly after that supremely psychodynamic stroll, I was plunged into the world of computer-aided behavioral research. Leichtman had emphasized that the children's behavior was highly variable in different contexts, that they didn't know how to listen and lacked social skills, and that Wediko's success with a child hinged on the child's success in the cabin group. (I thought of that later on when I met Sharon Foster, the behavioral researcher in San Diego.) This was my introduction to Jack Wright, a former Wediko supervisor now in the psychology department at Brown, who had set up the research program.

Wright, who worked in one of the clapboard cottages, told me that "one basic human tendency is to think about other people in global terms. If you ask people to describe someone, their first impulse is to use some global-trait term like 'He's conceited' or 'She's nuts.' Our kids are so extreme and some of their behavior is so unfamiliar, particularly to first-year staff, that the tendency to think about others in global terms becomes problematic. A lot of the kids' parents characterize them the same way, as 'good' or 'bad.' If your job is to produce behavior change, these categories are not helpful. We encourage everyone here to become more contextual. Instead of allowing staff to say, 'Johnny's aggressive,' or, 'Joey's withdrawn,' we encourage them to think when and where exactly he does it and when he does not do it.

"How do we do this? We collect detailed observations of the children to understand how their behavior varies over situations and over time. For each child at the end of each activity period, we have the staff provide information about the child's behavior during the period. That means for, say, a hundred and thirty children six to eight hours a day, a hundred staff or so are participating in the collection of data. It takes about ten minutes to fill out the form.

"So let's call a child Joey, in the Woodchucks, during archery period. I start with a global assessment of Joey's behavior during that activity. [Wright was using *global* as a technical term meaning "overall," while he and Leichtman had also used it in the looser, slangier sense of "way too cosmic and mushy."] I'd indicate whether he 'hit and physically aggressed,' 'bossed, provoked, or threatened,' 'teased or ridiculed,' 'argued or disapproved,' 'whined or cried.' There's a special category that includes hand-shaking, head-banging, eyebrow-pulling, rocking repetitively, highly repetitive scratching behaviors, and we get skin-pickers as well. These form a cluster under the heading of 'self-stimulation, self-abuse.' They're relatively rare in our population but highly diagnostic. Then there are three categories of 'prosocial' behavior: 'age-appropriate talk,' 'positive emotion,' 'attend-listen to others.'

"Then I move to the second level of analysis: specific events. If I gave Joey a time-out, a common intervention here, I would indicate which staffer did it and the child's response, using the behavior categories I described to you: did he hit me when I gave him the time-out? Then the staffer filling out the form checks off whether some other child in the group bossed, bullied, or threatened Joey, and what Joey did in return, and so forth. We collect these sheets, six or eight a day on every student in the setting, and our software processes the data in various ways to make it useful to administrators, supervisors, and staff. We can sit down in front of the computer with the staff and analyze how things are going with the students."

Wright's system can chart a child's progress throughout the summer, noting when surges of positive or antisocial behavior occur and tying them to incidents like visiting day. It can show which kids are getting the most attention and which are falling through the cracks. It can spot when the staff, fatigued, is being unduly harsh. It can tell which interventions seem to work best with a particular child in terms of the way the child behaved the rest of the day. It reveals "pockets of higher functioning" in a child that the staff can work with. And it helps staff to discuss Joey with his parents, showing them when Joey *isn't* just a pain in the ass.

The last part of my basic education was a talk with Jim Wade, an educational consultant who designed Think City, Wediko's school program. (During the winter he works for the State of Connecticut.) The children spend a couple of hours every day in the summer learning math and English, and they have a full school day in the winter. The point of Think City is Wediko's understanding that competence in school is fundamental to children's mental health; teachers aim to have the children think about school as a place where they can do well. "Any one of these kids can turn a whole elementary school upside down," Wade told me. "Even in many large school systems they still present very serious problems. We don't think school cures the kids, but it's essential for them. At some point in their lives, they will have to go out in the world with some skills to rely on. At the lowest level they have to be math literate and fill out a job application. And we have a lot of kids in the setting who are quite bright." Part of the curriculum is the Junior Great Books Program, which includes, for example, short stories by Doris Lessing and Langston Hughes that provide discussion topics pertinent to the kids' lives. Wade told me, "I've never met a kid who really believed school wasn't important. I've met a lot of kids who have been so unsuccessful in school that they've totally dissociated themselves from its purpose. The strongest paradox these kids present, which continues to amaze me, is how inordinately incompetent they are as individuals and at the same time how they yearn to be capable. You have this kid in front of you who wants so badly to be able to read but just cannot cooperate, cannot reciprocate, cannot engage in the give and take. We had a kid this winter who in two months went from barely being able to multiply two times three to complex multiplications. He left here to go to a psychiatric hospital."

The following summer I asked to follow two groups of children at ages I thought developmentally interesting. Luckily, two crack supervisors were heading such groups, so I hooked up with Caribou, Rossi's cabin of ten-to-eleven-year-old boys, and Chrysalis, a girls' cabin of fourteen-to-seventeen-year-olds supervised by Terry Landon, a veteran of ten years at Wediko who also did therapy in the Boston schools; I'd met her the year before. When I arrived—in time to watch the staff preparing for the kids' arrival—I found Rossi sitting on the porch of the bungalow that serves as summer quarters for him and for Hugh Leichtman.

Rossi was starting to review the files of the ten kids who would be in his group. The kids would have seven counselors—whoops, staff: four men who lived in the cabin and three women lodged in a dorm—and would stretch those seven young adults to the limits of their energy. Each child was preceded by a packet of detailed questionnaires designed by Wediko and filled out by the parent, the teacher, and the therapist, providing a case history and minute information on how the child responded to particular events. Rossi told me it might be educational to watch him review a file, so I settled down to learn about eleven-year-old Anthony Andrews.

A handwritten note had just been inserted on top of the file. It said, "A few weeks ago, after the first interview, Tony and three other boys cornered a small neighborhood boy, Monroe, and Tony sexually abused him by performing oral sex on him. Tony was able to talk about the incident leading up to the oral sex and his feelings about it. His foster parents were present. We discussed Tony's feelings of being coerced by the other boys, especially one, into doing it. Baby, the other boy, balled up his fist and threatened to beat Tony up unless he did it. Baby is denying any part in it. Tony feels responsible for what happened and also guilty, but he also feels everyone is blaming just him. Two pieces were emphasized: how he was coercive and threatening and unsafe to Monroe, and how he felt coerced into doing something he didn't want to do. Both are common problems for Tony. We talked about having counselors give him feedback when he is making people feel unsafe, and he will tell counselors when he is feeling coerced." The words *safe* and *unsafe*, like *appropriate* and *inappropriate*, are Wediko-speak: while adult observers may soon tire of them, for the kids they are easy to understand and comfortable to use.

Rossi said, "So this is the beginning of the treatment plan for the summer. It alerts me as supervisor, as the person who knows about these kinds of dynamics in kids from training and the past, to what details I'm going to pay attention to. I'm already wondering whether there was a history of his being sexually abused. Why is he with foster parents? What happened to his biological family?

"I'm also interested in the group composition. When I get to the medical form, I'll check out the height and weight, because it says he has oppositional behavior with adults, passive-aggressive and provocative behavior with peers, and depression as his top three problems that got him into special services in the first place. Some eleven-year-olds are quite big, and I want to figure out where he'll sleep so we don't get into trouble from the giddyap." We went on to "Will there be changes in the child's living situation after the summer program?" "I see 'maybe' checked, which is the worst possible answer for his sense of security," Rossi said.

He moved to the next topic. "Under 'family events which you think have been important to the child,' we have the bio mom's chronic substance abuse. Since when? 'Since birth.' "

"Has he got fetal drug or alcohol syndrome?" I asked.

"We don't know," Rossi said. "Multiple 51As filed for neglect and/or abuse by the mom. That was when he was aged three to nine. 51As are the official legal documents in Massachusetts. Tony and two sisters were placed in foster care when he was nine. A 51A was filed on the foster parents for abuse five months later, and the sisters were moved to another placement. This does not surprise me, after being in the field for so long, because kids that have been abused are kids that are abused in the future. How can this happen? we ask ourselves; we choose these foster families very carefully, but it happens over and over. There may be some of what Freud called the repetition compulsion at the kernel of this, setting up situations where it's likely to occur, like that recent incident, where he was coerced into doing something he professed he didn't want to do. Kids tend to do what they know. There's a certain security in repeat performances, even if they're aversive."

"Is there something cognitive here?" I asked. " 'This is how the world works, this is what mothers and fathers do, so I'm going to do what I do'?"

"Exactly," Rossi said. "Also, 'This is the only way I get any kind of attention at all. I don't like it, but I seem to kinda need it' . . . they don't *go through* all that, but it happens."

Last year Tony's mom was still on drugs, and a plan for him to move in with his grandmother fell through, a common pattern with Wediko children. Rossi was reading aloud to me from the therapist's form, what the therapist thought were the child's most serious problems. " 'Lack of trust'—no surprises there. 'Family history and current inconsistency of placement planning continue to impact Tony's ability to see adults as reliable and safe.' What else is new? 'Depression and low self-esteem.' Again, no surprises."

"Is the kid disturbed," I asked, "or is the kid eminently logical?"

"That's an eternal question that has enormous heuristic value when you're working with a kid, but for practical purposes it's insignificant. The kid was cornered, and inappropriate sexual activity occurred."

The depression was increasing, and Tony was acting the tough guy to ward it off. He had "poor expressive skills," and I asked Rossi what the file said about the boy's intelligence; Rossi said the anxiety and depression would probably depress test scores, so he wouldn't set much store by them. The therapist was asked to list Tony's good qualities, and these Rossi found auspicious: he could engage with adults over time, was good at sports, and had a sense of humor. On the symptom checklist, "running away" and "stealing" got top scores, also no surprise to Rossi: "He feels like he never gets enough, and he never has, so he steals. He's never really where he's supposed to be anyhow, and it never turns out, so why not run away? Why not take some control yourself, since you're going to be dumped anyway?"

Rossi read swiftly through the checklist and stopped at a zero rating for "Can identify choice points in stressful situations." This was a red flag, predicting impulsivity. The therapist's form suggested Tony had some ego strengths you could work with: oddly enough, he didn't sound a hopeless sociopath. "Not yet, anyway," Rossi said.

Then the therapist checked that Tony could "remember conversations about important problems," and Rossi raised an eyebrow. The therapist had a stake in saying this, he pointed out: didn't it reflect on her effectiveness? He would tell Jack Wright that this was a biased item that should go off the questionnaire.

The therapist's form, Rossi said, was generally the most positive, since she saw the child one-to-one; true to the contextual norm on these questionnaires, Tony's teacher almost always looked at things differently. Oddly enough, the teacher—who usually had no use for Tony at all— thought he sometimes *could* identify choice points in stressful situations. This was at first mysterious to Rossi, but then he said, "I think they're talking about *different* stressful situations. The teacher means when there's been an argument in the playground, and the therapist means when he lost his family." The disagreements continued, and I remarked on the distorted viewpoint that an outpatient therapist seemed to get. Rossi said, "That any one person will get. The viewpoint is significantly related to the context, and that's why we have the same form filled out by at least three people."

In reading Tony's file, Rossi continued to shift back and forth between the teacher's view, the therapist's view, the foster mother's view, and test results. "People will rarely go through these forms systematically, one page after the other," Rossi told me. "It's much more interesting to follow the things that become interesting to you." In watching him, I remembered a report I had read many years ago—before child therapy became an interest—about a psychological experiment in Amsterdam that analyzed the skill of grandmasters at chess: the grandmasters were not necessarily more brilliant than ordinary players, but they had learned to see the board in terms of remembered patterns instead of individual pieces. Thus they could zero in on significant moves. It seemed to me that

Rossi was a sort of therapeutic chess master—and what I saw of him throughout that summer confirmed that impression.

It was now time to look at Tony's performance on the WISC-R [Wechsler Intelligence Scale for Children–Revised], the standard intelligence test he had last taken three years before. With a child like Tony, whose life and emotional health were so variable, an old intelligence test was hardly gospel, but it gave some general indication of his turn of mind: overall he came out low-average in intelligence (probably an underestimation of his potential) with the verbal section higher than the performance section. Thus Rossi said, "I take the highest area of his recorded achievement, which is the 'average' verbal score, as indicative overall. Where the vein of gold is is important: higher verbal skills are related to ego strength, and that shows me he's likely to profit from intervention that involves language. In my experience kids who have higher nonverbal scores tend to be impulsive, because judgment always involves language. A kid who is high-performance and low-verbal is probably not going to understand when I try to explain what he was doing, so why waste my breath. With that kid I would do more behavioral interventions. With this kid, while the teacher says he responds well to behavioral interventions, I am also going to take the time to talk to him about what I'm doing."

The WRAT-R (for Wide Range Achievement Test–Revised), however, which assessed Tony's scholastic achievement, showed this eleven-year-old boy at a first-grade level in reading and math. He was a fourth-grader in special ed full time, because of "aggressive incidents with students and teachers, running out of the school building, destroying furniture and other things." Rossi told me that teachers, asked to list the child's most serious problem, almost always checked "following rules and regulations." Therapists, on the other hand, generally checked "poor self-image." Rossi didn't like this teacher because she'd also written "ignoring *orders* by adults." He said, "She's not writing 'directions,' she's not writing 'requests.' " Rossi looked through the forms for points of agreement between the teacher and the therapist, which would be significant, and finally, with the ironic laugh I came to recognize, he found one. "The first thing we get agreement on, the top of the charts, is that *this poor little kid seems unhappy*." As for the foster mom, she seemed a nice lady—the 51As may have come through other members of the household—and her view of Tony was right down the middle.

At a certain point the chess master—who also had a sense of where

Tony should sleep and how he would probably behave the first day— closed the file with a yawn. "I could probably fill the rest of this out myself, and so could you," he said. Tony would be subdued when he got off the bus. "We will expect this kid to begin the summer by acting out, getting into fights, being obnoxious and impulsive. As we make progress, he'll begin to look more depressed and less involved with things. My counselors will even begin to get the feeling he's going backward."

As I left Rossi to review other files, I thought Tony Andrews—whom we knew as well as one could know someone in anticipation—was a child that neither August Aichhorn nor Fritz Redl would have found unfamiliar.

I next waylaid Terry Landon, a round blond woman in her thirties with a fondness for funky clothes in wildly mismatched combinations, at one of the picnic tables on the lawn. The year before, Landon had told me about the Chrysalis program for teenage girls. Wediko had not been coed until the late seventies. Its founder had believed that mixing boys and girls would foster inappropriate sexual stimulation, and he envisioned a separate facility for girls that never got off the ground. Then Leichtman and Parad tried for some years to secure funding for a girls' program: it was not until 1978, when a little girl was beaten to death by her father, the headlines "screeching across the *Boston Globe*," as Leichtman put it, that the Massachusetts Department of Social Services recognized that girls suffer, too, and sent along enough of them to get a program going. The activities were unisex at first. The girls' programs had evolved later, Landon said, because the supervisors had felt the unisex programs weren't preparing them well.

"We wanted to give them skills for living life," she said. "A large portion of our population is inner city, and one of the inner-city patterns that emerges is that women are heads of households. These girls are having children young. So we interviewed girls and asked them, 'What do you need to know?' We taught them how to sew by hand and machine, how to cook on limited resources—which we had and which reflects what they'll be living with—and how to develop projects on their own. Both the women and the guys on staff here complained that it was limiting girls, but we said they've asked for this—give them the skills they really need."

Every year, Landon reminded me, many of the girls in Chrysalis have a history of sexual abuse. "The process of looking at their sexuality we start in the interview before they come here, trying to separate out the past sexual abuse from the notion of relationships. A few years ago I showed them a movie that had a big sex scene I'd forgotten about. They started hooting and hollering, so I turned it off and said, 'We're gonna fast-forward this because it seems you can't handle it.' One of the girls said, 'Terry, we've been having sex since we were four years old. We can handle this.' So we started to create the rift: this is not having sex, this is being molested and abused. They have to separate that experience from their own budding sexuality. In addition to body awareness and talking about pregnancy and birth control and safe sex around the AIDS issue, we're giving the girls feedback about how they're presenting to people, whether the image their clothing presents is appropriate. Probably every one of them has been sexually abused in some way if you define sexual abuse as being fondled, molested, or exposed to other people's sexual patterns in the family. That's some inappropriate exposure to sexual behavior, even if it wasn't perpetrated on them."

A common diagnosis among Wediko kids is what DSM-IV calls "Borderline Personality Disorder," whose "essential feature . . . is a pervasive pattern of instability of self-image, interpersonal relationships, and affects, and marked impulsivity . . . present in a variety of contexts." Borderlines, according to the manual, show "frantic efforts to avoid real or imagined abandonment . . . a pattern of unstable and intense interpersonal relationships characterized by alternating between extremes of idealization and devaluation . . . markedly and persistently unstable self-image . . . impulsivity in at least two areas that are potentially self-damaging (e.g., spending, sex, substance abuse, reckless driving, binge eating) . . . affective instability due to a marked reactivity of mood." While this disorder figures prominently in the work of Mahler and Kohut, the current inclination of DSM's framers is not to lay it on children and adolescents. Nonetheless, borderlines are all over Wediko, and they seemed to be particularly plentiful in Chrysalis. As Landon told me that first year, "You see behaviors that flip-flop real fast without much external warning. They'll have huge overblown reactions to things that we can't anticipate because we don't understand the internal structure. They see the world only in black and white."

This year, I learned, all of the Chrysalis girls would be either adopted or foster. "In reading the files," Landon said, "it's painful to see what has been done to this child and the child still loves the person who did it. The staff can't make any sense of it. But as you become a supervisor and work more with parents, you realize that first of all they didn't have it much better themselves. If we'd had contact with them when they were younger, perhaps we could have stopped the cycle. Our job is to help the children understand they were potential perpetrators of whatever had come their way: I make food the way my mother made food. We use that as an example. We try very hard never to put down families but to acknowledge, 'Boy, your mom has been having real hard times.' It allows the children to take a different step because they're not having to defend their families."

Instead of reviewing files, Landon gave me capsule biographies of all the girls in Chrysalis: I'll talk here about a couple who later drew my particular interest. Latisha James, a fourteen-year-old from Boston, had lived in many different homes during the first thirteen years of her life; she'd been with her current foster family for about a year. Her biological parents were drug addicts, her mother a prostitute; at first she had been bounced around her extended family, from grandparents to aunts to uncles, until they refused to have anything further to do with her and she moved into foster care.

Latisha was oppositional, sexually precocious, and subject to frequent mood swings. "She had a very rough April," Landon said. "Her foster parents separated, her biological cousin was murdered on the streets, she got pregnant and had an abortion. The biological family have now totally rejected any contact with her. The foster mom is wonderful: she says, 'I'm in it for the long term.' "

Cynthia Mercado was a year older than Latisha, a beautiful Latina who specialized in running away from one custodial older sister to the other. Her mother had been a gang leader. "She was incarcerated on drug charges," Landon told me, "but she always took care of the kids. There was probably some exposure to illicit activities of some kind, though everyone's in agreement that this woman did not abuse these children. Cynthia lived with different family members until she was nine and her mother got out of jail. And shortly after that the mother was stabbed to death on the street. Cynthia, who was the baby, is very poignant about her mother. Her older sister, Rosita, the adult in the family, is now in her twenties. She totally fell apart after her mother's death, became drug-addicted, and eventually had all five of her own children taken away. Now she's regained a couple of them. So Cynthia runs from sister to sister. They both love her, and everyone's unsure where she'll live. She's sort of walking in Mom's shoes, hanging out with delinquent friends and not using safe sex. She's interesting, articulate, and very defiant, but it's clear she has some learning deficit. It's hard to know what role this traumatic life history plays."

Each Chrysalis girl had a slightly different and equally horrific history. Several had been adopted by middle-class families and brought numerous snappy outfits, while others had two or three sweatshirts and a couple of pairs of sweatpants to their names, requiring the staff to run out for enough fill-ins to salvage minimal self-esteem. The staff consisted of four women full time, one part time, and an innovation this year: a male counselor, Dan, who had been carefully selected from returning staff to give the girls experience of a man "who's not going to hurt them, not going to take advantage of them, not going to betray their boundaries," as Landon put it.

Before the children came, Wediko force-fed the young staffers with copious printed material on subjects like "How attention deficits begin to shape a child's personality," and child abuse (how to define it, what the signs of it are, clarifying myths, what the families are like, what to do if a child discloses abuse to you). There were training sessions on how to keep battles from escalating, what to do when they do, and how to answer difficult questions. Parad, Landon, Rossi, and other experienced supervisors did many role-plays. The Basket Hold, which Parad demonstrated, might be needed when "a very cute little seven-year-old has finished her main course in seven minutes, waited four minutes for dessert, and the waitress came back one Popsicle shy." It—and other holds—looked like the carries I'd learned in junior life-saving. "Many children have been abused," Parad said. "Don't put your arm around the kid. Respect their space—it's not a friendly gesture. Say, 'If I need to help you, I will.'"

Rossi told the Caribou staff how to handle the cognitive side of a time-out. "Think of event, time and space," he said. " 'Why did I take you out of the clay cabin?' 'Because I told Kevin to shut up.' 'But why did you have to *leave* the clay cabin?' 'I didn't stop when you told me to stop.' 'Okay, that's right. Now how did all that start in the first place?' 'He told me I couldn't have the clay.' 'Okay, that's good. So when he told you you couldn't have the clay, you told him to shut up, right?' "

Landon told the Chrysalis staff, "We don't talk about our families. If you have gone through a similar life experience, you can't talk about it. It will haunt you. They'll think you're not together, like them. You can say, 'I come from a large family,' but telling private business scares the kids."

On the night before the kids arrived, Leichtman told the entire staff, "If you're not an adult now, you're going to be!" and Parad said, "Trust yourselves! You are wonderful people! Your mothers were right!" and finally Leichtman said, "Play ball!"

Late the next morning a fleet of buses from Boston and a line of parental cars disgorged sullen and shy new kids and brash reunioning returners, some looking ratty and some dressed to the nines. Latisha, in overalls and a white sweatshirt with "Gucci" on it, looked sad. Tony appeared to be a cool dude, a cheerful little black boy wearing his overalls one strap down, in the style of that year.

After a couple of days, I caught Rossi to get his first impressions of the boy I now felt an almost proprietary interest in. Tony, Rossi observed, was unusually concerned about his appearance. "Besides the overall strap off the shoulder, he's got the 'in' baggy length, almost like culottes. He tied his sneakers very carefully with four knots and arranged the way the laces would dangle and hang as he walked. He wore a rosary with a cross and chain, the rosary very deliberately outside his shirt, the chain on the inside but showing. I participated by telling him I would tuck his dangling overall strap in his pocket so it would be safe for kids walking behind him, and he liked that. That made it neater even."

"He's got a little pizazz," I said. "How do you turn that into something constructive?"

"That was my bit," Rossi answered. "The reason to tuck it in was more prosocial than strictly narcissistic, which the rest of it all is, very narcissistic. That kind of superficiality speaks to the way he lives his life and makes him ripe for gang involvement."

"If the incident we heard about is where three guys got him to do something, that suggests he's recruitable," I said.

"Recruitable is recruitable," remarked Rossi. "The gangs can get him, but we can get him too. What is spoken to by gang allegiance and leaders are needs for affiliation, recognition, safety, and power. We can offer him all those things. We've got a time limit, but we have a lot more people and a lot more commitment. They don't care who they don't recruit. We do."

"You've got to point out a more abstract future. They can look in their community and see . . . unless they also see the people that get shot and that sinks in," I said slowly, mulling it over.

"That's a sensational, *National Enquirer* kind of future."

"Then what's the future you offer?"

"The kind of future I can offer is one in which one feels a sense of stability internally, and a basis from which to make decisions you live with rather than go to. I'm offering the kind of freedom that comes from self-control, the knowledge that one can control oneself and resist temptations that are destructive. That's implicit in all this emphasis on *choices*."

But I wondered, considering the life Tony was going back to, whether Rossi was whistling in the dark.

Besides Tony, Caribou had, said the chess master, a full dramatis personae of basic Wediko types, such as Timmy Watkins, a skinny, agitated, hypervigilant coffee-colored boy whom Rossi called "the weathervane," ever alert to who might be the most powerful adult and child in the group; Jeff De Witt, a white boy with long brown hair who responded to stressful situations by acting provocative, so the staff would intervene and "ego boundaries are provided from without," as Rossi framed it; Lance Walker, who wanted to be called Jason—quite probably, Rossi surmised, in order to disown behavior he found inconvenient at the end of the summer, so the staff was ordered to keep calling him by his real name. I picked out Nicholas Foxe, a well-dressed, genial suburban boy whose presence at Wediko seemed mysterious until he lost the draw for a piece of Bazooka gum and let fly a long, loud stream of foul curses; and Ricky Appleton, a fragile, clinging, spooky-looking boy whose head seemed too large for his body. There was a lot of swagger among the Caribou, and fights broke out in the minute you turned your head. And whenever a kid said something the slightest bit "prosocial," a counselor would say, "Good asking, Jeff."

As the season began, Harry Parad was concerned about the minute structuring of feedback and incentives. "If there are eight children in a group and six get from the waterfront to athletics on time and participate without problems, while two kids come fifteen minutes late but do well once they get there, should those two children get the same incentive as the others? If we say the first fifteen minutes never happened, we're not giving accurate feedback, but if we say the other thirty minutes never happened, we're also not accurate," he said.

"That's an issue even for parents of ordinary kids," I put in.

"At times when you're overwhelmed as a parent, you tend to think in absolute terms," Parad told me. "You say to your kids, 'That's impossible, forget it, no discussion, no compromise.' A child can live with that if you've been overall a reasonable parent. They say to themselves, 'Mom is in a bad mood. She's had a hard day at work. I can live with that.' But if your experience is that this is the dominant way adults are, you build a sense of self that says either, 'I am okay,' or, 'I am not okay.' We need to get away from that division of self into good and bad and put in feedback systems that emphasize degree."

The other major push this summer was family therapy. It was important to avoid rivalry between staff and parents, a problem even in ordinary classrooms but a special concern "when the parents have had such a hard time being adequate. When you're competitors, you lose perspective as the helper. A question we have to ask ourselves is, 'What do we do that is so special that it justifies separating a child from the family system?' That's why we believe residential treatment should be short-term, not open-ended."

In working with parents, Wediko sought to provide the same finely grained feedback it gave the kids. "So Mum gets drunk and takes lousy care of the kids three times a week. If we say she must be cold sober tomorrow, she won't be successful. But if the goal is to help her see what leads up to the episodes where she loses control, and how her loss of control affects her children, whom she does love, and help her make a plan to decrease the frequency and intensity of these episodes, those goals are reasonable. If we're not working with the family, any progress the child makes during the summer, the *child* has to figure out how to incorporate into the family, which isn't realistic." There were several cases Parad described to me in which the child's admission depended on the parent's willingness to work with Wediko.

The first night—Friday of the July Fourth weekend—Parad was strolling the grounds at nine o'clock to head off bedtime crises. It was the twenty-fifth first night he had seen at Wediko, and he told me if tonight was this quiet, tomorrow night was sure to be a corker. It was pitch dark in the woods, and the ground was covered with slippery pine needles, rocks, and tree stumps. In the midst of a Mahlerian discussion of how a child might fall apart in a new situation without a sense of self to carry with her, Parad said, "How would you feel walking here tonight without me to guide you? It would be a different experience."

At that moment I remembered my visit the summer before, leaving a staff meeting at 1:30 in the morning trying to make my way to my temporary cabin without a flashlight in the pouring rain in these same pitch-dark woods. It was, I thought, what life is always like for Tony and Timmy and Cynthia and Latisha.

Before my first visit of the summer was over, I caught Leichtman and Parad together (a rare experience); part of our conversation dealt with the needs of traumatized children. "Once you've been damaged, it leaves a permanent injury," Leichtman said. "If you look at development as a spectrum, it influences so many different aspects of functioning. You can compensate. You're still dented, but you develop all sorts of compensatory mechanisms, ways of integrating this past experience so juvenile affects don't drive adult functioning. They influence it, but they don't *drive* it. We hope to provide the kids with adaptive tools they will be able to use for the rest of their lives."

Parad said, "You can get someone who's been physically abused to use cognitive and behavioral strategies 95 percent of the time, and they do fine. Then the child comes home, and the mom is with a new man, the new man goes out and gets blasted and comes home and knocks around the mom. That would be incredibly upsetting for any fifteen-year-old, but for this fifteen-year old, because it replicates patterns that Mom exhibited three, four, five times before, this is too affectively charged for the child to use the strategies she learned. The affective part just bursts into flames."

"The biological term for this is *kindling*, where you have certain areas of the brain that become activated through trauma, certain signals that set up these pathways, and you get an explosion," Leichtman said, raising what I later discovered is a cutting-edge idea in the world of biological psychiatry.

"I'm all for bringing as much science into this as possible," Parad countered, "but I also recognize this is an art. Any therapy is art. You can program to affect the way the kids form their relationships, the cues they pick up on, and the program reduces maladaptive behaviors, but you reach a certain point where the program can't do it all. In the moment, interacting with the children, you look for that balance of science and art. Your really expert clinicians always have that extraordinary balance."

Parad and Leichtman were simulating, intellectually, the existential tennis that modern clinical practice demands.

When I returned at midsummer, Rossi was on his porch giving haircuts to the Caribou—tails, spikes, and lowtop fades on request. Leichtman had told me there was a new boy in Caribou, an electrical genius with a family history of violence and mayhem. After the haircuts were finished, Rossi and I took a stroll, and there on the lawn outside Think City was a little blond boy with a crew cut, wielding a stick and looking murderous while a staffer held him by the left arm. "Put down the stick, and let's have a talk," Rossi said evenly. He introduced me to Earl Snow, and Earl said, "I don't want to be in this camp no more. I wanna go home for good and not come back, and I'm *gonna* go home for good and not come back if I don't get my way. I'll run over the bridge and hide in somebody's house."

"So let's figure out something you can get your own way about without having to leave," Rossi said. "How about we have you call home?"

"It won't work. I'm goin' home, and you can't stop me."

"It won't work? Well, I know you like it here, and I also know that when you start to feel frustrated and angry and provoked, every single time— the important thing is that I can't control everything about you. It really would be easier for you to just give up. Because it's hard to be doing as well as you've been doing. You wouldn't have to work so hard to keep in control and keep yourself from getting in trouble, and that'd be a lot easier."

Long silence. "I'm going home," said Earl softly.

"We'd better give a call to find out how your mother's car is," Rossi suggested.

"They shoulda done another system check and find out where the short is," Earl said. "Because my mom's caah—they thought it was the alternator, it was totally frying the batteries. You put a brand-new seventy-dollar caah battery in, the next day the battery's dead. There's a short in there, and I'm trying to find it, and I probably found it and fixed it."

They talked about Earl's worry that his mom couldn't get along without him and how they'd better call so he wouldn't worry so much, and they made a date to call after Earl's tutoring session. Sometime later I went up to the porch to watch this happen. Earl was sitting repairing a radio; its guts were spilled out on the table. When Earl went out to the toolshed to get a part, Rossi filled me in. "He wants to pull the ripcord and bail out every time there's a degree of stress that seems aversive. He has trouble focusing and limiting stimulation, so if there's a lot going on around him, it's all coming in at once. But when he looks at a radio with the parts spread out, he sees all of it, which is better for this kind of work—not to have the kind of focus where you just see one part as most important. If you have to focus on one at a time, it will take you three or four days.

"Earl was conceived in a gang rape. I believe that his uncle was a mass murderer who buried people in the front yard, and that uncle was more like a father figure to him than we might want. His grandfather, who just died, was also close to him. Mom has been hospitalized many times for physical ailments, so his impulse to run home is in many ways to protect her. That's how I kept reading it during the intervention. A month ago his uncle also died."

"The mass murderer?"

"I don't know how mass. I just said that for dramatic effect. I think it was just a few people."

"A *group* murderer."

When Earl came back, Rossi called his mother. "Hello, Mrs. Snow, this is Dr. Rossi at Wediko. There's nothing to worry about. We're just calling for a check-in. Earl's missing you and wondering about your car, and I thought I'd give him a chance to say hello. You doing okay? . . . He'll understand that better than I do. Earl, you want to talk?"

Earl got on. "Mom, is the caah fixed? Are the batteries tuned? Can you pick me up outside the liberry so I can leave here for good? I'm pissed off at this place. I'm *goin'* home, or else I have to *run* away home." Getting no immediate satisfaction, he asked some family questions, and then Rossi got on again. The radio, meanwhile, had been assembled, and there was static coming out of it.

"He's brought this dead radio *back to life*! He usually starts by saying he wants to go home, and I interpret that as his missing you, wanting to check and see how you're doing, and I think it's a test to see how we're going to respond. I think he's getting kind of nervous because he's actually been doing very well. . . . We can both tell Earl that he knows he has to be here to contain behaviors that are not good for him or anybody else. I think you can tell him we're all on the same team, to help keep him safe. I think he probably won't believe you'll say all that until you say it. Give him the message that you're safe and you still love him but it's important for him to stay here." This was essentially a family therapy session on the phone, in which Rossi, talking to Mrs. Snow in Earl's presence, was seeking to alter the dynamics; had it been a child guidance–style session, he would have spoken to her in private.

Rossi and Mom talked a bit more, and then he put Earl back on to listen silently and say good-bye. After the conversation Rossi told Earl he would take the radio and find some other broken radios and bring them all to Think City, to be used as a reward every time he did some schoolwork. Then he asked Earl to play back what he had just said. The incentive-and-contract side of Wediko takes the behavior management that Philip Kendall had found wanting in his graduate school days and refines it with sophisticated individual reinforcements—the radios were what Earl, and only Earl, would consider a big reward—and a background therapy that's both cognitive and psychodynamic, evidenced by the way Rossi interpreted to Earl and to his mother.

When Earl left, I asked for an update on Tony. It turned out Tony, because of his difficulty trusting adults and "a concrete learning style," had had to test the limits of every adult on the Caribou staff hierarchically, from Rossi himself down to the youngest woman counselor. "The kids have an uncanny sense of power," Rossi said. "They're far more accurate and alert than we might be." So then, after each staffer laid down the law, Tony began to open up and make attachments. He became the most popular member of the group. The least popular member was dorky little Ricky Appleton, who was trying to adjust by teasing everyone and acting weird. Rossi had been trying to get the other kids to help get him on track. One day, spontaneously, during the daily cabin meeting, Tony raised his hand and said, "Who likes Ricky? Raise your hand. I do. Let's shake." Then Tony led a sort of group encounter where almost the whole group filed past Ricky and said they liked him and shook his hand.

"There's an element of power in that, of course, but it was good for him and good for Ricky and good for the group. He did that stuff for a few days, and then he got to the next phase that often happens with a kid like Tony, where he begins to look depressed, irritable, and weepy. They usually have, and he did, a couple of days in a row where they wear two or three layers of clothing. Suddenly they feel naked and vulnerable. There's no going back. People are saying, 'You're not going to be able to punch people out anymore.'

"After that he had another short phase where he would run away on the grounds. He needs to get away at times, but that's not a productive way to cope. We have to know where the kids are."

At any rate after all these phases, Tony was kind of stuck with liking it, achieving things, and forming attachments. "He's always holding back the last ten percent of compliance," Rossi said. "Saving face with some defiance and swagger. But meanwhile he talks about what group he'll be in next year."

As I arrived at Chrysalis, Latisha was mouthing off at Terry Landon, "Get out of my face! Get *out* of my face!" slamming the screen door, storming down the path, and being nabbed for a time-out on a rock. Speaking globally, one might say she was one tough cookie. But in cabin meeting one day, Latisha had said, "I have been treated really badly by women, so I don't give women much of a chance." Landon told me Latisha's younger brother had been brought up for a visit the other day. "He makes her look like Mary Queen of Scots. He was so terrible that I stopped the meeting an hour earlier and said to the worker, 'This is insane.' Every time Latisha made a statement, he'd go, 'Oh, *right*,' in this sarcastic tone, and she'd hold her breath and count to five. She asked how their mother was, and he said, 'What do *you* care?' Afterward she cried, she said partly because her feelings were hurt and partly because it brought back the sarcastic way her mother had treated her, and partly because she was a lost child, and partly because her brother was a lost cause. Very few people here would be able to differentiate their feelings that way."

"Still, she can't get through life talking to people like that," I said.

"Right. Last Friday, when her brother picked at her for an hour, she saw what it felt like. She was able to go back and say, 'This really hurts. I don't want to treat people that way.' And for a couple of days she was able to behave differently. The flip side of her is how intelligent she is in cabin meetings—that's what we're fighting for. With girls who have been abused to the degree these girls have, there are only three roles they can play—the abuser, the abused, or some healthy side they strive to find. You watch them vacillate among these roles, back and forth, back and forth." Latisha and Landon had made a date to make a phone call; Landon, detained, sent another staffer to help Latisha, and Latisha blew up. Here was one more woman who wasn't there for her! "We are trying to move her from demand feeding—which is 'I need to do this right now with you!'—to 'Let's do it at this scheduled time with you,' to 'Let's do it at this scheduled time, even with somebody else.' It's kind of like weaning a baby." For good or ill, the volatile, hostile, but insightful Latisha was the leader of the group.

Meanwhile, Cynthia Mercado had had an epiphany. Cynthia, the chronically truant, promiscuous daughter of the murdered gang leader, had become more oppositional, balking at Wediko's structure but acknowledging in more rational moments that she felt happier. "One day last week I found her crying," Landon said. "She had been working with knives in the kitchen, and she was thinking, 'I wonder what it felt like for my mother to be stabbed. I wonder whether it hurt and whether she knew what was happening.' No one in her family has ever discussed their feelings about their mom, and it's taken Rosita, her big sister and guardian, a long time to get her act together. She sort of vacillates between being real strict like a parent and being a sister. Cynthia wants her to be one or the other—or the teenager in Cynthia wants a sister, and the child in her wants a parent.

"So the very same day when we happened to be here talking about the pain that only her sisters can understand but her sisters won't talk about, Rosita went to a meeting with her social worker, and they all determined that nobody was going to get any better until they talked about their mother. When we called Rosita the next day, Cynthia heard the message that if she didn't work on things, the state was going to have her placed in residential. Rosita said to Cynthia that when she got home, they had to talk about Mom. Cynthia thought I had told Rosita, but I hadn't—so it was fascinating to her that the two sisters, three hundred miles apart, had come up with the same plan to pull the family back together."

Cynthia was beginning to differentiate her own struggles for autonomy from her family problems: a summer away might, perhaps, help clear her thinking, but the solutions to her life's problems, Landon knew, lay within the family.

When I returned to Wediko to see the kids leave, the familiar defenses that ordinary human beings erect against separation and loss—that before-you-fire-me-I-quit syndrome—were out in full flower. Best friends were ridiculing each other and pushing each other away; children were glowering at their favorite counselors; at various award ceremonies the child whose name was called for a prize would pull his or her shirt over

his or her head, scowl, and clown when walking up to the platform. Jeff De
Witt, a boy with ADD whose father had been killed in a car crash, teased
his best friend Ralph Ward mercilessly for being overweight and encopretic, and then came over to Rossi and said that he, Jeff, was just a weird
demented kid who liked feeding wild animals to snakes. Tony said, "I
hate the whole place. I hate the counselors." And his friend Nicholas
Foxe said, "Hold on, there's something to be sad about. You're probably
never gonna see any of us again"—the first time Nicholas had ever really
mentioned feelings. Those four boys had made the most progress of the
Caribou, but Earl Snow had also managed to settle in with the group—
and would be back in the winter.

Tony had finally become the star. His street-thug veneer was melting
away. He had, Rossi said, "a highly efficient affect factory that manufac-
tures anything distressing into anger and menace." Most distressing to
Tony was the ubiquitous Wediko word *safe*. He came, after all, from an
unsafe neighborhood and would soon be returning to it. For several days
in a row, he kept saying "I hate your safety. It's too safe for me here. I can't
stand it!" His thuggy look wasn't working anymore, so as Rossi put it,
"You up the ante. When the defense system becomes a little weak, you
spend more and cut the budget for social services." He alternated between an impressive enjoyment of structured activities like archery
(where you had to wait your turn forever and behave perfectly so you
wouldn't lose it) and irritability at more chaotic games like Capture the
Flag. One evening this anger reached a climax. Tony was down on the
playing field holding three frightened counselors at bay with rocks he
threatened to lob at them.

Rossi, elsewhere, was summoned. The chess master deliberately am-
bled down to the field to defuse the crisis. By then, the counselors were
holding Tony, who had launched his missiles so as not to hurt anybody,
and so their arriving supervisor just took his arm gently and walked him
off the field and up to the porch of the house he, Rossi, shared with Hugh
Leichtman. "He was now clearly sad," Rossi remembered. "The face of
aggression was not there, so I wasn't angry at him, and he wasn't angry at
me. When Hugh came in, Tony put on his menacing face, and Hugh said,
'That's rude and inappropriate. People may have hurt you, but you're not
allowed to hurt other people. We're not going to tolerate that.' Tony broke
into tears and said, 'I'm sorry.' So then Hugh was very nurturing and
affectionate, dried his tears with his shirt-sleeve, and talked about how

Tony was really sad. Of course I had to kick Tony out of the Caribou cabin for the night because his display of violence required it for the group's safety.

"So Tony got to sleep on the porch. We set up a cot for him, and he was lying with his head on the pillow just sobbing and sobbing. So he sat on my lap like a little baby and just cried on my shoulder for a long time and allowed people to be kind to him. Some counselors came by and they too were supportive. But he said he was sad. He talked about the loss of his biological parents—his affect was integrated. You *always see*—I'm adamant about this—an increase in the sophistication of sentence structure, of language itself, when this kind of emotional integration occurs. It's a leap in development.

"The next morning Tony went back to the group and people noticed he was different. But all this spelled trouble if we kept it up because he had to be one of the kids again. And later he did start escalating: the road to goodies was to escalate the violence and get himself kicked onto Tod's porch. So I said, 'Tony, this was all very nice, but the next time you become violent you're going to the crisis center.' " That was one step more serious than the lawn—a few bare, solitary rooms in one of the buildings. Tony did get himself to the crisis center in custody of Brett, a staffer, with Rossi conspicuously absent. He said to Brett, "What if I scream in your face, what will you do?" and Brett said, "I'm not going to like it, but I'm not going to hit you. I'm just going to stay here as long as it takes. I don't really like this, but it's my job." And suddenly, after stamping around a bit, Tony just stopped.

After all this he became the most helpful boy in the group, calming the others down and continuing to stick up for Ricky Appleton, effectively, whenever the others teased him. It was a reenactment of what had happened to some of August Aichhorn's boys in Vienna in 1925. I asked Rossi what he thought Tony was capable of under the best of circumstances, and he said, "At best he's capable of what I'm capable of. He could go to college with a scholarship. He's got all the standard fare on his plate. He doesn't have brain damage. He's not predisposed to the oversensitivity to stimulation that schizophrenics have. He doesn't have the dramatic mood swings that may end up with manic depression, and he doesn't have the kind of rage responses that might be tied to seizures. He's got learned defenses that have been effective. He has a terrible struggle with loss and change, based on the fact that he's had terrible loss and change. Some people's environment is a product of their impulses; Tony is more a product of his environment."

Rossi was making a differential diagnosis on the basis of his own training and experience and a summer of observing Tony; later he did the same, minutely, for various other Caribou. Their prognoses hinged first on whether they were "playing with a full deck" and second on life circumstances, which were crucial; the ways these factors can combine, as I'd learned in reading Chess and Thomas, seems infinite. The same stuff was going on, at a more nuanced level, at Chrysalis: less violence and more verbal shafts, and at the same time an absolute bath of teenage-girl sentiment. Cynthia, who was studying to be a beautician, was creating elaborate coiffures for various cabinmates. Landon regularly terminated with an event called Chrysalis Spirit Week in which the cabin celebrated a different holiday every day, Valentine's Day, Halloween, and so on, ending with Birthday Party, a special dinner at which each girl got a red rose. The girls fought against having this party, but the staff insisted, and most had a good time (although one girl cried a lot because she'd never gotten flowers before).

Latisha, one of the most seriously disturbed, couldn't handle it and stayed away. Landon said it was amazing that Latisha could express any feelings at all, and she had been extremely insightful in differentiating her emotions on some previous occasions. She was highly intelligent: she read Alice Walker and Robert Ludlum and passed on to Landon a library copy of *Lord of the Flies*. "Her IQ tests out in the *upper eighties*," Landon said incredulously, "which is just not accurate. I think the data's not recent, and I would be curious to know exactly what was going on in her life when the testing took place. I can't imagine her scoring that low unless she was really oppositional or terribly tortured. We'll make a recommendation for further testing.

"We'll also recommend medication. We have been urging medication for depression, and Latisha herself has decided to pursue that. That's a step for her: prior to that she said, 'This is who I am, and if you don't like it, you can shove it.' After gaining her confidence, we said, 'Latisha, we can put up with anything for forty-five days, but we're talking about your life. You don't have to feel so bad.' We started to describe what depression is and how it manifests itself. She's in a wonderful foster placement now, and it gives her her best possible shot. I feel Latisha could go far—she's a wonderful writer—and I told her, 'The reason we're putting pressure on you is A, we cannot tolerate this stuff in our group and B, more important, when you start to go down the tubes and give up on yourself, all I can see is your books being pulled off the shelf.' " The value of, say, Prozac, for a girl like Latisha, who was utterly weighed down by the terrible experiences of her early life, was that she needed good experiences to modify her view of the world, but her depressed mood made it impossible to have those experiences. Medicine would not numb her but would enable her (if life cooperated) to see some better possibilities.

Another institution of Landon's was the tapings, which went on forever. The group made a tape for each girl, in which every cabin member and staff member recalled something good about her that they'd always remember. The girl then had the tape to take home and play whenever her life was grim (which was often): yes, she had once had friends; yes, she had once, in some small way, been competent; yes, perhaps it could happen again.

And on one of those last nights, when Landon was sitting in her room frantically grinding out reports, her staff burst in with a bowl of strawberries and began singing: "On the first day of Wediko, the children said to me: 'Fuck off, get out of my face.' On the second day of Wediko, the children said to me: 'You're not my mother, fuck off, get out of my face.' " The song went on through all twelve days of familiar imprecations, and then everybody dissolved in laughter and tears.

Finally it was time for the kids to go home. The departure scene looked not much different from six I had experienced as a camper, one as a counselor, and eight as a parent. I told this to Leichtman, and he was overjoyed.

I thought of Chrysalis and Caribou often during the years that followed that summer. During one visit I had found Leichtman in an uncharacteristically subdued mood. In putting together a presentation, he had been looking at slides from the late seventies. "What I was really struck by," he said, "is the number of children who died, children who were with us when they were ten. They would now be in their middle twenties, and some of these children are dead. Mostly in drug-related violence. I can have the most successful outcome, and the child will go to the Franklin Hill project and be shot to death. The kids we're able to follow and drape services around, their outcome is very good."

That summer Wediko was overflowing. It had 175 children. "If we were to predict how many would graduate from college, guess what the number would be? Ten," he said.

"Even from East Squeedunk State?"

"Twenty. Maybe more than that with some of the adopted kids, but I'm looking for kids who are functional. My goal with many of these girls is that they'll leave this program and not get pregnant till their twenties. Or for many of them, they'll have their babies and go back to school. We've seen this with a number of our children when they're thirty, and to me that's a successful outcome."

Two years later, in autumn, I returned to Wediko to learn what was new and what was old: that is, what had happened to the kids I followed, and whether Leichtman, Parad, Rossi, and Landon had anything more to point out. Parad said, "When I was in graduate school, people were talking about the invulnerable child: how were we to explain that within the same family system where factors seemed constant, one child would somehow grow up to be productive and another would have all kinds of difficulties. I've been at Wediko almost thirty years now, and the fact that there's not one theory model that explains all the children troubles me less and less. In one family system we might look psychodynamically at traumatic events in the family's history: one child was at a more vulnerable age than another. So the identified patient was seven months old when the parents went through a horrible breakup or a key person in the family was killed. The older sibs were two years seven months and four years seven months. "So one child would have had a chance to consolidate some basic trust, in Erikson terminology, and to work through attachment and separation issues, in Mahler terminology. Another child was in the midst of that and would be impacted differently. And that's simplistic because we know it's all mediated by issues like temperament and cognitive ability. One child is able cognitively to understand and make sense of something. Or one brother is a gifted athlete and gets the attention of coaches and support from peers, and that makes it easier for him to deal with losses that occurred early in life. Two sisters, one who's beautiful, one who's rather plain—that may or may not affect self-esteem during the adolescent years.

"The other thing about the invulnerable child concept is that family dynamics are important. When one child is in crisis and commands the family's attention, that changes the role of the other children in very complicated ways. So the child who is always mature and takes care of the siblings will look invulnerable, but that doesn't mean that child hasn't his or her own story to tell."

The fate of the children came out in driblets or not at all. Wediko had no formal mechanism for follow-up unless the children were part of its winter programs or returned in a subsequent summer: the staff were not allowed to stay in touch independently. Landon, in the Boston office, had a good handle on the Chrysalis girls because they kept up with each other. In general, some were doing well, others badly, and my ability to guess was fairly wanting: life intruded. After my last visit Landon had sent me some of Cynthia's writing, and her illiteracy had shocked me: how could this sixteen-year-old girl get through life when she couldn't communicate comprehensibly? Cynthia, however, seemed to be doing fine now: playing from her strengths, she had a job as a hairdresser. "Somehow Cynthia has the ability to connect to people and believe in what they are saying. Her mother, whatever her criminal activities, gave a stable base. Latisha, on the other hand, had had such a tumultuous early life that she couldn't trust anybody."

And so Latisha, for whom we had so many hopes, was now nearly seventeen and about to have a baby. The foster placement and several subsequent ones broke down. Landon would have liked to have her for three summers with therapy in the winter, but her life didn't allow for that—and Landon reminded me that "she has had to make her own way since two or three years old, when she remembers picking through the trash to find something to eat. She would definitely require long-term care." Both Landon and Leichtman thought Latisha's story wasn't over: with help she might still put her life together after having the baby. Or not.

Rossi, now directing the winter program in New Hampshire, had the best of the summer staff and the worst of the summer kids: that for him was hog heaven. The two winter sessions lasted most of the school year, with the kids going home for weekends and the counselors' schedule less intense. As Leichtman and I drove up to the main building, we saw a tall blond boy on a ladder doing repair work: I suddenly realized it was Earl Snow, who must now be almost thirteen. I immediately asked Rossi for an update.

"He's one of the oldest kids here. He still has a problem with soiling himself and has had that all his life, but he's on a program where he has to be more responsible for cleanliness. To many people's surprise, he is actually able to make it one day a week with a one-to-one aide in the public school in his home town. So he leaves here Thursday evenings, goes to school Friday, and takes some aikido or karate class that he likes. He's more conscious about his goals and more honest about his problems, though he still blames everybody but himself when he loses his temper and expresses his anger in the same stylized phrases. But we measure our success with him by the duration and intensity of his periods of acting out, and they are less intense. He hurts people less, he turns his aggression toward inanimate objects more often and he breaks fewer things. But he looks more and more unique as he gets older. He's on a lot of medication, and his facial expressions are a little more distant. He's not as cute as he used to be when he could be picked up with one arm."

I asked about the electrical side of Earl, and Rossi said, "We can rely on that to organize and focus him. I had a broken electric toothbrush and Water Pik, which I had not a clue how to deal with. . . . I don't know if there are those appliance fix-it places left anymore, but he could definitely run one of those."

If Earl had such a job, I asked, could he go to work every day? Rossi said Earl would love it—"it would be endlessly satisfying to him. . . . It's within the realm of possibility that he could have a workplace with two or three other people, and earn a decent living. The problem is if someone angers him in the moment, and the aftermath is he's behind bars for several years."

Earl also had some kind of attachment disorder—it took a day and a half for him to get over leaving his mother every single time. "The sign of progress is that he cries, he sobs, he's bitterly distressed in a way that is more clearly what it is, instead of running around attacking and throwing rocks at people, which he does less. He does not seem psychotic. His thinking remains relatively organized, which makes him far more dangerous because his energy is focused."

I asked Rossi if Earl could become a really vicious criminal, and Rossi thought he easily could. He would not be a serial killer stalking the Boston streets: "He's not an obsessive-compulsive about the act of violence. He doesn't ruminate about how he's going to get back at a person or a type of person. It's more impulsive, and if you short-change him in some way, literally or figuratively, he's enraged. You don't want to mess with him, basically."

The chess master's speculation about what might happen in Earl's life interested me. His mom had become increasingly competent: she was an asset. Wediko was working with the appropriate state and hometown officials, teachers, and aides to ensure continuity in Earl's case.

What Earl would need to keep him from a life of crime would be "really sophisticated medical care. His medications will have to be closely and carefully monitored. What I try to achieve, working with our consulting psychiatrist on medications, is to increase the moment between the impulse and the action, so judgment can enter in. Sometimes the kids have egregiously poor judgment as well, even when it does intervene. His judgment is improving. I would love the idea of his outgrowing the need for medication, though I'm dubious about that." Earl's mother, indeed, had been violent and impulsive until Earl was born, and she resolutely turned her life around: as Rossi romantically put it, "She fell in love with her unborn child. . . . Sometimes I think, What if Earl really fell in love with someone, and he was at risk of losing this girlfriend if he exploded one more time?"

Less romantically, I thought of domestic violence. I reviewed the possibility of his hooking up with one of those borderline Wediko girls who are easily battered and abused. Rossi said, sadly, it was a reasonable conjecture.

During this visit Rossi and Leichtman and I talked about various other children: some Caribou were doing better, but since adolescence lay ahead of them, they were more fragile than the Chrysalis girls. But many of the Caribou had vanished without a trace, swallowed up by agencies like the Massachusetts Department of Social Services, which was now in upheaval. One of those children, alas, was Tony Andrews.

One boy I had watched in session with Leichtman that summer, an appealing ten-year-old whose anger at his erratic mother was often displaced to everyone else, was now dead. He had been placed in some other treatment facility, where he died of a heart attack in the midst of a tantrum.

And the particular community of troubled children, committed professionals, and uneasy young staffers I had come to know and feel for that summer had vanished, like Brigadoon.

CHAPTER 17

TRIPLE BOOKKEEPING

To understand a given case of psychopathology you proceed to study whatever set of observable changes seem most accessible, either because they dominate the symptom presented or because you have learned a methodological approach to this particular set of items, be they the somatic changes, the personality transformations, or the social upheavals involved ... being unable to arrive at any simple sequence and causal chain with a clear location and a circumscribed beginning, only triple bookkeeping (or, if you wish, a systematic going around in circles) can gradually clarify the relevances and the relativities of all the known data.

—Erik H. Erikson,
Childhood and Society (1950)

Make way for Oedipus. All people said,
"That is a fortunate man";
And now what storms are beating on his head!
Call no man fortunate that is not dead.
The dead are free from pain.

—Sophocles,
King Oedipus (Yeats translation)

A REPORT ON HOW CHILD PSYCHOTHERAPISTS now work raises numerous questions. One set is pragmatic: given what we do and don't know about child psychotherapy, how does a parent decide a child needs treatment, choose a therapist, and evaluate whether the therapy is effective? Another set of questions is philosophical: while developments in pharmacotherapy have brought these questions new urgency and drama,

494

they've been around for a long time. Is therapy some kind of sinister social engineering that replaces worthy idiosyncrasies with brave-new-world docility? Is it a crutch for insecure or selfish parents seeking to evade their responsibilities? These questions are intertwined with the pragmatic questions, and I will address them together. A third set deals with public policy issues: which mental health services are necessary and which are frills, and how should such issues be decided; and how, with our current state of knowledge about psychological development, can we make our society more cordial to children?

As my research was beginning, I sat in a restaurant with my old friend Barbara Kane, a radiologist whose late husband had vanished under shattering circumstances when her three daughters were small. Barbara had been conscientious and thoughtful in raising the girls; now Laura, the oldest, was in graduate school, Alison, the middle child, was spending her junior year in Italy, and Valerie, the youngest, was a college freshman—and anorectic.

"Val was fifteen and a half when she started therapy," Barbara told me. "She was having difficulty participating in class and said she thought she'd like to see a therapist. She was more comfortable with the idea than teenagers usually are because I had been in analysis, so I went to the head of adolescent psychiatry at our hospital. He was too busy to see Val at that time and gave her a consult referral to another psychiatrist. I checked that man out with several other people at the hospital and with my own analyst, and I heard he was well-trained, had good judgment, and was not dogmatic—all of the things that give one confidence. He saw Val two or three times, and since he himself had no openings, he referred her to a psychologist he said was very good. At this point I assumed this woman was reliable and didn't check further. I knew she was analytically oriented, though Val wasn't going for analysis, but I had positive feelings about the psychodynamic approach. Later on I did learn that this woman had excellent credentials.

"During the first year Val didn't seem terribly plugged into the therapy, and she even thought of stopping. Since nothing drastic was going on and a feature of the analytic approach is not including the parent, I didn't mix in. I saw the positives in that, because one issue was independence. But after the first year and a half, Val began to be much more involved in the therapy. She felt she needed it more, and it seemed to turn things up rather than solve them."

There was the problem of Val's father: Barbara hadn't known any way to explain the full facts of his disappearance to a two-year-old, and as the years went on, there never seemed to be a right time. Now, however, she felt Val really ought to know: "She was old enough to understand, and you couldn't perpetually keep a secret. But it was very distressing and brought up a lot of feelings. Val became more dependent on the therapy. She seemed to have much more *faith*—a word chosen advisedly—in the process. She was amazingly strict, even rigid about keeping her appointments, even though adolescents characteristically are bad about that."

I asked Barbara if Valerie had given any warnings earlier in life that she might develop difficulties. "She always had problems separating, so I would expect leaving home would be a difficult process. But she had dealt with those issues very well before, would have brief difficulties and then emerge independent and strong. The only thing was the school anxiety, which wasn't major: she didn't have exam phobia, she just underperformed, so her grades were good, though not as good as they should be. She did very well on take-home exams, which made her less anxious.

"Before the anorexia there were increasing problems in her dealings with me. We had always been very close, which is not uncharacteristic with a single parent. My friends had said they thought she was overattached to me; teachers never said it. She began to act out of the ambivalence of her feelings about going away, absolutely stereotypical stuff. Things got very rocky between us, an enormous amount of hostility and contempt on her part engendering returned hostility on my part, I'm sure. Our whole family life was affected, and I was feeling powerless in dealing with it. I began to be rather regretful that she was so deeply into a form of therapy that didn't include me at all. We weren't talking things out. I felt that if we'd been having occasional sessions together with the therapist, that would be one hour of the week when we could talk. I could see that the child needed a hug, and she couldn't allow herself the comfort of a hug—but her fears about being on her own were unrealistic because she had enormous common sense and was always extremely competent in dealing with life.

"So things started to get worse. If one is sophisticated about therapy, one always knows things get worse when the defenses are down, but they just kept on being worse, and Val was going to go to college soon. Then came the anorexia. She had gained some extra weight and went on a diet and just kept going. She's a very controlled, restricting anorectic. I didn't figure it out at first, because there was a regular diet that made sense, she'd had a few extra pounds, she didn't lose that much weight, and she also had become a vegetarian, so I partly associated that with the continuing weight loss.

"Strangely enough, Val never denied the illness. She started fighting the disease early on. She knew she was sick but couldn't stop. After a couple of months of obsessive dieting, she asked to see her pediatrician about maintaining her weight; then I became concerned, and the school did too and asked me what was going on. The pediatrician and I were monitoring her, and after six months of barely maintaining the weight her behavior became even worse. First she was less than ten pounds below her ideal weight, then thirteen pounds below, and when she went away to school, she'd lost another eight or nine pounds. She started to prepare all her meals to eat alone and to pull back from all her friends. It was spring of her senior year. The therapy continued all this time, with no real change.

"The therapist wouldn't speak to me without telling Val everything that was said. I think she felt the issues had to do with me, but she never told me what she thought the issues were. I think she felt I wanted to keep Val home and dominate her life and Val needed to break away. I felt this was not a true construct. I *am* very involved in my kids' lives, but I'd been through Laura and Alison leaving, and I'd enjoyed dealing with adult daughters. I was excited about Val's going away, though she wanted to go to school on the West Coast and I expressed some reservations about that."

Given the anorexia, Valerie needed a therapist near school—she'd finally decided on a small college in the suburbs of a big midwestern city—and Barbara called the current practitioner for a referral. "She presented me with *one name*, she said the *only person* who could see Val there. That was a dogmatic statement, and it set my teeth on edge. With psychotherapy you can't get parental and say, 'This doctor gives you too much penicillin,' but I told Val it was a good time to get a consult. I'd called the therapist first, and the therapist screwed me. She said she wanted to talk to Val beforehand, and she set it up so Val got the feeling I'd been withholding something from her for some time. When I got to talking with Val, I didn't handle the discussion well, and as she was starting out the door, I said, 'You cannot go to college unless you see the consultant!' I was basically pointing out my economic power, but this produced the only summons I got to a joint session for the two and a half years Val was in therapy with this woman, and she interpreted my position openly as not wanting Val to go away.

"The consultant, the man at my hospital, said this therapist was well thought of but known to be very strict. He had a rather negative discussion with her because she wouldn't reveal anything, but he emerged with a sense that she was quite negative about me. He didn't think she had caused the anorexia. But he said not working with me had not been the best thing, that she was very dogmatic, that Val should not see a strict analyst.

"If you think about all this, my kid went into therapy with problems but was not sick. Now I have a kid who's sick. Choosing somebody now, I would look into what approach is used for this illness, but of course Val didn't have an illness then, just some trauma in the past and some mild dysfunction. She had lots of friends, she was doing well enough in school, she was interested in things, and she didn't look depressed. I think that therapy led her to push me away more than was necessary, which exacerbated her need for me. Then I began to feel almost pathologically involved with her. When your kid is sick, you start to analyze her smiles, how she sounds when she says hello. I was trying to read the tea leaves all the time."

The listener tried to read the tea leaves too, and while we had only one side of the story, it was clear that Barbara Kane was, at minimum, a loving, intelligent, and sophisticated parent, and that this therapist, however distinguished, at minimum failed to communicate a convincing rationale for her approach to treating Val. Obviously the chemistry between clinician and parent was bad; but engaging a teenage patient's family (assuming they aren't monsters) is the clinician's responsibility. After watching what happens in good therapy, it is time to consider failure, an experience to which even the best practitioner is not immune. The experience Barbara and Valerie had is, obviously, the sort that parents most fear. Was it built in to the therapist's orientation or to her personality? Could it happen to anyone? Is there a way of preventing it, or do parents simply adopt a vigilant stance once the therapy has begun?

I asked the clinicians who lead off the parts of this book to describe a success and a failure that would shed light on their way of thinking and therapeutic approach. I will report these without interposing my own reactions, except for questions I asked them; moreover, since by now it should be familiar, I will let them use their tribal language in full throttle.

Charles Sarnoff (who, while recognizing the importance of adolescent privacy, would have been less rigid with Barbara Kane) told me about two cases: one where he decided in a few weeks that the child was beyond his purview and referred him out; and one where the child required several tries to benefit from therapy but finally did. In a sense this case was a matter of snatching victory from the jaws of defeat.

"The first youngster was brought in because he'd been thrown out of every school he'd been to for talking back to the teacher and other authorities, throwing a ball back and forth in the classroom without paying attention to the teacher, and holding conversations with other children. Within a short period of time, I was able to tell the parents he didn't deal with me with any of the calm moments and ability to attend to what I'm saying that show any respect for someone else's words. He had a deep sense of entitlement, manifested in opening a window and chewing up pieces of my stationery and spitting it on the cars below. There was no way to enlist his ability to develop a self-reflective awareness."

"Was there," I asked, "any possibility that the kid had underlying AD/HD or some intellectual difficulty?"

"Certainly that was a possibility," Sarnoff said. "This would be in the differential diagnosis, but it's also true that no matter what happened, if he ran into trouble in school, his mother would write a note in support of his lies. Clearly what was happening was a family system situation in which the mother's interaction with the child had less to do with his reality and more to do with intrusions from her own past. This required that her contributions be analyzed while mother and child were in the room at the same time. Family therapists are far more trained to do that than I, so I referred this case to one of them."

The second child was with Sarnoff, on and off, from age six to age ten. "This youngster would bite other kids, crawl over to them across the seats in the back of the classroom. At six years old he had the urge to kiss other boys, and he bit them because he was defending against his own erotic wishes. He would curse in class and looked as if he was trying to shock people. You could work through with him certain thoughts and attitudes, not the least of which was that he thought he came from a place that was different from where everyone else came from, which probably had to do with the fact that he was adopted. He had a fantasy that he had a different set of rules.

"But it turned out he had a thin boundary between the system unconscious and the system conscious. [In early Freudian terminology the *system unconscious* applies to material that is repressed and "not capable of becoming conscious in the ordinary way."] You could say that the primarily autonomous function of the ego to the id would be erased under pressure of somebody else knowing what he didn't know, in the classroom or anywhere else. When you think about it, that's not too severe a stressor, but this everyday thing would really set him off. He had such narcissistic vulnerability.

"My therapy was psychodynamically informed, but it wasn't that I was interpreting. I had to help him develop a way of dealing with the anxiety long enough to slow down his reactions and realize what he was doing. But he had some musical talents and began to develop tremendous pride because he could play an instrument and be admired. He also could read very well. So the most important thing there was the encouragement and development of sublimations."

In the beginning the boy would just applaud Sarnoff's interpretations and regard them as approval, so Sarnoff worked with him to examine his reactions and the consequences of his behavior, often doing role-plays. "You'd get somewhere, and then the whole thing would fall apart. You'd have a teacher who'd be not particularly understanding. He'd be sent down to the principal, and it would humiliate him and set off this reaction." A couple of times Sarnoff, thinking the therapy successful, terminated, telling the parents to feel free to come back if problems recurred. As it turned out, the child did need more therapy, and the family returned to Sarnoff, who concluded, "There was an underlying character deficit that required me to go more deeply into the triggers that were setting him off. But he matured and developed a greater facility for verbalization and insight, which contributed mightily to his improvement. He was able to say, 'Why do I do these crazy things?' Some cases fail that could have succeeded if the children had been brought in at a different time, or if the parents, like these parents, had been willing to try again."

Philip Kendall's perception of success, he points out, is buttressed by teacher ratings and other data. The client, in Kendall's private practice, was a thirteen-year-old boy "with anxiety disorder co-morbid with depression, highly perfectionistic, fussy, pedantic, and prissy. The presenting problem was basically school avoidance with anxiety and distress. He couldn't sleep, he was getting, as he called it, 'busted' by the other kids. He was the grandson of a well-known high-tech entrepreneur. Every day his parents would drive him to public school, dressed preppy to the nines, in one of their fancy cars.

"A key ingredient was that I was a significant other adult who presented another way to look at things. 'Why do you think they busted on you? What are some other ways we could explain that? Do you ever bust on other kids? Do you ever see other kids getting busted? How do they react? Ah, so when some kids get busted, they bust back, and when other kids get busted, they laugh and bust back, and when you get busted you kind of clam up and don't say anything, and they keep going. I wonder if there's anything you could do different that might have an impact on that?'

"He told me he'd just talk to the teachers, because adults are safe, they don't bust up kids. I said we were not going to do that." They got into an analysis of tone of voice and the difference between fun teasing and mean teasing. Kendall worked on the primness and fastidiousness and "had many meetings with the father, a good half dozen of them about how to deal with the child. I wanted the father to develop a playful fatherly relationship, not a controlling governing relationship. This kid didn't need 'sit still, use your fork, be proper, say please.' The father shaped up on that. He himself was fastidious, compulsive, and entitled, with all the qualities the child was developing. But the mother had major, very deep-rooted behavior patterns that weren't very changeable. Any suggestion that she do something different she would take as an attack. So she became a peripheral player, and the child began a much better relationship with the dad.

"Very early on there had been a sort of suicide attempt. He took a bunch of medications that were in the house. The confidence is ninety percent that it *was* a suicide attempt but not one that he wanted to end his life. He was given some medications for pain and for distress, and he took a few more than he should have because he was feeling really bad. I thought it was more of a suicidal gesture to get attention, but it still required monitoring, and we had him temporarily hospitalized.

"At the end of the therapy—one way we evaluated his outcome—was that he was able to go on a three-week tour of the country with other teenagers. This was a kid who was socially avoidant. The mom said he couldn't go on this trip, but I said no, he's got to go on this trip, and he went. He did call home every day for a while and probably spent more money than the other kids, but he could not have done that when he started. Two or three hobbies have come and gone, each with a peer involved and each with some growth."

I asked Kendall how he accounted for the success, and Kendall said, "My gut reaction is that this was a very distressed kid about to do himself in, and he found a friend. The friend didn't say, 'You're sick,' the friend said, 'Let's look at this differently.' Another explanation, though I don't have the hard data, is that he got a more rational and flexible view of peer relations. And we changed the family system: Dad doesn't treat him like a baby. I think he's still going to be a fastidious prissy kid, but bohemian prissy. He's going to line up his magazines on his desk, but there'll be more diversity in the magazines. He's not going to be upset if someone borrows one, and he won't look down on people who can't afford to buy them. I suspect he'll call me up in a year or two to say he's having a hard time with this or that, and we'll kick it around, and he'll hang up and not call me back again for another two years."

And the failure? "A hyperactive boy, also thirteen. The mom worked for the fire department, the father managed a Seven-Eleven store. The mom had spent a portion of her income on private school, a portion of her income on private therapy and medications, and it was getting nowhere and the kid was going to be thrown out of school. In a sense it wasn't all that much of a failure, because we got him through the year without getting thrown out. But he wouldn't come back, and his relationship with his mom deteriorated, and he did not go away with the skills I tried to teach him.

"I take a little responsibility because I think I didn't orchestrate a few things the way I would now. I would say the father's total disengagement was a bad influence and that the mom persisted in making things difficult. The boy and I worked at problem-solving and self-instructions and controlling himself, and he did well in the private office for fifty minutes. It didn't generalize well to school, even though we worked with the teacher and got a little bit of improvement. But as soon as the mom would come to pick him up—or stay for part of the time, which I invited her to do—with the tension and the anger and the fighting between the two of them, I couldn't get anything done. If you could change the world, I would separate the mom and the dad and have the child live with the mom for a while and possibly later live with the dad. The parents' conflict was played out in the kid."

In essence, what we have heard from both Sarnoff and Kendall is that they work well with parents who just need some guidance, but they are not trained to deal with children whose problems are driven by such serious family conflict that the therapist must alter the dynamics of the system in order to help the child. What, then, does a failure look like for Richard Chasin, who *is* trained to deal with these situations? (Chasin cited the two tapes we looked at in depth in Chapter 10 as successes, one a full-fledged case and the other a consult.)

Chasin's failure has haunted him for more than a decade. It was nearly twenty years ago when he got the case, which started well enough. "A six-year-old child was having a lot of learning difficulties," he remembers. "At a family meeting the parents behaved in a thoughtful, understanding way, and I could see no connection between why this kid was not paying attention and what the parents were doing. But when I talked with them about anything except their parenting behavior, they were very guarded." Chasin asked the parents if they would talk more freely at a session without the child, and he got a mixed response. "They described themselves as having a lot of difficulties in their relationship but that when things were calm, the child didn't get into the middle of it. I asked them on which subjects did things get not calm, and the laundry list was unbelievably long."

The parents' backgrounds were very different. The mother, Jewish, came from a nouveau-riche Detroit family that had lived ostentatiously until her father's speculative investments crashed, her mother became an alcoholic, and the family plunged into seedy poverty. The father, Irish, came from a working-class family with a hot-tempered father who suddenly dropped dead, whereupon his mother insisted he go to his after-school job the day of the funeral and not talk about feelings. He was an intelligent and effective businessman as long as you didn't cross him, and "his idea of making it was to have lots and lots of friends and a respectable wife and family, while she wanted to reconstitute the grand old high life and didn't care if she had any friends at all. He could pal around with professors, industrialists, and the postman, but there was very good evidence that he'd been brutally treated by his father, and he had a wild, almost violent temper when she irritated him. It was definitely scary.

"So their idea of what should happen with this kid couldn't have been more divergent. He just wanted the kid to plug away; she wanted evidence of giftedness and didn't care whether he worked or not. The kid got extraordinarily mixed signals." Chasin decided to focus on the couple and had them get the boy a tutor. It took ten candidates to find someone the parents could agree on, "someone who had high aspirations but felt that plugging was just a part of life whether you were a genius or a nincompoop."

But Chasin's sessions with the parents got out of hand, because the wife became obsessionally indecisive on every subject they discussed and set off her husband's temper so he would scream and shake his fists at her, making her even more uncertain. Chasin said, "The therapy seemed to have an antitherapeutic effect": the wife decided to get what she wanted for herself and went on shopping binges and had affairs, which drove the husband wild with rage till the wife threatened to kill her child and herself, which got the husband to relent for the time being. Not surprisingly, the child began to deteriorate: the mother enlisted him as an ally; the father "appreciated the boy's intelligence and his artistic ability, but the kid wouldn't do his schoolwork and so he was trash. So the boy was rejected by the father and fell into the depressed arms of this woman who lived in a fantasy world."

"Where were you during all this?" I asked.

"I'm getting lots of consultations," Chasin said. "Three people were brought in in various ways. The boy was put into a group. I got the woman into individual therapy and the man into individual therapy, but there seemed to be no way to get a purchase on this case." The boy, now teenaged, took refuge in drugs, stealing cars, and dropping out of school, and finally, about ten or twelve years too late, the parents split up. In reflection, Chasin said, "I never figured out a way to make a joint session go, to keep it out of the skids. Things happened with tremendous speed. I watched other people working with them, and they all seemed to have the same problem." Then in a most Chasin-like comment, he added, "I think their style of dealing with each other pushed buttons with me. Neither of them seemed to feel there was any value in peace." But the husband, taking the wife's threats seriously, wouldn't leave until the boy moved out on his own. The end of this story is that the mother now lives alone in boozy indigence, the son is marginally self-supporting, and the father, plugging away, has made a fresh start and is considered an eligible bachelor. But he has declared himself interested only in working-class women.

This is an old case, and Chasin is more authoritative now: he might try another technique, but in essence he would strongly support the couple's moving toward an early divorce. He also believes that the child, who had some "biological disadvantages," had tried to ease his pain with drugs. To some extent Chasin shared the father's values, and the boy seemed to feel that cooperating with the therapist was disloyal to his mother.

Perhaps failures in family systems work are themselves systemic, and once the therapist is sucked into the vortex, he can't get out; certainly even the best therapists have bad chemistry with some clients; and perhaps, since nobody else fixed this family either, some cases may just be unusually difficult. This particular family, of course, does not sound coordinated enough to cut its losses and try an entirely new practitioner, but it's worth keeping in mind that no specialist's qualifications guarantee a perfect record; everybody fails sometimes.

We have already met two clear-cut successes of Harold Koplewicz: Amy Ratner, the bereaved teenager on Prozac, and Andrea Moss, the AD/HD girl whose school life and relationship with her parents improved on Ritalin. He now told me about Jason, a case in which time, in Koplewicz's phrase, became the enemy.

"Jason was an adopted child, and he had a behavioral problem. He was in treatment, as many of these kids are, with a psychoanalyst twice a week for two or three years, which included being in the room with his mother, and he would hit his mother with a pillow and the psychoanalyst would make interpretations. The situation got worse in school, although he was very bright, and his behavior became more and more problematic.

"He was eleven by the time he came to me. It was clear that he didn't just have AD/HD, he also had a lot of co-morbid problems: anxiety and some pervasive developmental delays. He didn't look you in the eye, he didn't shake hands, and he had some difficulties with learning style. All this had a tremendous effect on his self-esteem, and he was very impulsive and provocative and at times very violent. He would torture and try to hurt his younger brother. Ritalin certainly helped this boy to sit longer, to become a much better student, and to have tremendous success in school, and his parents said he was a different child: less irritable and less provocative.

"But by the time the treatment really took hold, he was already twelve years old. There were many family problems: a mother so enraged that she couldn't help herself—or wasn't willing to stop saying very provocative things to the kid; and these are the kinds of kids where you clearly need lots of patience, you have to be able to give a warning and then institute a punishment. The parents were so focused on school and what friends would say that they compromised constantly, and the kid started developing conduct disorder problems as well. They were living in fear that he was going to threaten them with a knife. He was cheating on his medicine.

"I worked together with the psychologist, who was doing cognitive-behavioral approaches with them, and clearly they couldn't control this kid and his environment. The straw that broke the camel's back was he shot a BB into someone's house and shattered a window, and they kept saying somebody else had put the gun in his hand, which very possibly was true. This was the kind of kid who wasn't the mastermind but the one who always got caught.

"He was a fiasco at one of the less restrictive boarding schools, where he set a fire and his father did not make it clear to him that he would have to go away to *some* school. By the time they got him into a special school with a behavior therapy approach, he was fifteen. The child is now on lithium. He came home to visit and was so noncompliant with his medicine and so violent that his parents were afraid to leave him alone. They were petrified of his doing something illegal. The father had to stop working during those few days to stay with the child and supervise him, and now Jason's back there. I've spoken to the school doctor, and I'm not sure if the medication is working or not. He's doing better in school, but I'm quite concerned. Will time become our friend?

"This situation would have required earlier intervention. He's stable but not symptom-free: he's very provocative, he's shaved his head, and there's the combination of conduct problems, judgment problems, and anxiety symptoms, compounded with very poor parenting for this kind of child."

"Is he perhaps bipolar?" I asked.

"That's why we hoped the lithium would work. My recommendation now is to try Tegretol, which is an antiseizure medicine found to be effective for certain bipolar patients when they don't respond well to lithium. I think one of the main problems was that I got the parents when they already seemed pretty burned out and remained part of the problem, though not necessarily the etiology of it. The mother makes provocative statements like, 'You'll be dead on a slab, that's what's going to happen—and that's what I wouldn't want.' This is defective parenting, yet she's fine with the other children."

The parents are unwilling to try family therapy or to change their behavior. "Whether it was my failure, not being able to make an alliance with these people to follow through on recommendations, or whether the mother is intractable, I'm not sure."

Picking up on his earlier comment, I asked Koplewicz whether maybe these problems had just been marinating too long, and whether he'd have been more successful had he gotten the child at six or seven. He said, "I would have had a much better shot. The cognitive-behavioral social-skills training has worked well with kids like this, and we could have modified some of his peculiar behaviors: when he looks at someone he squints a lot, he grimaces, it makes him less likable to authority figures and to peers. And by the time I started to see him, I think his mother disliked him intensely. Ten years ago these people were opposed to seeing a psychopharmacologist: there was a different mindset, and a psycho-analyst made more sense."

Hugh Leichtman of Wediko was able to give me a long-term success and a failure who were brothers. "Peter Millett was with us from 1978 to 1983," he told me. "He is now twenty-seven years old, with a degree in marketing from a college in the Midwest. He couldn't find a marketing job, and the last time we heard from him, a year ago, he was working as a computer programmer. He came from a very bright family, incredibly high-risk and riddled with alcoholism and explosive parenting style. The father was in a civil service job, was in and out of the home, and did the family a favor by dying of cirrhosis of the liver. The mother was a secretary at Tufts. We were able to get the kid out of the family and into alternative placements. This was before we fully understood how foster and adopted children are torn by conflicting loyalties to birth parents, even when the birth family is as chaotic as Peter's: he could never stick with a foster family, even though he had two very good ones. He ended up going back to his group home placement, where he could see his mother but not be in the family. We followed this kid up with services till he graduated from high school, where he was able to get college scholarships. You don't get a better outcome with what you have there. He's married and has a stable job, not the career of his choice, but he's dealing. He learned guitar at Wediko, and he's an accomplished musician.

"We got our hands on Peter when he was ten. Today he would be diagnosed with oppositional defiant disorder, a major impulse control problem, major depression. Peter is very interesting because the use of labeling behavior, being able to develop these symbolic categories, was an important piece. [When Leichtman uses the word *labeling*, he does so in the cognitive sense of teaching children to identify and label their own feelings and actions, a central feature of Wediko's therapeutic techniques. Other therapists and critics of therapy sometimes use *labeling* in the completely different sense of tagging a child with a diagnosis that haunts him for life.] He was quite talented in ceramics, but he'd take ceramic pieces and throw them against the wall when they came out of the kiln. As we watched him, and because he was so bright and articulate, this seemed like a classical case of 'undoing' [a Freudian defense mechanism in which one repeatedly "removes" an act that is dangerous, forbidden, or offensive]. The more he was succeeding, the more he'd start to change the center of gravity of his self-concept, because you define yourself in relation to what you're able to master. To keep the same 'unsuccessful' self-concept, you destroy all the things you do well.

"I remember very well—I did this one myself—*Peter* spelled backward is *Retep*. So we had a T-shirt for him that said 'Peter' on the front, and on the day he had a success everyone would sign it. And the back of the shirt said 'Retep,' and every success he had tried to undo was listed on the back. I'd do my daily rounds and grab his hand and have him walk backward with me for a while. He didn't understand why he was balling up his projects, and I called him Retep, and it was all very compelling and he got it. When he talked to us many years later, he said he used to think about these dramatic interventions, and he remembered Retep and walking backward ten years later, as he said—'the time you put in to treat us all so differently.'"

This is an old case, and Leichtman digressed for a minute: "To break a child out of a monstrous depression, we have to know what's happening biochemically. Just to form a psychological hypothesis whenever there's a sudden change in behavior isn't enough. Good diagnosticians always ask, 'Do we have a biological explanation?' That's the first thing that needs to be checked out."

Peter's older brother Richard arrived at Wediko at age thirteen. "These events accumulate until they reach a critical mass, and Richard had a couple of strikes against him. He wasn't as bright as Peter, though he was bright enough and had a good work ethic. But he was a brittle diabetic, and as he got older, drinking played havoc with his health and his diabetes. We were able to get him out of the house, but everything was about two or three years later than with Peter, and he had that much more damage. We were not able to construct the same type of follow-up treatment package around him. He was never able to finish high school, was incarcerated for drunken driving, and there was also some question, although I never found out definitely, of his embezzling money from his employer. So the last time I heard he was out of jail, struggling with his diabetes—and the diabetes influenced his growth so he was very short, and you had all these things together. He was absolutely enraged that his younger brother had left him behind. When he started feeling depressed he would drink and the drinking led to lapses in judgment and would activate his diabetes. The matrix was so complicated, with all the variables."

I asked Leichtman if the brothers had broken with each other, and he said, "They kept the connection, but Peter made sure he was not pulled into Richard's life. He said, 'I have to work hard just to keep my head above water,' and he did."

Besides whatever light they shed on each clinician's approach, these stories seem to yield up a few leitmotivs. One is that children always return to an environment, and the best therapeutic efforts will fail if the family is ridden with conflict or in some way determined to sabotage the therapy, or even if they're just not very helpful: indeed, as Charles Popper pointed out in Chapter 15, the patient's ability to manage his or her disorder and seek help when it's needed can be more important than the seriousness of the biological disability. Another theme is the significance of timing: success depends partly on the child's being at the right age to benefit from therapy, but problems left to marinate very often get worse, not better. A third theme is the salutary effect of talents, hobbies, and mastery at school.

A final leitmotiv is that therapists are human beings and subject to the same defenses as the rest of us in accounting for their mistakes. How therapists explain their failures, I learned, is a subject of interest to Philip Kendall too: he and two of his graduate students polled 315 clinical psychologists—psychodynamic, humanist, cognitive-behavioral, and eclectic, in this case meaning practitioners who combined two of the other orientations—who were members of the American Psychological Association and the American Association for Behavioral Therapy. None were psychiatrists, social workers, or child therapists, but that doesn't matter here, as we are talking about a basic human process. What did turn out to matter somewhat was their theoretical orientation.

About 11 percent of each therapist's patients were not making progress. The authors classified these cases as mild or severe according to DSM diagnosis or previous hospitalization, and they concluded, logically, that severity is a major correlate of failure to make progress in therapy. Interestingly enough, however, not one of the polled therapists chose what would seem to be an obvious explanation for the lack of progress by his or her own client: that the client's symptoms were so severe as to be intractable or at least very difficult to clear up. In general, they didn't much blame themselves either. Psychodynamic, humanistic, and eclectic therapists were most likely to fault the client's inability or lack of motivation; cognitive-behaviorists, though they also blamed the client first, were more willing to cite bad luck. The cognitive-behaviorists threw up their hands in six months, while the psychodynamic practitioners slogged along for more than a year, and the other orientations were in between the two.

Some two-thirds of the therapists were about to refer the clients out (or had already done so). Only a quarter of them had an alternative treatment plan, while 41 percent were going to (as I would paraphrase it, using that old definition of *fanaticism*) redouble their enthusiasm the further they got from their goal, and the rest admitted they ultimately would refer the clients out.

Kendall and his co-authors deplored the absence of objective criteria for failure (or success), and that the "lack of acceptance/use of alternate techniques places the therapist in the position of having to explain 'failures' by blaming their clients." Kendall and all the other lead therapists in this book were at least willing to acknowledge the limitations of their own approach or seek consultations; they didn't just push on alone. But it is important for parents to recognize that clinicians, like Valerie Kane's therapist, may have too large an emotional investment or too little flexibility or strength of character to acknowledge defeat. For this reason it behooves the parents to inform themselves sufficiently about therapeutic approaches that they will not be intimidated by the practitioner's credentials. They should feel enough self-confidence to tell the therapist that the child seems to be making no progress after a reasonable amount of time—or that the child seems *more* reclusive or distressed—and it's time to get a consult.

The obvious first question that lay people (whether choosing a therapist for their own children or making a referral) ask is, What is known about the effectiveness of therapeutic outcomes for children? In two words, not much. In the book *Child Psychotherapy: Developing and Identifying Effective Treatments,* the psychologist Alan Kazdin, then of the University of Pittsburgh and now of Yale, cites a 1985 meta-analysis of smaller outcome studies that established that the average child who is treated is better off at the end of talk therapy than 76 percent of those who did not receive treatment. This figure is slightly less optimistic than an accepted figure of 80 to 85 percent better off for treated versus untreated adults. At the same time Kazdin notes the absence of sufficient satisfactory empirical data to compare techniques of therapy. In varying degrees all types of child therapy are understudied.

According to Morris B. Parloff, clinical professor of psychiatry at Georgetown and retired chief of the Psychosocial Treatments Research Branch, Division of Extramural Research Programs at the National Institute of Mental Health, what studies exist tend to cover cognitive-behavioral therapy because of that school's interest in measurement and because the duration of cognitive-behavioral therapy is short enough to be a manageable dissertation subject. On the other hand, psychodynamic therapists find outcome studies "reductionistic"; and since they were so long the establishment, they haven't felt the need to prove themselves.

Parloff, an adult psychologist, has written frequently about the implications of the "nonspecificity" hypothesis—that "since different forms of psychotherapy, using quite different 'specific' techniques and procecedures, nonetheless achieve equivalent effects, then such effects may be attributed not to the specific techniques but to some 'nonspecific' elements common to these therapies."

In discussing what these nonspecific common factors are, Parloff notes the work of Jerome Frank, who held that all therapy treats the patient's "acute sense of demoralization" and does it in four different ways: it offers "a trusting, confiding, emotional relationship"; it does this in a setting which has a special "safe" aura; the therapist offers an explanation for "bewildering subjective states and behaviors"; and there is a "prescribed set of procedures based on the conceptual scheme."

We have seen the measure of professional therapists' skills throughout this book, and they clearly are in a different league from those of amateurs like sympathetic Aunt Susie and semipros like Ms. Brooks, the fifth-grade teacher, and Parson Brown. The nonspecificity hypothesis is not supposed to be simplistic. It doesn't obviate the need for talent, skill, and experience on the part of the therapist, who is more than just a paid chum. As Parloff points out, "The expert therapist knows when to turn down the rheostat and do something else. The novice, however, who is uncertain of what to do, has no justification for doing anything other than being 'a nice guy.' " The hypothesis also doesn't apply to severe psychoses, for which therapy is neither the cure nor the sole treatment but simply a rehabilitative measure. But as we have also seen throughout this book, there are usually several ways for a talk therapist to define a problem, and with little hard evidence that one is better than another, parents have some freedom to choose what seems most comfortable for the child and for themselves. The more minute internecine theoretical differences among, say, family systems therapists or psychodynamic therapists make interesting reading for parents who are so inclined, and it will help them understand why their child's therapist is following a particular tack; but what is most important is how from moment to moment this clinician connects with this child.

As for the pharmacotherapy that applies to a particular disorder, it is essential to give it informed consideration: failure to do so can lead a child on a long hike down the wrong road, with a risk of secondary complications.

Outcome studies deal mostly with behavior therapy and pharmacotherapy. Short-term tests might assess whether the treatment helps children do better at certain school tasks; long-term tests study such empirically based results as whether fewer treated patients, compared with controls, were arrested or hospitalized or divorced or flunked out of school. This information is, unfortunately, of limited value for parents deciding whether to get therapy for their children and which therapy to choose. It is hard to find a rigorous objective quantitative measure for self-esteem and satisfying relationships with family and friends, although an individual set of parents might be able to figure one out for their own child. Finally, all but the narrowest and most immediate measures of psychotherapy are limited because circumstances affect lives, and it's difficult to assign credit or blame to the therapy.

Neither Parloff nor Kazdin believes that comparisons of therapeutic outcomes are impossible: both suggest that by abandoning global questions we might eventually find out more about "*what* treatment, by *whom*, is most effective for *this* individual with *that* specific problem, under *which* set of circumstances." Since the net of all this is that parents are still, to a large measure, on their own, that is a good first question for them to ask.

Pharmacotherapy, as far as it goes, offers the most rigorous evidence for or against a particular treatment: that is, a body of literature reports that if a patient has a certain set of symptoms, a given medicine is more or less effective than placebo in removing or modifying some or all of these symptoms. Psychopharmacologists, as a group, are cautious to a fault in documenting their claims: indeed, when one such psychiatrist states that patients who turn out to have a particular disorder tend toward a certain type of dream, others are likely to push him to the wall saying, "As compared to whom? Where's your documentation?"

Still, in pharmacotherapy as in all therapies, some things happen in individual cases that no one predicted. Information on the long-term effects of particular medicines is limited chiefly by the newness of the drugs: some drugs—Prozac and its peers, for example—have not been around for very long or may be fairly new as a treatment for children or for a specific disorder. One always weighs the risks of taking the medicine against the risks of not taking it: that is, a child is a developing organism, and a disorder that impairs the child's functioning may have lifetime consequences that far exceed a D in history. This dictates that a careful clinical diagnosis is the minimum requirement for the use of psychiatric medicine, and after that the decision depends on the individual case.

The most thoroughly studied drug used for children is Ritalin, which, as we remember, as been around since the mid-fifties. There is an extensive body of literature on its effects and side effects over both the long and short term; parents and other nonprofessionals who need to make decisions should read up before forming an opinion. Harold Koplewicz says, "We've had kids who have been on Ritalin for many, many years, and we know that it affects weight and there seems to be some delay in growth, and maybe even the kids may not be as tall. These are minor effects long term considering the fact that the kids who don't take it might have a higher rate of problems in being maintained in school.

"The tricyclic antidepressive medicines," Koplewicz continues, "have been used for enuresis and depression for a long time. We know at least that kids who took them for several years for enuresis have not had severe side effects later in life. But I think it's noteworthy that we really don't have the answers to a lot of questions. I think we hold ourselves—and the public holds mental health professionals who use medicines—to a higher standard, because after all, the medicines have a spooky quality. Some parents are very concerned. 'How is it possible that a medicine is going to give my child longer attention? Is it going to change their personality? Am I going to have a different adolescent? Is it somehow going to control their brain?' No, but you have to sit down and explain why.

"You don't think of psychiatric medicines as causing situations like DES, but certainly one has to be very careful in monitoring medicines for young children. In conventional pediatrics, it has always been customary to start the antibiotic before you get the culture back. That's something we don't do in psychiatry. You try to have high confidence in the diagnosis before you give them."

How, then, should parents go about choosing a therapist, and what should they do if the therapy doesn't seem to be working? I assume readers have absorbed some of this information osmotically through the earlier chapters; still, a more directive wrapup is useful and incorporates my own conclusions after three years of research.

Parents who are unsure of the seriousness of their child's symptoms might find it helpful to go to the library and consult DSM-IV. If behavior described in the manual sounds familiar, that's one signal to seek diagnostic help, although the therapist's conclusion may be different from what the parents inferred after reading the manual. DSM comes with a caveat: as Wediko's Harry Parad points out, "The diagnostic nomenclature unfairly dumps children into categories that deemphasize the affective component in their lives and emphasize the behavioral. We find that children we work with who fall into the conduct disorder categories need to be rediagnosed once a therapist has worked with the child for six months or so. The child looks more dysthymic or depressed." What this means is not necessarily that the therapy has changed the disorder but that the therapy can itself be a diagnostic exploration. DSM, in other words, is a point of departure, not a conclusion, and only a clinician can make individual diagnoses. Many symptoms of AD/HD are by now familiar, but if there is a question of OCD or eating disorders, DSM is a good way to point oneself in the right direction by seeking a therapist with particular knowledge of the problem.

Not all children who are reacting to stressful situations—a move, a divorce, a death in the family—necessarily require help. But parents should be vigilant, and if there seems to be no progress in healing or adjustment (or if there is a sudden onset of symptoms) after several months, it makes sense to consult a professional. A child can, as readers now know, have a chronic condition exacerbated by stressful events.

When a child is having school problems—which may be academic or social—the first step is usually a parent-teacher or parent-principal conference, often initiated by the school. Good questions to ask are whether the difficulties occur with one teacher or several, and whether there are also problems with classmates. Sometimes a change of teacher or even a new school might solve the problem; obviously, if this happens more than once, it's time for parents to seek a different explanation.

If the school and the parents decide the child might have a psychological or learning disorder, parents may prefer to seek out their own testers: then they, not the school, are in charge of the case. Michael Thompson, the psychologist and school consultant in Chapter 6, notes that "if you have a kid who's not doing well in high school and has never done well in school, is there a primary learning disability that's never been diagnosed and now the kid's failure-ridden and depressed? Or is this in fact a child who has no learning disability but has been depressed all along and was never able to mobilize her energy? This is what psychological and learning-disability testing studies."

Whether the issue is school problems or something else, a good source of referral is the child's pediatrician (although he or she should not be the one to prescribe psychiatric medicine). So are friends whose children have had similar problems, provided the parents themselves check out the therapist's credentials. In general, besides academic and institutional credentials a therapist should have treated many children with similar conditions. Children with eating disorders need to begin with a medical workup and continue to be monitored by a physician, since these are life-threatening illnesses. In a case that does not require hospitalization, however, psychologists and social workers—provided they specialize in eating disorders—often do excellent therapy.

Only a *pediatric* psychiatrist or neurologist—preferably a specialist in psychopharmacology—should prescribe medicine, and only after a thorough diagnostic workup that includes not only a physical examination but educational tests, information from the school and the parents, and a long session or several with the child.

The diagnosis should be delivered in clear lay English. As Koplewicz says, "Parents should ask, 'What is the diagnosis? What is the prognosis? What can you tell me about the different types of treatments that are available? What are the successes and failures of each treatment? And what is the risk to the child of not having any intervention?' This is what they would do if they were going for surgery or for any kind of intensive procedure for their child." Medication should be accompanied by some amount of talk therapy, which can be done either by the psychiatrist or in tandem with a psychologist or family therapist who, in each of their particular spheres, may surpass the psychiatrist. Even so, a biological psychiatrist should not be brusque: he or she should display both the skill and the patience to talk helpfully and at length with the child and the family.

Even if parents are not aware of particular family or marital difficulties (and some soul-searching is definitely in order), a symptomatic child disturbs the family system and some family therapy can be helpful.

In Erikson's phrase therapists ought to be doing triple bookkeeping, paying attention to the child's biology, his internal psychology, and the family and school worlds in which he lives. Parents should be on guard for rigid formulations or the suggestion that a certain set of symptoms inevitably has one etiology. For example, in a recent lawsuit in which a therapist convinced a young woman and her mother that the young woman was repressing memories of incest by the father, according to the *New York Times* report, the therapist told the family that bulimia is usually caused by incest. This is absolute nonsense: as any specialist in eating disorders would point out, bulimia has many possible causes.

The next question—an absolutely crucial issue—is the reaction of the parent and the child to the therapist. While we don't necessarily have to like our ophthalmologists or dermatologists, mental health professionals are people we do have to like. Under no circumstances should children be dragged to therapists they hate: many of the horror stories I heard involved such incidents. The therapist will accomplish nothing, and the child's unpleasant memories will poison the efforts of future practitioners. As for the parents, they should feel the therapist has some rapport with their values—note the nine entry points cited by the family therapist Betty Karrer in Chapter 12. They should not feel intimidated or diminished; they should feel some relief and at the same time have something to chew over when they leave.

Koplewicz says parents should ask themselves, " 'How was the person able to share with me information that could have been very upsetting? And was it done so that I could really understand the information?' Some people will say, 'The doctor speaks too slowly, there's too much silence,' and others might say, 'The doctor is too frenetic and high-paced and too pressured for me. I have trouble with that style.' You have to trust this person, and you have to work with them: if their style makes it difficult for you to hear what they're saying, or if they seem either too rigid or too loose, it's going to make the task harder."

Parents should avoid hastiness, Koplewicz says. "During the first or second session, when there's a diagnostic evaluation, someone is giving you information about your child that may be very upsetting to you, even if the prognosis is good. Parents should take some time to think before making a decision, so they might actually say to the doctor, 'I'd like to come back and see you for another session to discuss the findings after I've thought them over,' and see how they feel after the second session. If the parents feel comfortable and the child is just resistant to anybody, one of the things to do is tell the child, 'Look, you have to see someone and we feel comfortable with Dr. A and Dr. B. You can choose which of them you want, but you have to see somebody.' If the child still refuses, it's a terrible bind, and you may have to ask the doctor, "Are you willing to work with our child even though our child doesn't want to work with you?' Some doctors can't do that, and others will say, 'We'll work together as a family, or we'll work together for brief periods with the child alone.' "

It's essential to set goals for the treatment in advance (Stanley Kutcher, in Chapter 15, is especially good on this) and get some realistic notion of how long the therapist thinks it will take to reach them. To avoid situations like Barbara Kane's, parents and therapist need to fix ground rules in advance. As Koplewicz observes, "What the fees will be is minor compared to: Will the doctor speak to the parents? Will the doctor talk to the school? Is the doctor willing to visit the school and have a conference with the child's teachers? What are the guidelines for confidentiality? When the child is twelve or over, this information should be shared with the child."

Moreover, Koplewicz says, "anytime in a treatment that's moving on, if the child's symptoms are not getting better or something is going on that makes the parents uncomfortable, the first thing to do is to go to the mental health professional and state your concerns." I asked him about a situation in which the child is adolescent and her privacy is important but the parents, feeling the buck stops with them, want to know how things are going. "It's a major problem if the child is really doing poorly and you have no way of getting that information to the therapist. The problem is more subtle where the kid is doing well and the parent is just curious and the patient is in a dynamically oriented treatment where the therapist feels somehow it will affect the patient's trust."

The point is that these issues should be resolved as treatment starts. "A concerned parent will feel the need to get report cards," Koplewicz says, "and it would be helpful if the therapist would state, 'These are the things we'll be looking at, and if things are going well, these things will be diminishing and those things will be increasing. Then we'll know we're going in the right direction. If you insist on an update, I could do this every six months, or every quarter I can give you a brief summary without giving the details of the case. It would also be helpful at that time if you could give me feedback as to how you think things are going and information I may have been missing.' " If this sort of relationship is established at the outset, a good therapist should not object to a consult when the therapy seems to be stuck.

In Chapter 5 we encountered the theories of Thomas S. Kuhn on how scientific revolutions proceed: while I reported them as applied to the psychodynamic world, I found Kuhn's theories also cited in historical accounts of cognitive-behavioral therapy and family systems therapy. In sum, Kuhn describes the reevaluation and controversy that ensue when anomalous discoveries force scientists to reconsider the assumptions under which they have done their work: there follows a period of uncertainty and even crisis while new sets of assumptions (paradigms, in academic language) compete to dominate the field. The revolutionary process described by Kuhn takes many years.

It seems very clear that the field of mental health is in the process of a Kuhnian revolution. Psychological research with infants in laboratories and with victims of accidents and strokes and brain disease, new brain imaging technology, animal studies, neuroendocrinology, and the effects of psychotropic drugs are overturning many of our previous assumptions about mental processes, and researchers are still on the trail of a cohesive set of assumptions to replace them, beyond the very broad notion that biological predispositions are evoked by environmental conditions. Selection theory, for example, a complex formulation described in a recent book by Michael S. Gazzaniga, director of the Center for Neurobiology at the University of California at Davis, is just one example of the ideas now competing in the intellectual marketplace. It holds that "all we do in life is discover what is already built into our brains," that "an organism comes delivered to this world with all the world's complexity already built in. In the face of an environmental challenge, the matching process starts, and what the outsider sees as learning is actually the organism searching through its library of circuits and accompanying strategies for ones that will best allow it to respond to the challenge." Researchers who espouse selection theory, for one small illustration, discount the unconscious but seek other explanations for psychological complexity. Noting that humans alone among animals have the adaptive capacity to assume deceptive facial expressions, they suggest we gradually sharpen our ability to deceive others, and in the process we learn to deceive ourselves.

The real message of the excellent but controversial book *Listening to Prozac* is that there are no givens. Not only the effects of the drug on patients—as perceived and reported by the psychiatrist Peter D. Kramer, who wrote the book—but a body of pertinent research done in the past few decades (which Kramer also describes) may overturn our notions of the nature-nurture balance in the etiology of mental illness. Clinicians have already come to regard major depression and AD/HD as biological illnesses not fundamentally different from ulcers and diabetes: perhaps your sour personality is as medically treatable as your sour stomach. It may be, as suggested in the "kindling" model of mental illness (which Kramer describes, Leichtman and Parad mention in Chapter 17, and Kruesi and Kutcher give nods to in Chapters 14 and 15), that minor depression unmedicated makes the patient increasingly vulnerable to ever-milder stressors, resulting in a major episode later in life; if this is the case, Prozac is not what Kramer calls "cosmetic psychopharmacology" but sound preventive medicine. On the other hand, as a result of Prozac perhaps, a patient with minor depression lifted is able to succeed at school, work, friendship, and family life, and these supports may buffer her against the effects of later stress.

Psychiatrists who treat children deal with issues somewhat different from those with adult patients, because a child's personality is still being formed. Harold Koplewicz, for example, still strongly believes you cannot medicate self-esteem: it comes indirectly from the experiences of success and mastery that healthy children enjoy. These experiences are to varying degrees blocked for a child with obsessive-compulsive disorder, AD/HD or clinical depression. Once the obstacle is removed by Ritalin or Prozac, the child appears more self-confident and outgoing, but life, not medicine, has produced that effect.

As Gabrielle Carlson, the diagnostician we met in Chapter 2, points out, if an AD/HD child gets Ritalin in elementary school and turns out to be among the 50 percent who outgrow the disease in adolescence, when you discontinue the drug you have still given him a childhood of benign experiences that can't but help him in later life. If, however, the child is among the other 50 percent who retain their symptoms (particularly in the group at the far end of the spectrum that goes on to develop conduct disorder), when you discontinue the drug you will be back at square one.

If all this is so, the belief that self-knowledge acquired by visits to a talk therapist twice a week is a brand of healing morally superior to that of taking a pill is not only harmful but silly; we seem to be having an onrush of Luddism. But while I would submit that perceived (and equivocal) moral issues are a poor basis for devising treatment plans in any case, we have not sorted out the nature-nurture questions yet, and we will not do so tomorrow. Theories are battling, and and no one knows which combination of them will ultimately prevail.

This is healthy and normal, part of the historical pattern of scientific progress. But it is harrowing for lay people who want definite answers. It won't directly help Mr. and Ms. Jones find the best treatment for their troubled son Brian. But if the Joneses remain sensible and open-minded, it offers them some choice and power: they need not defer to an authoritarian expert, and they can inform themselves and select what seems applicable. This doesn't mean any therapy will do for any patient, but it does mean there are no absolutes in the way a therapist may properly assemble the treatment package. Depending primarily on the nature of the problem, there are usually several helpful ways to see a case.

This book is not a tract on public policy, but some issues leap out after a study of theory and practice in psychotherapy. It is surely time we thought about making our society friendlier to children. In April 1994 the Carnegie Corporation of New York published a report called *Starting Points: Meeting the Needs of Our Youngest Children:* it offers numerous compelling suggestions for dealing with the effects of social change and poverty on children under three. Several clinicians have pointed out to me that we do very badly with adolescents also: at just the time when teenagers are beginning to separate from their parents and need to form close relationships with other adults, we plunge them into large impersonal schools, where students move from class to class and each teacher has a clientele of at least 150. We cut after-school activities and sports programs in communities, close libraries, and in general reduce opportunities to get to know those supportive adults who often serve to buffer children from the stresses of life. (Once again, let's ask that ubiquitous question, Do psychotherapists give children anything they can't get from Aunt Susie, the scout leader, or the sixth-grade teacher? One answer: What Aunt Susie? What scout leader? What sixth-grade teacher?) There is much more we can do in simple low-tech services to keep kids healthy: if, as the African proverb suggests, it takes a village to raise a child, what sort of villages have we set up?

We now know the different tribal worlds therapists live in and that informed parents must become case managers for their children. What happens when parents haven't the skills to do this? Harry Parad told me what happened when Wediko's school-based program needed to refer children and their families for hospitalization: the children, who were saying they wanted to hurt themselves or others, clearly met the criteria. "When we sent the child and the parent into the hospital by themselves, very few would be admitted, no matter how convincing," Parad said. "The children wouldn't tell their story to the person doing the screening interview, in part because they didn't know the person but partly because they had to repeat that story, which was embarrassing, the same number of times that anyone does if they go in for a physical problem. You have an aching knee, and the first thing they do is take your temperature.

"If you're facing some pressing psychological issue, going through all those different filters makes it less and less likely that by the time you actually reach the psychiatrist, a total stranger, you're going to feel sufficiently respected to tell your story. The admitting process took from five to seven hours from arrival in the emergency room to a decision being made.

"When we sent a Wediko therapist or a school guidance adviser who knew the family, the rate of admission was very high. The family would let that professional help tell their story, but you had to free someone up for the entire day and give them a lot of quarters to keep everyone in candy bars and sodas while they waited endlessly in an emergency room. We figured out how to make that chunk of the system more responsive, but it is incredibly time-consuming and expensive. Then, when the child is in the hospital for seven to ten days and gets discharged, the continuity of service has become increasingly important. If you go one place for this chunk of service, another place for this, and a third place for that, how do a troubled child and his parents integrate all that? The hospitals need to have working relationships with the professionals who refer the children. When we keep the same people available and make a commitment to the family to help them through the maze, these parents are much more amenable to working with us than we thought—or than the field as a whole thought."

The most important issue in providing mental health care, then, is to diminish the fragmentation. This also applies to social services: everybody at Wediko, not to mention other professionals in residential treatment, told me the ability to put together a continuous package of services for a child is crucial to successful results.

The scientific revolution I discussed earlier in the context of parental decisions has public policy implications too. For example, when and if we ever sort out conclusively the biological and environmental components of homosexuality, somebody will be very unhappy and the knowledge is bound to affect policy. To the extent that we find biological factors in violent behavior, the questions of when to intervene will be difficult and important. Other genetic discoveries in the field of mental health will also raise hard questions both for individuals and for society. While my own religious belief that the truth shall set us free is tempered slightly by middle-aged experience, I still believe that inevitable decisions are made better from a solid base of knowledge than from primitive emotional prejudices. As Gabrielle Carlson remarks, "We used to think thunderbolts were hurled by Zeus, but now we know better." Let us, then, get on with the research that needs to be done. After reading various articles about the probable social consequences of Prozac, I am also skeptical of efforts to guess the effects of scientific and technological development on mass behavior: look up predictions about automobiles, television, and computers, and you discover they have always been at least a little off.

I have spent the past three years focusing my attention on the numberless varieties of human suffering. One is bound to be affected by this: as the research neared its end, my patience with lay people sitting at the dinner table moralizing about pharmacotherapy and other mental health issues began to wear thin. If nonprofessional readers close this book less sure of the causes of mental illness than they were when they opened it, I will feel satisfied. Whether a patient needs therapy, and what kind of therapy, is a most personal decision between that patient (and if the patient is a child, the child's parents) and the clinician who has evaluated that case. Since therapy costs money, we must, realistically, have gatekeepers: but the only gatekeepers I trust are those with everyday experience in treating the sick.

As for tribal viewpoints, they follow two paths: empirically focused therapists—those in the behavioral and biological groups—say, "We won't deal with what we can't see and thus at least try to prove"—and thus must disregard much of the texture of human anguish. The psychodynamic therapists say, "We will make our best guess." Thus they alone confront our dark side. If we can no longer quite call them scientists, they are surely poets, and we need the poet as much as we need the scientist. While it is perilous to mistake poetry for science, we must also know that science has its limits.

Let us, then, think back to Hector Lopez, the seven-year-old "dinosaur boy" who challenged the diagnostic conference in Chapter 2. Science can tell us that Hector has attention-deficit/hyperactivity disorder and will be able to focus better on his life with the help of Ritalin: to deny him that would be callous indeed. But science cannot tell us about the dinosaur games Hector has developed to cope with the chaos of his brain and his family. With luck, talk therapy will do that. Science cannot teach Hector that in order to make a life for himself and find friends he can turn to when the world is frightening, he will need to act differently; behavior modification can do that. And science cannot make a plan for Hector's life or help his family manage the problems they have; family therapy and social work can try to do that.

And when (and if) all of these professionals have done their job, Hector will still be Hector, the sum of his biological endowment and his social experiences in his family and his culture. He will still be unique.

NOTES

CHAPTER 1: HOW DO OUR CHILDREN GET SICK?

page

7. But recent community . . . *mal du siècle*.: Elizabeth J. Costello, Ph.D., "Developments in Child Psychiatric Epidemiology," *Journal of the American Academy of Child and Adolescent Psychiatry* 28 (1989), p. 836.

8. In 1988 . . . childhood ailments.: Elizabeth J. Costello, Ph.D., et al., "Psychiatric Disorders in Pediatric Primary Care," *Archives of General Psychiatry* 45 (December 1988).

8. The suicide rate . . . 1988.: "From the Centers for Disease Control, Attempted Suicide Among High School Students—United States, 1990," *JAMA* 266, no. 14 (9 October 1991).

8. The suspicion . . . Catherine T. Howell.: Thomas M. Achenbach, M.D., and Catherine T. Howell, M.S., "Are American Children's Problems Getting Worse? A 13-Year Comparison," *Journal of the American Academy of Child and Adolescent Psychiatry* 32, no. 6 (November 1993), pp. 1145–54.

10. In 1989 a special section . . . *Psychiatry*.: Costello, "Developments."

10. A good example . . . in 1988.: David Shaffer, F.R.C.P., F.R.C. Psych., et al., "Preventing Teenage Suicide: A Critical Review," *Journal of the American Academy of Child and Adolescent Psychiatry* 27, no. 6 (1988), pp. 675–87.

11. While drug overdose . . . substance abusers.: While guns are the preferred method of both teenage boys and teenage girls, the study points out that "there seems to be a complicated association between sex, substance abuse (which in the New York Study is a common correlate among male suicides but not among females) and suicide by firearm."

13. As practitioners . . . "factor analysis.": Stella Chess and Alexander Thomas, *Origins and Evolution of Behavior Disorders: From Infancy to Early Adult Life* (Cambridge, Mass.: Harvard University Press, 1987), pp. 61ff.

13. But as they observe . . . reservations.: Ibid., pp. 64ff.

15. In a 1989 . . . "stress or turmoil.": Eric Ostrov, J.D., Ph.D., Daniel Offer, M.D., and Kenneth I. Howard, Ph.D., "Gender Differences in Adolescent Symptomatology: A Normative Study," *Journal of the American Academy of Child and Adolescent Psychiatry* 28, no. 3 (1989), pp. 394—98.

18. Criminality is not . . . have here.: Cathy Spatz Widom, "Childhood Victimization and Adolescent Problem Behaviors," in *Adolescent Problem Behaviors*, ed. M. E. Lamb and R. Ketterlinus (New York: Lawrence Erlbaum, 1994).

page
19.   The result . . . a British psychiatrist.: Norman Garmezy, Ph.D., and Michael Rutter, M.D., eds., *Stress, Coping, and Development in Children* (Baltimore: Johns Hopkins University Press, 1988).

20.   To do so . . . "factors in the environment.": Garmezy and Rutter, *Stress*, p. 49.

22.   "It was evident . . . their environment.": Ibid., p. 69.

23.   "Whether the concepts" . . . have written.: Chess and Thomas, *Origins and Evolution*, p. 14.

23.   Theories that recognized . . . "for culture.": Ibid., p. 19.

23.   Both the research literature . . . these ideas.: For this account of how the NYLS began, I have also drawn on *Fifty Years Together*, a privately printed memoir by Stella Chess, M.D., Alexander Thomas, M.D., and Penny Colman.

24.   According to this . . . "and distorted development.": Chess and Thomas, *Origins and Evolution*, p. 21.

30.   (In his book *Child Psychotherapy* . . . emerge and disappear.): Alan E. Kazdin, *Child Psychotherapy: Developing and Identifying Effective Treatments* (New York: Pergamon Press, 1988), p. 7 regarding problems that go away, and p. 8 for problems that are precursors of adult problems.

30.   Those who believe . . . "Z-process.": Ibid., pp. 41–44.

31.   While most clinicians . . . the challenge differently.: D. W. Winnicott, *The Piggle: An Account of the Psychoanalytic Treatment of a Little Girl* (New York: International Universities Press, 1977), p. 2.

34.   And as the psychologist . . . used to be.: Judith S. Wallerstein, Ph.D., and Sandra Blakeslee, *Second Chances: Men, Women, and Children a Decade After Divorce* (New York: Ticknor & Fields, 1989), p. 297.

36.   To compare . . . demographics of therapy.: The estimated number of child and adolescent psychiatrists, as of 1994, comes from the American Association of Child and Adolescent Psychiatrists. The number of psychologists and social workers comes from a National Institute of Mental Health Report, "Mental Health, United States 1990," ed. Ronald W. Manderscheid, Ph.D., and Mary Anne Sonnenschein, M.S. The estimated number of child clinical specialists comes from the American Psychological Association.

CHAPTER 2:   FINDING THE LESION

41.   (While current definitions . . . outer world.): This definition comes from *Psychoanalytic Terms and Concepts*, edited by Burness E. Moore, M.D., and Bernard D. Fine, M.D., and published by the American Psychoanalytic Association and Yale University Press in 1990. Although Carlson and the others in the case conference are not psychoanalysts, this is one analytic term that is in general use.

52.   "[A] specifiable course . . . and biological correlates.": G. A. Carlson and J. Garber, "Developmental Issues in the Classification of Childhood Depression," in *Depression in Children: Developmental Perspectives*, ed. Michael Rutter et al. (New York: Guilford Press, 1986), p. 400.

53.   It is not the tool . . . in the United States.: This historical account is taken from DSM-IV, pp. xvi–xviii.

54.   In 1989, Carlson . . . issues in AD/HD.: G. A. Carlson and M. D. Rapport,

page
     "Diagnostic Classification Issues in Attention-Deficit Hyperactivity Disorder, *Psychiatric Annals* 19, no. 11 (November 1989), pp. 576–83.

54.   ([S]uch as clumsiness . . . dyscoordination): Also described by Charles W. Popper, M.D., "Disorders Usually First Evident in Infancy, Childhood, or Adolescence," in *American Psychiatric Press Textbook of Psychiatry*, ed. R. E. Hales, J. A. Talbott, and S. C. Yudofsky (Washington, D.C., American Psychiatric Press, 1988), chap. 21.

55.   But this next . . . "of a disorder.": Carlson and Rapport, "Diagnostic Classification Issues."

59.   Carlson herself . . . subsequent disorders.: Carlson and Garber, "Developmental Issues." p. 427.

60.   Back in the sixties . . . *Psychoanalytic Study of the Child*.: Three papers by Anna Freud, "Assessment of Childhood Disturbances" (1962), "The Concept of Developmental Lines" (1963), and "The Symptomatology of Childhood" (1970), along with work by others at Hampstead, were collected in *Psychoanalytic Assessment: The Diagnostic Profile*," ed. Ruth S. Eissler, Anna Freud, Marianne Kris, and Albert Solnit (New Haven: Yale University Press, 1977).

63.   As Brooks wrote . . . "child's development." Robert Brooks, "Projective Techniques in Personality Assessment," in *Developmental-Behavioral Pediatrics*, ed. Melvin D. Levine et al. (Philadelphia: W. B. Saunders, 1983), p. 974.

64.   This is what Brooks . . . "personality characteristics.": Ibid., p. 983.

CHAPTER 3:   THE PLAYING CURE

72.   The American Psychoanalytic . . . "motivational forces.": Moore and Fine, *Psychoanalytic Terms and Concepts*, p. 152.

72.   A child who has undergone . . . "unexpected places.": Charles A. Sarnoff, *Psychotherapeutic Strategies in the Latency Years* (Northvale, N.J.: Jason Aronson, 1987), p. 145.

73.   Freudians aren't . . . "to a unity.": *A General Selection from the Works of Sigmund Freud*, ed. John Rickman, M.D. (New York: Anchor Books, 1957), p. 124.

73.   When feelings . . . "are reinstated.": Sarnoff, *Strategies in Latency*, p. 74.

75.   Sarnoff, like most psychodynamic . . . "being left out.": Ibid., p. 103.

76.   Sarnoff, as he has written . . . "therapist or analyst.": Ibid., pp. 107–8.

77.   "People with emotional" . . . he writes.: Ibid., p. 96.

77.   "Learning is only one . . . sense of inadequacy.": Ibid., p. 109.

CHAPTER 4:   ROOTS (PART ONE)

88.   The comments of Martin Leichtman . . . "formulated and evaluated.": Martin Leichtman, "Developmental Psychology and Psychoanalysis: I. The Context for a Revolution in Psychoanalysis," *Journal of the American Psychoanalytic Association* 38, no. 4 (1990). My thinking has also been influenced by the yet-unpublished second part of this account, "Developmental Psychology and Psychoanalysis: II. The Emergence of a Revolution in Contemporary Psycho-

page

analysis," presented at the fall meeting of the American Psychoanalytic Association, Miami Beach, Fla., 8 December 1990.

88. "Despite decades. . . seems possible.": Peter Gay, *Freud: A Life for Our Time* (New York: Anchor Books, 1989), pp. xvi–xvii.

89. Two particular live children . . . through Hans's father;: Sigmund Freud, "Analysis of a Phobia in a Five-Year-Old Boy," *The Sexual Enlightenment of Children*, ed. Philip Rieff (New York: Collier Books, 1963).

89. And Ernst, the boy with . . . not a patient.: Sigmund Freud, "Beyond the Pleasure Principle" (1920), in Rickman, *A General Selection*, pp. 145–48.

93. These observations . . . "alter something.": Rieff, *Sexual Enlightenment*, p. 141.

93. In "The Sexual . . . interests him most.": Ibid., p. 21.

94. The second important . . . therapy techniques.: Rickman, *A General Selection*, pp. 145–48.

95. "In the play-analyses . . . loss he fears.": D. W. Winnicott, *Through Paediatrics to Psycho-Analysis* (New York: Basic Books, 1958, 1975), p. 69.

95. At first . . . producing pleasure.: Freud, "Beyond the Pleasure Principle," in Rickman, *A General Selection*, p. 141.

96. The uncontrolled operation . . . "road to pleasure.": Ibid., pp. 142–43.

96. Freud had two successive theories . . . "ordinary way". Sigmund Freud, "The Ego and the Id" (1923), in Rickman, *A General Selection*, p. 210.

96. In 1923 . . . "contains the passions.": Ibid., p. 210.

97. ". . . the need to resolve . . .": Phyllis Tyson, Ph.D., and Robert L. Tyson, M.D., *Psychoanalytic Theories of Development: An Integration* (New Haven and London: Yale University Press, 1990).

97. "The super-ego . . . threats and punishments.": Sigmund Freud, "The Dissection of the Psychical Personality," in *New Introductory Lectures on Psycho-Analysis*, trans. and ed. James Strachey (New York, London: W.W. Norton & Co., 1965).

98. Primary process . . . at birth.: Freud, "The Ego and the Id," in Rickman, *A General Selection*, p. 213.

98. "With a few notable . . . secondary process thinking.": Tyson and Tyson, *Psychoanalytic Theories*, p. 164.

98. Numerous writers . . . scientific phenomena.: Ibid., p. 42.

99. Heinz Hartmann pointed out . . . "ego development.": *Ego Psychology and the Problem of Adaptation*, quoted in Leichtman, "Developmental Psychology I," p. 920.

99. An *object* is . . . "achieve its aim.": Moore and Fine, *Psychoanalytic Terms and Concepts*, p. 129.

100. She continued to practice . . . of her discovery.: Melanie Klein, "The Psycho-Analytic Play Technique: Its History and Significance," *The Selected Melanie Klein*, ed. Juliet Mitchell (New York: Free Press, 1987).

102. (According to Juliet Mitchell . . . prosaically spelled fantasy.): Ibid., p. 22.

102. "[T]he oral-sadistic relation . . . the superego.": Ibid., p. 50.

102. "[O]bject relations start . . . the beginning of life.": Ibid., p. 52.

103. Klein did not treat . . . three to six.: "Early Stages of the Oedipus Conflict," ibid., p. 69.

103. "It does not seem clear . . . bites, devours and cuts.": Ibid., p. 71.

105. In 1940, Winnicott . . . "an infant.": Winnicott, *Through Paediatrics*, p. xxxvii.

105. Described in the introduction . . . psychiatric writing.: Introduction by M. Masud R. Khan, in ibid.

page
105. While Winnicott did . . . base his beliefs.: "The Observation of Infants in a Set Situation," in ibid. p. 62.
108. The good-enough mother . . . "with her failure.": "Transitional Objects and Transitional Phenomena" (1951), in ibid., p. 238.
109. At the same time . . . "out for ever.": "Hate in the Countertransference" (1947), in ibid., p. 201.
109. And he insists . . . let her grow.: "Pediatrics and Psychiatry" (1948), in ibid., p. 161.
109. Winnicott (and his contemporaries) . . . relatively healthy neurotics.: "Metapsychological and Clinical Aspects of Regression within the Psycho-Analytical Set-Up" (1954), in ibid., p. 291.
109. An example of . . . epidemic of stealing.: "Symptom Tolerance in Pediatrics: A Case History" (1953), in ibid., p. 101.
111. Winnicott is particularly . . . is not other.: "Transitional Objects and Transitional Phenomena," in ibid., p. 229.

CHAPTER 5: ROOTS (PART TWO)

113. Erikson had been trained . . . "ego to society": Erik H. Erikson, *Childhood and Society* (New York: W.W. Norton & Co., 1950), p. 12.
113. [I]t studied . . . "social organization.": Ibid., p. 11.
114. A good example . . . in northern California.: Ibid., pp. 21–34.
117. But "It was clear . . . therapy nor theory.": Ibid., p. 60.
117. First Erikson put Freud . . . arranged horizontally.: Ibid., pp. 44–92.
119. "[T]he field of psychiatry . . . has his being.": Harry Stack Sullivan, *Conception of Modern Psychiatry*, excerpted in *The History of Psychotherapy*, ed. Jan Ehrenwald, M.D. ed. (Northvale, N.J.: Jason Aronson, 1976), pp. 305–13.
121. The relationship between . . . and his client.: Harry Stack Sullivan, *The Psychiatric Interview* (New York: W.W. Norton & Co., 1954), p. 4.
121. "If you will pause . . . happen to have.": Ibid., pp. 28–29.
122. In 1955, Mahler . . . "in normal development.": This account comes from Margaret Mahler, Fred Pine, and Anni Bergman, *The Psychological Birth of the Human Infant* (New York: Basic Books, 1975), p. ix.
123. "At one extreme" . . . her colleagues wrote.: Ibid., pp. 14–15.
124. "We observed infants . . . needs demand it?": Ibid., pp. 24–25.
125. Like Freud, Klein, Winnicott . . . Freud's thermodynamic metaphors.: Tyson and Tyson, *Psychoanalytic Theories*, p. 92.
125. Newborn infants . . . "common boundary.": Mahler et al., *Psychological Birth*, pp. 42–44.
126. "[B]reast feeding . . . smiling response very early.": Ibid., p. 49.
126. If symbiosis goes well . . . "differentiation" or "hatching.": Ibid., pp. 54–64.
128. The next Mahlerian subphase . . . by actual walking.: Ibid., pp. 65–75.
130. "One could see . . . life cycle.": Ibid., pp. 99–100.
131. In an appraisal . . . "of the 20th century.": Richard D. Chessick, M.D., Ph.D., *Psychology of the Self and the Treatment of Narcissim* (Northvale, N.J.: Jason Aronson, 1993), p. 5.

page

132. Back in the thirties . . . "lengthening of the analyses.": Ibid., p. 19.
133. In treating an unusually tall man . . . "a psychological fact.": Ibid., pp. 108–9.
133. The emphasis . . . this particular person.: In addition to Chessick's interpretation, I have derived some of my understanding of Kohut from an interview with Richard Marohn, M.D., who appears in Chapter 6 of this book.
133. The essence of the therapy . . . "baby or patient.": Ibid., p. 118.
133. The therapist . . . "a modicum of internal structure.": Ibid., p. 110.
133. Very briefly . . . "shortcomings of maternal care.": Ibid., p. 113.
134. Finally it is interesting . . . psychoanalytic world.: Ibid., pp. 146–47.
134. Kuhn says . . . new paradigm becomes orthodox.: Thomas S. Kuhn, *The Structure of Scientific Revolutions*, 2nd ed. (Chicago: University of Chicago Press, 1970), pp. 4–19.
135. At the beginning . . . "end-product backwards.": John Bowlby, *Attachment*, 2nd. ed. vol. 1 (New York: Basic Books, 1982: first published by the Tavistock Institute of Human Relations in 1969), pp. 3–23.
137. But while the world . . . infant's inner world.: Martin Leichtman, "Developmental Psychology II."
137. In 1985 there appeared . . . at Cornell University Medical Center.: Daniel N. Stern, *The Interpersonal World of the Infant: A View from Psychoanalysis and Developmental Psychology* (New York: Basic Books, 1985).
138. Stern wants to know . . . "as development proceeds?": Stern, *Interpersonal World*, p. 3.
138. And in outlining . . . formulations of DSM-IV.: Ibid., pp. 7 and 69–71.
140. The first thing that is essential . . . "the most central.": Ibid., p. 15.
140. Here he reports on . . . what infants know.: Ibid., pp. 38–42.
141. From this volume of . . . "events, sets, and experiences.": Ibid., pp. 41–42.
144. Thus in play therapy . . . mother doll.: Ibid., pp. 166–67.
145. What happens to . . . in Stern's world?: Ibid., pp. 256ff.
146. As Leichtman writes . . . "in its history.": Leichtman, "Developmental Psychology II," p. 40 of manuscript.
146. Certainly most therapists . . . "development proceeds.": Tyson and Tyson, *Psychoanalytic Theories*, p. 37.

CHAPTER 6: IN THE SERVICE OF THE EGO

157. Spiegel sent me . . . New York office.: Stanley Spiegel, *An Interpersonal Approach to Child Therapy: The Treatment of Children and Adolescents from an Interpersonal Point of View* (New York: Columbia University Press, 1989).
157. But it is most useful . . . in his book.: Ibid., pp. 1–25.
158. Spiegel says that . . . directly from Sullivan.: Ibid., p. 304.

CHAPTER 7: "SHOW THAT I CAN"

175. Perhaps the most characteristic . . . *Adolescent Psychiatry*.: John Scott Werry, M.D., and Janet P. Wollersheim, Ph.D., "Behavior Therapy with Children and

page

    Adolescents: A Twenty-Year Overview," *Journal of the American Academy of Child and Adolescent Psychiatry* 28, no. 1 (January 1989), p. 2.

176. Because pure behavioral . . . article defines it.: Ibid., p. 3.

177. "Consider the experience . . . when they occur.": Philip C. Kendall, ed., *Child and Adolescent Therapy: Cognitive-Behavioral Procedures* (New York: Guilford Press, 1991), pp. 9–10.

180. The essence of . . . for anxious children.: The treatment manuals are available from Philip Kendall, Ph.D., Head, Division of Clinical Psychology, Department of Psychology, Temple University, Philadelphia, PA 19122.

CHAPTER 8: REBELS AND REVISIONISTS

201. For an understanding . . . Rutgers University: Daniel B. Fishman and Cyril M. Franks, "Evolution and Differentiation Within Behavior Therapy: A Theoretical and Epistemological Review," in *History of Psychotherapy: A Century of Change* ed. Donald K. Freedheim (Washington, D.C.: American Psychological Association, 1992).

202. In "Psychology as the Behaviorist" . . . territory.: cited in ibid., p. 162.

202. Twelve years later . . . stimulated by stroking.: John B. Watson, "Experimental Studies on the Growth of the Emotions" (1925), in *The Process of Child Development*, ed. Peter B. Neubauer, M.D. (New York and London: Jason Aronson, 1983), pp. 55–74.

203. I have chosen . . . thirty-six years to evolve.: B. F. Skinner, *About Behaviorism* (New York: Knopf, 1974).

203. The source of . . . Watson himself.: Ibid., pp. 5–7.

204. Earlier "methodological" behaviorists . . . "what people do.": Ibid., pp. 12–23.

204. As Skinner points . . . "out of consideration.": Ibid., p. 17.

204. For example, the old . . . approaches a fire.: This example is my extended paraphrase of one of Skinner's. See ibid., p. 52.

205. The feelings are "merely collateral.": Ibid.

205. It is useful . . . "if at all.": Ibid.

205. "It is then easy . . . free to choose.": Ibid., p. 59.

205. "It is often said . . . induces self-observation.": Ibid., p. 169.

205. For example, in the chapter . . . "to the mind.": Ibid., p. 115.

207. Finally he reiterates . . . "to explain behavior.": Ibid., p. 269.

208. A representative sample . . . in graduate school.: Albert Bandura, *Principles of Behavior Modification* (New York: Holt, Rinehart and Winston, 1969).

208. Bandura starts . . . "spirits of ancient times.": Ibid., chap. 1.

209. The idea of symptom . . . "symptom will take.": Ibid., pp. 48–49.

209. He attacks the notion . . . "source of gratification.": Ibid., p. 78.

210. Thus: "behavior that is harmful . . . the medical domain.": Ibid., p. 10.

210. An interesting example . . . "the nursery school.": Ibid., p. 26.

211. "There exists . . . environmental stimulus events.": Ibid., p. 39.

214. Ellis had been trained . . . ineffective and unscientific.: Albert Ellis, "Rational-Emotive Therapy," in *Psychotherapist's Casebook*, ed. Irwin L. Kutash and Alexander Wolf (Northvale, N.J. and London: Jason Aronson, 1993), pp. 277–87.

page

214.   Since as Ellis . . . emotional and confrontational.: Ibid., p. 277.

214.   Ellis held that . . . "of their lives.": Ibid., p. 278.

214.   Ellis even drew up . . . "sustain emotional disturbance.": This is taken from a summary written by Ellis (A. Ellis, *The essence of rational psychotherapy: A comprehensive approach to treatment* (New York: Institute for Rational Living, 1970), and reprinted in Michael J. Mahoney, *Cognition and Behavior Modification* (Cambridge, Mass.: Ballinger, 1974), pp. 171–72.

216.   Mahoney launched his 1974 book . . . "but ethically prescribed.": Mahoney, *Cognition*, p. 1.

216.   But "humans do . . . system of rules.": Ibid., p. 15.

217.   "The principle . . . accuracy or conceptual breadth.": Ibid., pp. 22–32.

217.   "Subjects asked to imagine . . . an aversive stimulus.": Ibid., p. 40.

217.   "The average television viewer" . . . have never flown.: Ibid., p. 45.

217.   As Bandura . . . "receiving a paycheck.": Bandura's observation is reported in Mahoney, *Cognition*, p. 44.

218.   "They need not . . . by their owner.": Ibid., p. 51.

218.   "The skull becomes . . . of private experience." Ibid., p. 61.

220.   Mahoney repeats . . . "won't be Cheerios!": Ibid., pp. 163–64. The source of the story is G. C. Davison.

220.   "Extensive investigations . . . problem-solving options.": Ibid., p. 165.

221.   Mahoney suggests . . . respected cognitive therapists.: Ibid., p. 174.

221.   The next step . . . is self-instruction.: Ibid., p. 184.

222.   Mahoney observed that . . . we think caused them.: Ibid., p. 213.

222.   Mahoney's experience working . . . "he countercontrolled.": Ibid., p. 245.

222.   Mahoney remarks that . . . better than others.: Ibid., p. 227.

222.   He asks what . . . "and believing it?": Ibid., p. 232.

223.   There is, he says . . . beliefs change gradually.: Ibid., p. 240.

223.   It is, he says . . . "a technical consultant.": Ibid., pp. 274–75.

223.   Meichenbaum's particular interest . . . "of the product.": Donald Meichenbaum, *Cognitive-Behavior Modification: An Integrative Approach* (New York: Plenum Press, 1977), p. 13.

224.   Meichenbaum, like Mahoney . . . evaluates those events.: Ibid., p. 108.

225.   Meichenbaum neatly differentiates . . . "skills and responses.": Ibid., p. 194.

CHAPTER 9:   ENLARGING THE REPERTOIRE

230.   A recent book . . . and the behavioral.: Eva L. Feindler, "Cognitive Strategies in Anger Control," in Kendall, *Child and Adolescent Therapy*.

230.   And she cites . . . "self-reported physical aggression.": Ibid., p. 67.

231.   Feindler reports, among . . . by their peers.: Ibid., p. 70.

231.   While research thus favors . . . "delivered is high.": Ibid., p. 76.

232.   In one study . . . waiting-list control group.: Eva L. Feindler et al., "Group Anger–Control Training for Institutionalized Psychiatric Male Adolescents," *Behavior Therapy* 17 (1986), pp. 109–23.

241.   Before talking to Foster . . . Heidi Inderbitzen-Pisaruk.: Heidi Inderbitzen-Pizaruk and Sharon L. Foster, "Adolescent Friendships and Peer Acceptance:

page

Implications for Social Skills Training", *Clinical Psychology Review* 10 (1990), pp. 425–38.

247. When I asked Schreibman . . . book on child psychotherapy.: For a taste of the controversy, see *Harvard Mental Health Letter* (July and December 1993).

247. In a book . . . "repetitive behavior.": Laura Schreibman et al., "Infantile Autism," in *International Handbook of Behavior Modification and Therapy*, 2nd ed., ed. Alan S. Bellack et al. (New York: Plenum Press, 1990).

249. During the forties . . . needless grief.: Ibid.

CHAPTER 10: GETTING UNSTUCK

263. While Alan Kazdin . . . defines the patient.: Kazdin, *Child Psychotherapy*, p. 25.

CHAPTER 11: "BEING TOM IS DIFFERENT FROM BEING A WAGNER"

291. I had boned up . . . disparate strands.: For this account of the history of family therapy, I have drawn on Michael P. Nichols, Ph.D., and Richard C. Schwartz, Ph.D., *Family Therapy: Concepts and Methods*, 2nd ed. (Boston: Allyn & Bacon, 1991).

293. While contemporary family . . . shudder of familiarity.: Gregory Bateson et al., "Toward a Theory of Schizophrenia," *Behavioral Science* 1 (1956), pp. 251–64.

293. (Another example that . . . "your own initiative."): Carlos E. Sluzki, M.D., and Eliseo Veron, Ph.D., "The Double Bind as Universal Pathogenic Situation," *Family Process* 10, no. 4 (1971), pp. 397–410.

297. The book I read . . . for nearly a decade.: Salvador Minuchin, *Families and Family Therapy* (Cambridge, Mass.: Harvard University Press, 1974).

297. Traditional therapy . . . "his social context.": Ibid., pp. 2–3.

297. It brought three . . . "significant in change.": Ibid., p. 9.

297. Moreover, structural family . . . "interpret the past.": Ibid., p. 14.

298. "Moral and emotional . . . have been lost.": Ibid., p. 19.

299. He then offers . . . "socialization and support.": Ibid., p. 50.

299. It is, incidentally . . . "crossing a boundary.": Ibid., p. 57.

300. But when the family . . . will always seek.: Ibid., p. 60.

300. "To join a family . . . within the family.": Ibid., p. 123.

301. The goal of therapy . . . "of all systems.": Ibid., pp. 143–44.

302. A family therapist is . . . "social manipulation.": Ibid., p. 140.

302. How might a structural . . . "effective parental unit.": Ibid., pp. 99–100.

305. His style of therapy . . . is called "symbolic-experiential": August Y. Napier, Ph.D. with Carl A. Whitaker, M.D., *The Family Crucible* (New York: Harper & Row, 1978).

305. After Don fails . . . "the one to stay home,": Ibid., p. 7.

305. Napier describes . . . "own unconscious agenda.": Ibid., p. 6.

306. In the course . . . "delivering babies and stuff.": Ibid., p. 33.

306. As Napier describes . . . "the therapy hour.": Ibid., pp. 92–93.

page

306. But Napier also says . . . "the social environment.": Ibid., pp. 38–41.

307. The Brice family conforms . . . "inadequacy in men.": Ibid., pp. 13–14.

308. Summing up, Napier . . . "trouble the person.": Ibid., pp. 274–75.

309. It would if . . . in the field.: For this account of Bowenian therapy, I have drawn on Nichols and Schwartz, *Family Therapy*.

311. The first, "Family Rituals" . . . updated,: M. Selvini Palazzoli et al., "Family Rituals: A Powerful Tool in Family Therapy," *Family Process* 16, no. 4 (1977), pp. 445–53.

315. The second paper . . . a rundown here.: M. Selvini Palazzoli et al., "Hypothesizing-circularity-neutrality: Three Guidelines for the Conductor of the Session," *Family Process* 19 (1980), pp. 3–12.

317. In the field in general . . . influence each other.: This assessment draws on Nichols and Schwartz, *Family Therapy*, pp. 135–41.

319. White emphasizes that . . . "anyone of anything.": Michael White, Family Therapist, Dulwich Centre, "The Process of Questioning: A therapy of literary merit," in *Dulwich Centre Newsletter* (Autumn 1988).

321. In 1988, Marianne . . . family problems.: Marianne Walters et al., *The Invisible Web: Gender Patterns in Family Relationships* (New York: Guilford Press, 1988).

321. "A major conceptual . . . and thus devalued.": Ibid. This excerpt appears on page 19, but I have reversed the two passages separated by ellipsis to make them more comprehensible here.

CHAPTER 12: JOINING THE CULTURE

324. Before we met . . . "Across Cultures.": Paulette Moore Hines et al., "Intergenerational Relationships Across Cultures," *Families in Society: The Journal of Contemporary Human Services*, CEU Article no. 23 (1992), pp. 323–37.

325. Strong and far-reaching . . . a family's life.: See Nancy Boyd-Franklin, *Black Families in Therapy* (New York: Guilford Press, 1989), for a detailed view of these and other issues. McGoldrick and Hines wrote the foreword to the book.

330. The commonalties are . . . relation to the therapist's.: Betty Karrer, "The Sound of Two Hands Clapping: Cultural Interactions of the Minority Family and the Therapist," in *Minorities and Family Therapy*, ed. G. W. Saba, B. M. Karrer, and K. Hardy (New York: Haworth Press, 1989), pp. 209–37.

331. These dimensions . . . cultural transition.: Karrer credits this idea to C. J. Falicov, "Learning to Think Culturally," in *Handbook of Family Therapy Training and Supervision*, ed. H. Liddle, D. Breunlin and D. Schwartz (New York: Guilford Press, 1988).

334. In studies . . . their adoptive sisters.: Michael Bailey, Ph.D., assistant professor of psychology, Northwestern University, and Richard C. Pillard, M.D., professor of psychiatry, Boston University School of Medicine, "The Innateness of Homosexuality," *Harvard Mental Health Letter* 10, no. 7 (January 1994).

334. And a researcher . . . of the X chromosome.: "Report Suggests Homosexuality is Linked to Genes," *New York Times*, July 16, 1993.

335. Moreover, psychological research . . . men in a bedroom.: Chandler Burr, in "Homosexuality and Biology," *Atlantic* (March 1993), reports the work of Evelyn Hooker.

page

335. A 1987 article ... its first year.: Emery S. Hetrick, M.D., and A. Damien Martin, Ed.D., "Developmental Issues and Their Resolution for Gay and Lesbian Adolescents," *Journal of Homosexuality* 14, nos. 1–2 (1987).

337. But among 137 ... made several tries.: Gary Remafedi, M.D., MPH, James A. Farrow, M.D., and Robert W. Deisher, M.D., "Risk Factors for Attempted Suicide in Gay and Bisexual Youth," *Pediatrics* 87, no. 6 (June 1991).

348. One family therapist ... family therapy textbook.: Nichols and Schwartz, *Family Therapy*.

348. As he later ... "unaware of her cure.": Richard Schwartz, "Our Multiple Selves," *Family Therapy Networker* (March–April 1987).

349. This view, as readers will ... the four selves.: See Chapters 4 and 5 of this book.

353. I remembered that ... in biological psychiatry,: See Chapter 15 of this book.

353. ... not all families ... to this pattern.: Joan Jacobs Brumberg, in *Fasting Girls: The Emergence of Anorexia Nervosa as a Modern Disease* (Cambridge, Mass.: Harvard University Press, 1988), uses *anorectic* as a noun to designate patients with the disorder and *anorexic* to designate behavior that may or may not derive from anorexia nervosa (p. 275). I follow and extend her rule, using *anorectic* also as an adjective applied to a person with the disorder: an anorectic person has anorexic symptoms.

CHAPTER 13: "WITH A MOTHER LIKE THAT ..."

361. The epigraph for this chapter comes from Harold S. Koplewicz and Daniel T. Williams, "Psychopharmacological Treatment," in *Clinical Assessment of Children and Adolescents—a Biopsychosocial Approach*, ed. C. Kestenbaum and D. Williams (New York: New York University Press, 1988), p. 1084.

366. But Koplewicz ... grand rounds that day.: The authoritative text in lay language on obsessive-compulsive disorder is Judith Rapoport's *The Boy Who Couldn't Stop Washing* (New York: New American Library, 1989).

CHAPTER 14: BREAKING THE CODE

403. A summary written ... development and skills.: Barbara Fish and Edward R. Ritvo, "Psychoses of Childhood," in *Basic Handbook of Child Psychiatry*, vol. 2, ed. Joseph D. Noshpitz (New York: Basic Books, 1979).

404. An overwhelming percentage ... optimum career achievement.: This pair of quotations comes from a chapter called "To What Extent is Early Infantile Autism Determined by Constitutional Inadequacies?" originally published in *Genetics and the Inheritance of Integrated Neurological and Psychiatric Patterns*, ed. D. Hooker and C. C. Hare (1954). But this formulation appears in other papers of Kanner's published in the forties and fifties, and these and later papers were collected in *Childhood Psychosis: Initial Studies and New Insights* (Washington, D.C.: V. H. Winston & Sons, 1973), which is where I read them.

404. Bender believed there was ... the age of eleven.: Lauretta Bender, "Childhood Schizophrenia," *American Journal of Orthopsychiatry* 17 (1947), pp. 40–56.

page
405. Bender offered a different . . . "process and development.": Ibid.

406. In 1967 the British psychiatrist . . . nonpsychotic disorders.: Michael Rutter and Linda Lockyer, "A Five to Fifteen Year Follow-up Study of Infantile Psychosis," *British Journal of Psychiatry* 113 (1967), pp. 1169–99. David Greenfeld co-authored the second paper in this series.

406. The next significant . . . team of colleagues.: I. Kolvin et al., *British Journal of Psychiatry* 118 (1971), pp. 381–417.

407. Meanwhile, genetic studies . . . going on.: Seymour Kety et al., "Mental Illness in the Biological and Adoptive Families of Adopted Schizophrenics," *American Journal of Psychiatry* 128, no. 3 (September 1971), pp. 302–306.

408. By 1968, even Kanner . . . played some role.: Kanner, *Childhood Psychosis*. This comes from a paper called "Early Infantile Autism Revisited," which first appeared in *Psychiatry Digest* 29 (1968), pp. 17–28.

408. Indeed, they observe . . . children very sick.: See Chapter 5 of this book.

409. As for schizophrenia . . . adult, hallucinating kind.: Recent research on adult schizophrenia using magnetic resonance imaging has found abnormalities in the left temporal lobe of the brain among fifteen chronic schizophrenic men. This study was described in *New England Journal of Medicine* 27 (August 1992) and reported in *Harvard Mental Health Letter* (May 1993).

409. The second line . . . surprisingly long history.: For this account I have drawn on Jerry M. Wiener, M.D., and Steven L. Jaffe, M.D., "Historical Overview of Childhood and Adolescent Psychopharmacology," in *Diagnosis and Psychopharmacology of Childhood and Adolescent Disorders*, ed. Jerry M. Wiener (New York: John Wiley & Sons, 1985).

410. Ritalin, now the stimulant . . . hyperactivity and impulsiveness.: Mina K. Dulcan, M.D., "Information for Parents and Youth on Psychotropic Medications," *Journal of Child and Adolescent Psychopharmacology* 2, no. 2 (Summer 1992), provides a useful summary of how the different medicines act.

411. Before going further . . . mental disorders: In understanding brain processes, I have found Roland Ciaranello, M.D., "Neurochemical Aspects of Stress," in Garmezy and Rutter, *Stress*, to be helpful. I have also been helped by Paul H. Wender, M.D., and Donald F. Klein, M.D., *Mind, Mood and Medicine* (New York: Farrar, Straus & Giroux, 1981), and by Richard M. Restak, M.D., *Receptors* (New York: Bantam Books, 1994).

413. While he was at the NIMH . . . *Archives of General Psychiatry*.: Markus J.P. Kruesi et al., "Cerebrospinal Fluid Monoamine Metabolites, Aggression and Impulsivity in Disruptive Behavior Disorder of Children and Adolescents," *Archives of General Psychiatry* 47 (May 1990); and Markus J.P. Kruesi et al., "A 2-Year Prospective Follow-Up Study of Children and Adolescents with Disruptive Behavior Disorders," *Archives of General Psychiatry* 49 (June 1992).

CHAPTER 15: LIVING WITH THE PUZZLE

420. The epigraph for this chapter appears in Rickman, *A General Selection*, pp. 59–60.

421. A review of adolescent . . . to set the scene.: S. P. Kutcher, M.D., and P. Marton,

page

Ph.D., "Parameters of Adolescent Depression," *Psychiatric Clinics of North America* 12, no. 4 (December 1989), pp. 895–918.

422. Another paper Kutcher . . . his clinical approach.: Stanley P. Kutcher, M.D., et al., "The Pharmacotherapy of Anxiety Disorders in Children and Adolescents," *Psychiatric Clinics of North America* 15, no. 1 (March 1992), pp. 41–67.

435. But since 90 percent . . . about gender issues.: Prevalence information comes from DSM-IV and from Katherine A. Halmi, M.D., "Eating Disorders; Anorexia Nervosa, Bulimia Nervosa and Obesity," *American Psychiatric Press Textbook of Psychiatry*, 2nd ed., ed. R. E. Hales, S. C. Yudofsky, and J. Talbott (Washington, D.C.: American Psychiatric Press, 1994), pp. 857–75; and Katherine A. Halmi, "Anorexia Nervosa and Bulimia," *Annual Review of Medicine* 38 (1987), pp. 373–80.

435. A book chapter . . . Saint Catherine of Siena.: Halmi notes this in ibid. For an interesting and intelligent long analysis of the history of anorexia nervosa with an emphasis on sociocultural factors, see Brumberg, *Fasting Girls*.

439. I asked her if . . . "problems in front of you.": See Chapter 1 of this book.

446. But after our talk . . . women but not men.: G. M. Goodwin, C. G. Fairburn, and P. J. Cowen, "Dieting Changes Serotonergic Function in Women, Not Men: Implications for the Aetiology of Anorexia Nervosa?" *Psychological Medicine* 17 (1987), pp. 839–42. Also I. M. Anderson et al., "Dieting Reduces Plasma Tryptophan and Alters Brain 5-HT Function in Women," *Psychological Medicine* 20 (1990), pp. 785–91.

CHAPTER 16: "ALIVE WITH PATHOLOGY"

461. While Bruno Bettelheim . . . in the United States,: Bruno Bettelheim and Emmy Sylvester, "The Therapeutic Milieu," *American Journal of Orthopsychiatry* 18 (1948), pp. 191–296.

461. August Aichhorn's work . . . by Freud himself.: August Aichhorn, *Wayward Youth* (Evanston, Ill.: Northwestern University Press, 1983).

461. The first to apply . . . visible at Wediko: Ibid., p. 8.

461. . . . while much has been . . . we met in Chapter 14.: Ibid., p. 40.

462. His friends and peers . . . Pioneer House reborn.: Fritz Redl and David Wineman, *Children Who Hate: The Disorganization and Breakdown of Behavior Controls*. (New York: Free Press, 1951).

466. (I thought of that . . . in San Diego.): See Chapter 9 of this book.

471. Thus they could zero . . . significant moves.: The original report of this experiment comes from Herbert A. Simon and William G. Chase, "Skill in Chess," *American Scientist* (July–August 1973). My account of the experiment, cited here, appears in Katharine Davis Fishman, *The Computer Establishment* (New York: Harper & Row, 1981).

483. The incentive-and-contract . . . in his graduate school days: See Chapter 8 of this book.

CHAPTER 17:   TRIPLE BOOKKEEPING

page
510. How therapists explain ... American Association for Behavior Therapy.: P. C. Kendall, D. Kipnis, and J. Otto-Salaj, (1992). "When clients don't progress: Influences on and explanations for lack of therapeutic progress," *Cognitive Therapy and Research* 16 (1992), pp. 269–281.

511. In the book ... did not receive treatment.: Kazdin, *Child Psychotherapy*, p. 36.

511. This figure is ... versus untreated adults.: Morris B. Parloff, "Psychotherapy Research and Its Incredible Credibility Crisis," *Clinical Psychology Review* (1984), p. 98.

511. In varying degrees ... are understudied.: Kazdin, *Child Psychotherapy*, p. 37 and passim.

511. Parloff, an adult therapist ... "common to these therapies.": Parloff, "Psychotherapy Research," p. 99.

512. In discussing what ... "on the conceptual scheme.": The source for Frank's work is ibid., pp. 99–100.

515. If the school ... charge of the case.: Parents whose children are candidates for special education programs should check the Individuals with Disabilities Education Act (PL 94-142) and Section 504 of the Rehabilitation Act of 1973, which provide for due process to ensure that the children get services they need and do not get services they don't need. Among the former are evaluation and testing, at least some of which must currently be paid for by the school.

516. For example, in a recent ... caused by incest.: Jane Gross, " 'Memory Therapy' on Trial: Healing or Hokum?" *New York Times*, 8 April 1994.

519. Selection theory ... the intellectual marketplace.: Michael S. Gazzaniga, *Nature's Mind: The Biological Roots of Thinking, Emotions, Sexuality and Intelligence* (New York: Basic Books, 1992), pp. 2, 4.

BIBLIOGRAPHY

Aichhorn, August. *Wayward Youth*. Evanston, Ill.: Northwestern University Press, 1983. (Originally published in German, 1925; second German edition, 1931. English translation revised and adapted from the second German edition.)

American Psychiatric Association. *Diagnostic and Statistical Manual of Mental Disorders*, 4th ed. (DSM-IV). Washington, D.C.: American Psychiatric Association, 1994.

———. *Diagnostic and Statistical Manual of Mental Disorders*, 3rd ed., rev. (DSM-III-R). Washington, D.C.: American Psychiatric Association, 1987.

Bandura, Albert. *Principles of Behavior Modification*. New York: Holt, Rinehart and Winston, 1969.

Bettelheim, Bruno. *Truants From Life: The Rehabilitation of Emotionally Disturbed Children*. New York: Free Press, 1955.

Bowlby, John. *Attachment*. 2nd ed. New York: Basic Books, 1969, 1982.

Boyd-Franklin, Nancy. *Black Families in Therapy*. New York: Guilford Press, 1989.

Brooks, Robert, Ph.D. *The Self-Esteem Teacher*. Circle Pines, Minn.: American Guidance Service, 1991.

Brumberg, Joan Jacobs. *Fasting Girls: The Emergence of Anorexia Nervosa as a Modern Disease*. Cambridge, Mass.: Harvard University Press, 1988.

Chess, Stella, and Alexander Thomas. *Origins and Evolution of Behavior Disorders: From Infancy to Early Adult Life*. Cambridge, Mass.: Harvard University Press, 1987.

———. *Temperament in Clinical Practice*. New York: Guilford Press, 1986.

——— and Penny Colman. *Fifty Years Together: Researchers, Psychiatrists, Professors, and Parents*. Privately printed.

Chessick, Richard D., M.D., Ph.D. *Psychology of the Self and the Treatment of Narcissism*. Northvale, N.J.: Jason Aronson, 1993.

Combrinck-Graham, Lee, M.D., ed. *Children in Family Contexts: Perspectives on Treatment*. New York; Guilford Press, 1989.

Ehrenwald, Jan, M.D., ed. *The History of Psychotherapy*. Northvale, N.J.: Jason Aronson, 1976.

Erikson, Erik H. *Childhood and Society*. New York: W.W. Norton & Co., 1950.

Freud, Sigmund. *A General Selection from the Works of Sigmund Freud*. Ed. John Rickman, M.D. New York: Anchor Books, 1957.

———. *An Outline of Psycho-Analysis*. Translated and edited by James Strachey. New York: W.W. Norton & Co., 1969. (Originally published in German, 1940.)

———. *New Introductory Lectures on Psycho-Analysis*. Translated and edited by James Strachey. New York: W.W. Norton & Co., 1965.

———. *The Sexual Enlightenment of Children*. Edited by Philip Rieff. New York: Collier Books, 1963.

Friedman, Lawrence J. *Menninger: The Family and the Clinic*. New York: Alfred A. Knopf, 1990.

Garmezy, Norman, Ph.D., and Michael Rutter, M.D., eds. *Stress, Coping, and Development in Children*. Baltimore: Johns Hopkins University Press, 1988.

Gay, Peter. *Freud: A Life for Our Time*. New York: Anchor Books, 1989.

Gazzaniga, Michael S. *Nature's Mind: The Biological Roots of Thinking, Emotions, Sexuality and Intelligence*. New York: Basic Books, 1992.

Goldstein, Joseph, Anna Freud, and Albert J. Solnit. *Beyond the Best Interests of the Child*. New York: Free Press, 1973, 1979.

Kaysen, Susanna. *Girl, Interrupted*. New York: Vintage Books, 1994.

Kazdin, Alan E. *Child Psychotherapy: Developing and Identifying Effective Treatments*. New York: Pergamon Press, 1988.

Kendall, Philip C., ed. *Child and Adolescent Therapy: Cognitive-Behavioral Procedures*. New York: Guilford Press, 1991.

——— and Lauren Braswell. *Cognitive-Behavioral Therapy for Impulsive Children*. New York: Guilford Press, 1985.

Klein, Melanie. *The Selected Melanie Klein*. Edited by Juliet Mitchell. New York: Free Press, 1987.

Koplewicz, Harold S., and Emily Klass. *Depression in Children and Adolescents*. Chur, Switzerland: Harwood Academic Publishers, Monographs in Clinical Pediatrics, vol. 6.

Kramer, Peter D. *Listening to Prozac*. New York: Viking, 1993.

Kuhn, Thomas S. *The Structure of Scientific Revolutions*. 2nd ed. Chicago: University of Chicago Press, 1970.

Kutash, Irwin L., and Alexander Wolf, eds. *Psychotherapist's Casebook*. Northvale, N.J.: Jason Aronson, 1993.

Mahler, Margaret S., Fred Pine, and Anni Bergman. *The Psychological Birth of the Human Infant: Symbiosis and Individuation*. New York: Basic Books, 1975.

Mahoney, Michael J. *Cognition and Behavior Modification*. Cambridge, Mass.: Ballinger, 1974.

Malcolm, Janet. *Psychoanalysis: The Impossible Profession*. New York: Vintage Books, 1982.

Meichenbaum, Donald. *Cognitive-Behavior Modification: An Integrative Approach*. New York: Plenum Press, 1977.

Minuchin, Salvador. *Families and Family Therapy*. Cambridge, Mass.: Harvard University Press, 1974.

Moore, Burness E., M.D., and Bernard D. Fine, M.D., eds. *Psychoanalytic Terms and Concepts*. New Haven: The American Psychoanalytic Association and Yale University Press, 1990.

Napier, Augustus Y., Ph.D., with Carl Whitaker, M.D. *The Family Crucible*. New York: Harper & Row, 1978.

Neubauer, Peter B., M.D., ed. *The Process of Child Development*. New York: Jason Aronson, 1976, 1983.

Nichols, Michael P., Ph.D., and Richard C. Schwartz, Ph.D. *Family Therapy: Concepts and Methods*. 2nd ed. Boston: Allyn & Bacon, 1991.

Psychoanalytic Assessment: The Diagnostic Profile. An anthology of *The Psychoanalytic Study of the Child*. Edited by Ruth S. Eissler, Anna Freud, Marianne Kris, and Albert J. Solnit. New Haven: Yale University Press, 1977.

Rapoport, Judith L., M.D. *The Boy Who Couldn't Stop Washing: The Experience and Treatment of Obsessive-Compulsive Disorder*. New York: New American Library, 1989.

Redl, Fritz, and David Wineman. *Children Who Hate: The Disorganization and Breakdown of Behavior Controls*. New York: Free Press, 1951.

Restak, Richard M., M.D. *Receptors*. New York: Bantam Books, 1994.

Sanders, Jacquelyn Seevak. *A Greenhouse for the Mind*. Chicago: University of Chicago Press, 1989.

Sarnoff, Charles A., M.D. *Latency*. Northvale, N.J.: Jason Aronson, 1976, 1989.

———. *Psychotherapeutic Strategies in the Latency Years*. Northvale, N.J.: Jason Aronson, 1987.

———. *Psychotherapeutic Strategies in Late Latency through Early Adolescence*. Northvale, N.J.: Jason Aronson, 1987.

Skinner, B. F. *About Behaviorism*. New York: Alfred A. Knopf, 1974.

Spiegel, Stanley. *An Interpersonal Approach to Child Therapy: The Treatment of Children and Adolescents from an Interpersonal Point of View*. New York: Columbia University Press, 1989.

Stern, Daniel N. *The Interpersonal World of the Infant: A View from Psychoanalysis and Developmental Psychology*. New York: Basic Books, 1985.

Sullivan, Harry Stack. *The Psychiatric Interview*. New York: W.W. Norton & Co., 1954.

Trieschman, Albert E., James K. Whittaker, Larry K. Brendtro. *The Other 23 Hours: Child Care Work with Emotionally Disturbed Children in a Therapeutic Milieu*. New York: Aldine De Gruyter, 1969.

Tyson, Phyllis, Ph.D., and Robert L. Tyson, M.D. *Psychoanalytic Theories of Development: An Integration*. New Haven: Yale University Press, 1990.

Wallerstein, Judith S., Ph.D., and Sandra Blakeslee. *Second Chances: Men, Women, and Children a Decade After Divorce*. New York: Ticknor & Fields, 1989.

Walsh, Froma and Monica McGoldrick, eds. *Living Beyond Loss: Death in the Family*. New York: W.W. Norton & Co., 1991.

Walters, Marianne, Betty Carter, Peggy Papp, Olga Silverstein, and the Women's Project in Family Therapy. *The Invisible Web: Gender Patterns in Family Relationships*. New York: Guilford Press, 1988.

Wender, Paul H., M.D., and Donald F. Klein, M.D. *Mind, Mood, and Medicine*. New York: Farrar, Straus, Giroux, 1981.

Winnicott, D. W. *The Piggle: An Account of the Psychoanalytic Treatment of a Little Girl*. Edited by Ishak Ramzy, Ph.D. New York: International Universities Press, 1977.

———. *Through Paediatrics to Psycho-Analysis*. New York: Basic Books, 1958.

ACKNOWLEDGMENTS

This book would not exist without the kindness of those parents and children who, in hopes of helping others, agreed to talk with me and/or to let me watch them in therapeutic session; my thoughts and hopes for the future go with them.

The clinicians who lead the parts of the book were notably generous with their time and both patient and engaging in their explanations. In addition, they steered me toward useful research and introduced me to colleagues who in turn proved accessible and informative.

I am most grateful to all the therapists who took time to discuss their practice with me. Some of their names appear in the text; the names of others—whose work was equally impressive and who taught me a lot—do not, mostly because writing the book was like assembling a stew that required a certain balance and distribution in the ingredients. Special thanks go to Efrain Bleiberg, Maureen Donnelly, and David Waters, who went out of their way to be helpful when I visited. Jacqueline Taylor helped choreograph my repeated visits to Wediko, setting up conversations with therapists whose days and evenings were especially complicated and stressful; she also tracked down a load of information.

No one was given control over what would be published about his or her work, but in the interests of accuracy, someone knowledgeable in each therapeutic orientation read the relevant parts of the manuscript. Thus Gabrielle Carlson, Richard Chasin, Daniel B. Fishman, Harold Koplewicz, Richard Marohn, Sallyann Roth, and Michael Thompson read descriptions of theory and research in their therapeutic schools and the work of their colleagues, and Rosalind Miller read the whole manuscript. Their comments were valuable and mostly put to good use; what sins remain are my own.

C. Michael Curtis, a senior editor at *The Atlantic Monthly*, first suggested I look into child psychotherapy. I am immeasurably grateful to him, not only for thoughtful editorial guidance while I was writing the original article, but for assigning me a piece that pointed me toward what became five exciting years of work. My thanks go also to William Whitworth for approving that assignment and to Sue Parilla for the thorough, fastidious fact-checking for which the magazine is known.

Barbara Frank transcribed tapes with speed and skill.

I am thankful to Joy Harris, my agent, for fruitful work, involvement, and support, particularly during a time of tragedy in her own life.

If a writer could invent an editor, she would invent Ann Harris, whose intelligence, experience, knowledge, energy, and enthusiasm made the process of bringing out this book one of high intellectual challenge, fellowship, and shared goals. Janet Biehl proved to be a deft and able copyeditor.

Finally, I am grateful to my own tribe: most particularly to Joseph Fishman; and also to Dan, Claire, Maggie, and Nancy Fishman, and Yiftach Resheff, for good cheer, interest, reading, and useful insight from their various disciplines—psychology, sociology, anthropology, and the law.

INDEX